No Words fo

Alexithymia is a multifaceted constr
one's feelings, difficulties describing
style. In the long term, higher alexithy
outcomes. There is, however, a lack of
these vulnerabilities.

This book shows that the facets of alex
to neutral and emotional situations, by im
language, and behavior). The effects are i
emotion responding and others that contri
ance of drawing better connections among m
early processes have impacts on later processe
alexithymia facets, is expected to lead to ineffec
risks for physical and mental illness.

The chapters in this book were originally publis

Olivier Luminet is Full Professor at UCLouvain a
Research (FRS-FNRS), Belgium. His main areas of int
and health, and the links between emotion, identity,
lective levels). He has published more than 50 papers
book *Alexithymia: Advances in Research, Theory, and Cl*
Memories: New Challenges and Future Perspectives (Routle

Kristy A. Nielson is Full Professor at Marquette University, M
and neuropsychologist whose research targets the neural sub
and sensorimotor changes in aging and Alzheimer's disease;
role of individual differences, such as sex, sexual orientation, a
on cognition and "successful aging"; early biomarkers predictin
exercise, for preventing, reducing, and adapting to cognitive decl

Nathan Ridout is Senior Lecturer at Aston University, Birminghar
the primary aim of his research is to understand cognitive and affe
ology, most notably depression and eating disorders. His areas of inte
ical memory) and social cognition (especially processing of facial em
alexithymia (particularly in association with psychopathology, and influe
tive changes observed in older adults.

No Words for Feelings

Alexithymia as a Fundamental Personality Dimension at the Interface of Cognition

Edited by

Olivier Luminet, Kristy A. Nielson and Nathan Ridout

Routledge
Taylor & Francis Group
LONDON AND NEW YORK

First published 2025
by Routledge
4 Park Square, Milton Park, Abingdon, Oxon OX14 4RN

and by Routledge
605 Third Avenue, New York, NY 10158

Routledge is an imprint of the Taylor & Francis Group, an informa business

British Library Cataloguing in Publication Data
A catalogue record for this book is available from the British Library

ISBN13: 978-1-032-73133-9 (hbk)
ISBN13: 978-1-032-73135-3 (pbk)
ISBN13: 978-1-003-42690-5 (ebk)

DOI: 10.4324/9781003426905

Typeset in Myriad Pro
by Newgen Publishing UK

Publisher's Note
The publisher accepts responsibility for any inconsistencies that may have arisen during the conversion of this book from journal articles to book chapters, namely the inclusion of journal terminology.

Contents

Citation Information

The chapters in this book were originally published in *Cognition and Emotion*, volume 35, issue 3 (2021). When citing this material, please use the original page numbering for each article, as follows:

Introduction

Introduction: Having no words for feelings: alexithymia as a fundamental personality dimension at the interface of cognition and emotion
Olivier Luminet, Kristy A. Nielson and Nathan Ridout
Cognition and Emotion, volume 35, issue 3 (2021), pp. 435–448

Chapter 1

Cognitive-emotional processing in alexithymia: an integrative review
Olivier Luminet, Kristy A. Nielson and Nathan Ridout
Cognition and Emotion, volume 35, issue 3 (2021), pp. 449–487

Chapter 2

Adaptive and maladaptive emotion processing and regulation, and the case of alexithymia
Georgia Panayiotou, Maria Panteli and Elke Vlemincx
Cognition and Emotion, volume 35, issue 3 (2021), pp. 488–499

Chapter 3

Negative valence specific deficits in judgements of musical affective quality in alexithymia
Joel L. Larwood, Eric J. Vanman and Genevieve A. Dingle
Cognition and Emotion, volume 35, issue 3 (2021), pp. 500–509

Chapter 4

Alexithymia and reaching group consensus
Hila Zahava Gvirts and Lihi Dery
Cognition and Emotion, volume 35, issue 3 (2021), pp. 510–523

Chapter 5

The role of alexithymia in memory and executive functioning across the lifespan
Anthony N. Correro II, Elizabeth R. Paitel, Steven J. Byers and Kristy A. Nielson
Cognition and Emotion, volume 35, issue 3 (2021), pp. 524–539

Chapter 6

The influence of alexithymia on memory for emotional faces and realistic social interactions
Nathan Ridout, Jade Smith and Holly Hawkins
Cognition and Emotion, volume 35, issue 3 (2021), pp. 540–558

Chapter 7

Alexithymia disrupts verbal short-term memory
Nicolas Vermeulen
Cognition and Emotion, volume 35, issue 3 (2021), pp. 559–568

Chapter 8

Alexithymic traits predict the speed of classifying non-literal statements using nonverbal cues
Lorna S. Jakobson and Pauline M. Pearson
Cognition and Emotion, volume 35, issue 3 (2021), pp. 569–575

Chapter 9

Getting lost in a story: how narrative engagement emerges from narrative perspective and individual differences in alexithymia
Dalya Samur, Mattie Tops, Ringailė Slapšinskaitė and Sander L. Koole
Cognition and Emotion, volume 35, issue 3 (2021), pp. 576–588

Notes on Contributors

Steven J. Byers, Department of Psychology, Marquette University, Milwaukee, WI, USA.

Anthony N. Correro II, Medical College of Wisconsin, WI, USA.

Lihi Dery, Department of Industrial Engineering and Management, Ariel University, Ariel, Israel.

Genevieve A. Dingle, School of Psychology, The University of Queensland, St Lucia, Australia.

Hila Zahava Gvirts, Department of Behavioral Sciences and Psychology, Ariel University, Ariel, Israel.

Holly Hawkins, Department of Psychology, School of Life & Health Sciences, Aston University, Birmingham, UK.

Lorna S. Jakobson, Department of Psychology, University of Manitoba, Winnipeg, Canada.

Sander L. Koole, Department of Clinical Psychology, VU University Amsterdam, Amsterdam, The Netherlands.

Joel L. Larwood, School of Psychology, The University of Queensland, St Lucia, Australia.

Olivier Luminet, Research Institute for Psychological Sciences, UCLouvain, Louvain-la-Neuve, Belgium; Fund for Scientific Research (FRS-FNRS), Brussels, Belgium.

Kristy A. Nielson, Department of Psychology, Marquette University, Milwaukee, WI, USA; Department of Neurology, Medical College of Wisconsin, Milwaukee, WI, USA.

Elizabeth R. Paitel, Department of Psychology, Marquette University, Milwaukee, WI, USA.

Georgia Panayiotou, Department of Psychology and Center for Applied Neuroscience, University of Cyprus, Nicosia, Cyprus.

Maria Panteli, Department of Psychology and Center for Applied Neuroscience, University of Cyprus, Nicosia, Cyprus.

Pauline M. Pearson, Department of Psychology, University of Winnipeg, Winnipeg, Canada.

Nathan Ridout, Department of Psychology, School of Life & Health Sciences, Aston University, Birmingham, UK.

Dalya Samur, Department of Clinical Psychology, VU University Amsterdam, Amsterdam, The Netherlands.

Ringailė Slapšinskaitė, Greenpeace International, Amsterdam, North Holland, The Netherlands; Department of Clinical Psychology, VU University Amsterdam, Amsterdam, The Netherlands.

Jade Smith, Department of Psychology, School of Life & Health Sciences, Aston University, Birmingham, UK.

Mattie Tops, Developmental and Educational Psychology, Leiden University, Leiden, South Holland, The Netherlands.

Eric J. Vanman, School of Psychology, The University of Queensland, St Lucia, Australia.

Nicolas Vermeulen, Psychological Sciences Research Institute, UCLouvain, Louvain-la-Neuve, Belgium; Fund for Scientific Research (FNRS-FRS), Brussels, Belgium.

Elke Vlemincx, Vrije Universiteit Amsterdam, The Netherlands.

Introduction – Having no words for feelings: alexithymia as a fundamental personality dimension at the interface of cognition and emotion

Olivier Luminet, Kristy A. Nielson and Nathan Ridout

ABSTRACT

This special issue brings together two important reviews and seven cutting-edge empirical papers concerning the influence of alexithymia on cognitive and emotional processing. Alexithymia is a multifaceted construct that is characterised by difficulties identifying one's feelings; difficulties describing one's feelings to others; and an externally focused, utilitarian cognitive style. In this paper, we begin by considering how emotion science has evolved in its understanding of personality traits, before highlighting the potential importance of alexithymia research for the field of cognition and emotion. After summarising the historical context of alexithymia research, we consider the contributions of the featured papers to the literature of cognition and emotion. The collected works highlight that alexithymia influences several aspects of how one perceives and responds to neutral and emotional situations, by impacting upon multiple processes (attention, appraisals, memory, language and behaviour), showing the importance of drawing better connections amongst multiple processes, toward disentangling the effects of early processes on later ones. A lack of correspondence between processes, as well as amongst alexithymia facets, is another central finding of the special issue. This pattern is thought to lead to ineffective and inflexible emotion regulation and to pose significant risks for physical and mental illness.

The field of cognition and emotion has led to major advancements in understanding the importance of detecting, identifying, understanding, labelling and regulating emotions (see Koole & Rothermund, 2019). These functions represent a complex interplay of developmental, experiential and cognitive processes that are fundamental to adaptive individual and social functioning. As a complementary perspective, the study of disruptions of emotion processing is also key to understanding the role and meaning of emotions in everyday life. The aim of this special issue is to examine the cognition–emotion interface through the lens of disrupted emotion processing in alexithymia, which literally means having no words for one's feelings. More specifically, alexithymia is a multi-dimensional personality construct that has three major facets, (1) difficulty identifying one's feelings and distinguishing them from bodily sensations; (2) difficulty describing one's feelings to others; and (3) an externally oriented cognitive style, that is utilitarian and without including affective responses when facing stressful situations (Taylor et al., 1997; 2016).

We begin by showing how emotion science has evolved in its understanding of personality traits, and then highlight what can be learned about the cognition–emotion interface from experimental research on alexithymia. In the second section, we situate the evolution of alexithymia research in the historical context of psychosomatic medicine and overview the early research on the construct. In the third section, we provide a review of the papers that are part of this special issue and their contributions to both the literature on alexithymia and to understanding the cognition–emotion interface. In the final section, we highlight dissociations in emotion processes that were revealed by the papers in this issue, and discuss the ways in which the heterogeneity of functioning in alexithymia can inform future studies and theory about the cognition–emotion interface.

1. Personality and the cognition–emotion interface

Emotion psychology has evolved considerably in explaining the role of personality traits in emotion processing (Kuppens et al., 2009). Initially, personality theories of emotion focused on traits reflecting general tendencies to experience certain emotions with higher or lower intensity and/or frequency. This approach obscured the emotional processes underlying the trait(s) because each trait is more likely to manifest in situationally specific ways (Mischel & Shoda, 1998). Current perspectives adopt an explicit interactionist framework, which assumes that individual differences in emotional responses are explained by the concomitant effects of the person (including his/her antecedents or history), the situation (including its novelty or controllability) and time (including updating as a function of changes in both context and person) (Kuppens et al., 2009). One important goal of this approach is therefore to identify the conditions under which individuals with higher scores on a specific trait like alexithymia evidence modulations in their emotional responses.

The goal of identifying conditions where alexithymia results in modulated emotional response fits perfectly with a process-oriented approach that has recently been developed in personality psychology (Quirin et al., 2020; Robinson et al., 2019). In the Dynamics of Personality Approach (DPA), Quirin et al. (2020) emphasise the need for investigating personality processes in an integrated manner, involving large classes of psychological functions that include cognitive and emotional dimensions. DPA models involve objective measures explaining how different functions interact for producing cognition, emotions and behaviours. Following the perspective developed by Shoda and Mischel (2000), these new approaches contend that within-person variations across different types of stimuli (e.g. emotional and neutral) are essential for understanding information processing (Quirin et al., 2020; Robinson et al., 2019). Furthermore, a central aspect is that mechanisms involved in personality traits can be modelled through the use of cognitive and behavioural tasks that directly investigate processes such as attention, perception, appraisals, cognitive control or behaviours (Robinson et al., 2019). These new approaches integrate the descriptive richness of the trait perspective with the explanatory power of process-oriented models. The goal is to capture personality tendencies in vivo together with high degrees of experimental control to provide explanatory frameworks of the personality process (Baumert et al., 2017).

The field of cognition and emotion is also essential in illuminating and empirically validating the clinical significance of emotion. Perhaps most important is the translation of experimental paradigms from cognitive psychology to study the processing of emotional information in clinical disorders (Oatley et al., 2011). A major contribution of clinical cognition–emotion research has been the development of tasks that reveal and characterise information processing of emotion, and specify the distinct features of those with emotional disorders, particularly when salient material is applied (Joormann, 2019).

The central aim of this special issue is to advance the scientific understanding of how alexithymia alters emotional processing. To do so, cutting-edge studies are presented that employ novel empirical approaches to characterise which processes of the cognition–emotion interface are crucially involved. Several papers specifically examine information processing paradigms and sensitivity to salient material. The special issue represents two particularly compelling shifts in this literature. First, these studies examine what can be learned about the cognition–emotion interface from experimental research on alexithymia and in so doing, they challenge alexithymia research on the very nature of the emotional response. From the early work in the 1970s, the dominant perspective was to view alexithymia as an overall *deficit* of emotion processing (e.g. Sifneos et al., 1977; Taylor, 2000). While this view is occasionally challenged by findings showing *excessive* emotional responding, there is a lack of empirical research or integrative theory that intentionally distinguishes the conditions and contexts under which different, nuanced responses occur. Moreover, these distinctions are of critical importance for the cognition–emotion literature, illustrating previously overlooked nuances of emotional responding and dysfunction, and potential dissociations in emotional responding that need clarification. These clarifications are likely to have fundamental influences on the understanding of emotion processing. The papers in this special issue give attention to specifically evaluating these distinctions.

A second substantial shift that this special issue reveals is the beneficial role of a facet level analysis toward better understanding the nuances of alexithymia, and through it, the cognition–emotion interface. Although most studies have examined alexithymia as a unitary construct (i.e. using the total score), recent studies have given much more attention to evaluating the influence of individual facets of alexithymia through subscale scores. Total scores remain preferred for clinical purposes (Reise et al., 2013). However, for research purposes, considering facet scores allows clearer identification of which processes are particularly related to specific alexithymia features, and thus, how those features might influence individual's mental and somatic vulnerabilities.

All except one of the empirical papers in this special issue adopted a facet-level analysis, and the review by Luminet et al. (2021) combined a facet-level analysis with a process perspective. Their findings provide clear support for important differential influences of the facets on specific processes, as well as indicating dissociations in emotion processing effects in alexithymia. Thus, immersion in the theoretical and empirical paradigms of cognition and emotion using such an approach can substantively broaden understanding of the fundamental processes underlying alexithymia. Furthermore, these studies of alexithymia highlight the benefits of process-level analyses in more generally understanding emotion processing, particularly in delineating when and under what conditions (e.g. affective vs. non-affective) dissociations occur.

Although systematic research examining the cognition–emotion interface did not begin until the mid 1990s, the foundations of alexithymia and the study of the clinical significance of emotion are rooted in earlier work. Yet, it was not until the mid-1990s that validated assessment of alexithymia became broadly available. Thus, the two fields evolved rapidly and in the same era. We next provide an overview of this historical context in alexithymia to set the stage for understanding how the papers in this special issue fit within this context and how they advance it.

2. Alexithymia research: from clinical observations to controlled experiments

The notion of alexithymia originates with the observation that people with specific somatic diseases were unable to experience and identify their emotions as subjective feelings, had a lack of fantasies about feelings and instinctual drives, and exhibited a preoccupation with external events (e.g. Groddeck, 1923; Wittkower, 1938). These observations were the foundational steps of psychosomatic medicine. The 1940s' ushered in more systematic emotional and cognitive observations of these individuals, with the basis for somatic disease attributed to unconscious psychological conflicts (Alexander, 1950) or stunted development of personality and symbolic expression (Ruesch, 1948). MacLean (1949) proposed psychosomatic illnesses occur through physiological stress resulting from deficits in verbal emotion expression. Subsequent study further described psychosomatic patients as lacking introspection and fantasies (Horney, 1952; Kelman, 1952), with a utilitarian, concrete way of thinking (i.e. "pensée opératoire"; Marty & de M'Uzan, 1963). Overall, these clinical reports indicated a pattern of symptoms including disturbed verbal and symbolic emotion expression, low imaginative ability, and a tendency toward solving stressful situations by physical action instead of mentalization. In the early 1970s, Nemiah and Sifneos (1970) systematized these observations and drew direct links between difficulty perceiving, understanding, describing and expressing feelings and proneness for various somatic diseases. A turning point came when Sifneos (1973) coined the term "alexithymia" and began testing its validity and using methods for assessing its severity.

Most of the research in the following two decades focused on understanding somatic illness, and physiological and behavioural responding during emotion, but progress was impaired by the lack of a reliable instrument to assess alexithymia severity. By the mid-1990s, however, a first carefully researched instrument became available that allowed valid assessment of alexithymia, which is now the most widely used assessment scale (TAS-20; Bagby et al., 1994a, 1994b; see Luminet et al., 2021, this issue, for a review of the current knowledge regarding TAS-20 validity). The initial research on alexithymia specifically examined the relationship of alexithymia with somatic illness (e.g. Parker et al., 1993a; Schmidt et al., 1993), suggesting vulnerability to illness in alexithymia through deficits in the cognitive processing of emotions (Taylor, 2000; Taylor et al., 1997) and the arrested development of affective regulation and interpersonal outcomes (e.g. Krystal, 1988). Other studies examined dissociation (i.e. "decoupling") of physiological from cognitive-experiential components of emotional responses (e.g. Papciak et al., 1985), neurobiological bases of alexithymia (e.g. Hoppe & Bogen, 1977; Lane et al., 1998), and interventions aimed at reducing alexithymia (e.g. Beresnevaite, 2000).

Although there were attempts in early alexithymia research to address the cognition–emotion interface (Mann et al., 1994; Parker et al., 1993a, Parker et al., 1993b), the studies were limited by small samples and the lack of a valid alexithymia assessment instrument. In 1997, Taylor et al. highlighted the need for a shift towards studies examining the cognition–emotion interface in order to fully understand the underlying mechanisms involved in high alexithymia scores: "Investigations that systematically evaluate differences in attention, retrieval, recognition, and recall of emotional and non-emotional stimuli have the potential to delineate more clearly the mechanisms underlying failures in affect regulation" (p. 268). By definition, each facet of alexithymia characterises disturbance of the interaction between cognitive and emotional processes. Nevertheless, it is only in the last 25 years (1995–2020) that more systematic research, using methods and tools originating in cognitive psychology, has begun to elucidate the specific pattern of impairments associated with alexithymia.

This new line of research has examined the types of processes and the degree of deficits in the processing and regulation of emotions associated with alexithymia severity. Those data helped to reveal the complex (and possibly causal) links between mechanisms underlying the central facets of alexithymia and subsequent negative mental and physical health outcomes. They also contributed to defining some of the specific circumstances in which the impairments happen. For instance, studies revealed that people scoring higher on alexithymia exhibit emotion processing deficits particularly when task difficulty is increased, such as under short time constraints or degraded stimulus quality (e.g. Ihme et al., 2014a, 2014b; Kätsyri et al., 2008; Prkachin et al., 2009). Deficits might also be dependent on the type of material used. If we consider the ability to detect, identify and recognise emotions in oneself and others, deficits in alexithymia mainly occur for negative states such as anger, sadness or fear (Luminet & Zamariola, 2018). Yet, the specific papers included in this special issue, which we overview next, advance knowledge and add compelling new nuances to our understanding of the circumstances and possible mechanisms involved in alterations of the cognition–emotion interface in alexithymia.

3. Overview of the special issue

Luminet et al. (2021): The special issue begins with a review of the empirical research in alexithymia that directly addresses the cognition–emotion interface across the domains of attention, appraisals, memory, language and behaviours (Luminet et al., 2021). The paper importantly and uniquely analysed the literature towards identifying and distinguishing specific patterns of *deficits* in alexithymia, in contrast with findings of excessive responding, which they dubbed *"over-responding"*, together with delineating the specificity of the effects as a function of the type of material, and the context involved (i.e. affective vs. non-affective). Although there was a primary pattern of deficits in processing across domains, over-responding was also frequently found, with a particularly striking predominance in the domain of behaviours. These patterns were further evaluated relative to specific alexithymia facets, wherever a facet-level analysis was available, providing a clearer and more nuanced picture of what to expect in emotion processing studies in alexithymia.

Importantly, the facet "externally oriented thinking" was consistently linked to deficits, while the facets "difficulty identifying feelings" and "difficulty describing feelings" were more typically linked to over-responding, sometimes even to beneficial over-responding. Furthermore, these patterns of deficits and over-responding were not limited to emotive contexts and materials but were found also for some neutral contexts and materials. Finally, the paper discusses how the preponderance of the findings fit with several contemporary emotion theories, indicating that impaired or biased attentional processing and cognitive control, during both early and late processing, along with impaired emotion schemas, contribute to downstream effects on appraisal, memory, language and behaviours. This framing was used to show how future alexithymia and emotion research can guide each other, and how clinical interventions in alexithymia might be informed by cognitive findings.

Panayiotou et al. (2021): The second paper of the special issue is a review of disruptions of physiological reactivity and emotion processing in alexithymia, which contextualised the findings in the attention domain. Panayiotou et al. (2021) draw on a selective literature review of valence, arousal, attention, memory, executive control and interoception to evaluate the inflexibility of emotion regulation as a catalyst for elevating allostatic load (McEwen, 1998). Specifically, maladaptive emotion regulation is conceived to lead to frequent stress, inadequate reactivity, failed shutdown and failed habituation, which can ultimately result in physical and mental illness. They advocate for alexithymia investigations that extend beyond simple reactivity to emotional stimuli, proposing instead a dynamic-phasic model of emotion regulation focused on five stages of processing (anticipation, response, recovery, habituation and rest), toward evaluating emotion regulation flexibility and its role in alexithymia.

Notably, in considering physiological reactions, disruptions at the anticipation and response stages of emotional processing were proposed to correspond to alexithymia-related dysfunction in attentional deployment. In support of the proposal, electrophysiological evidence was presented indicating reduced early processing of emotional material in alexithymia, suggestive of dysfunctional attentional engagement and attentional control that underpin slow or inadequate recovery from emotional stressors. Although this important review did not consider alexithymia facets, the proposal offered is nevertheless fitting with the other review paper in this issue (Luminet et al., 2021), which consistently showed attention and appraisal deficits, with "externally oriented thinking" as the primary facet associated with these deficits.

Larwood et al. (2021): In their paper, Larwood et al. (2021) examined the influence of alexithymia on ratings of intensity and valence for a series of musical excerpts designed to represent anger, fear, joy, sadness and tenderness. This paper thus addresses appraisals processes, which is the act of subjectively evaluating stimuli or situations and is central to the generation of emotional feeling states in response to provocative stimuli (e.g. Ellsworth & Scherer, 2003; Frijda, 1986). Appraisals can take multiple forms, but in alexithymia, valence has been the focus of study to date (see Luminet et al., 2021). The results of Larwood et al. (2021) showed that participants with higher alexithymia rated pieces depicting negative emotions as more neutral than did participants with lower alexithymia. In contrast, no influence of alexithymia was found when pieces depicted positive emotions. These results fit with studies evaluating the recognition of non-verbal emotions (i.e. auditory vocalizations, such as laughs or cries), in which alexithymia was related to reduced accuracy for negative, but not positive stimuli (Bayot et al., 2014).

Moreover, Larwood and colleagues also found that participants with higher alexithymia rated more extreme emotions (i.e. anger and fear) as less intense than did low alexithymia scorers. Yet, they rated less extreme emotions (i.e. sadness) as *more* intense than did those with low alexithymia. These results highlight an overall blunting effect of alexithymia on the appraisal of negative stimuli, as well as an inability to distinguish among emotional states that vary in terms of intensity. This is consistent with the theory that alexithymia-related deficits in responding to emotion are due, at least in part, to poor evaluation of stimulus valence or intensity resulting from poor early processing for stimuli that have a high demand for processing resources (Luminet et al., 2021; Panayiotou et al., 2021). By investigating emotional responses to music, the study by Larwood and colleagues represents an important extension of the literature examining appraisal processes in alexithymia, which has tended to focus only on emotional responses to personally experienced events (e.g. Luminet et al., 2000) or to visually presented affective words or images (e.g. Aaron et al., 2018; Koven, 2014; Luminet et al., 2004).

Given the evidence of poorer emotional awareness and differentiation (da Silva et al., 2017) and less well-developed emotion schemas (e.g. Luminet et al., 2006; Lundh et al., 2002; Vermeulen et al., 2006), it is not altogether surprising that people with higher alexithymia scores would be less likely to benefit from the typical salience effects of emotion, where attention is captured and directed toward emotive content (e.g. Yiend, 2010). It is well-understood that memory is assisted by these salience effects (e.g. Mather & Sutherland, 2011; Nielson & Correro, 2017). As such, we might expect that memory deficits would be common in those with higher alexithymia, at least in emotive contexts. While literature examining memory in alexithymia has grown quickly in recent years, there is a lack of study of the intersection of these processes that would better characterise the contexts and sources of memory deficits in alexithymia. The next three papers that examine memory processes answer these important gaps in current knowledge.

Correro et al. (2021): In their paper, Correro et al. (2021) examined episodic memory (i.e. immediate and delayed recall for stories and words) and executive functioning (i.e. cognitive control, complex attention) in three independent, large sample cross-sectional studies. They furthermore explicitly examined memory using neutral rather than emotive memoranda, hypothesising that with strong statistical power, subtler general relationships between alexithymia and memory might be apparent. Contrary to Larwood et al. (2021), who only examined total alexithymia scores, this paper, together with all the subsequent papers, also include an analysis at the facet level of alexithymia. The paper by Correro and colleagues provides compelling evidence about the cognition–emotion interface on three fronts. First, it importantly revealed that alexithymia contributes to *general* cognitive deficits, particularly those associated with aging. Second, it extended the existing literature to affirm that alexithymia contributes substantively to memory deficits, even for neutral material or contexts, including after delayed retention testing, which has not been well-studied so far. Finally, this study highlighted distinct contributions of the alexithymia factors "difficulty identifying feelings" and "externally oriented thinking" in memory functioning.

Correro et al. (2021) found that "difficulty identifying feelings" was linked to executive functioning deficits, suggesting reduced processing resources available for complex tasks in alexithymia. Executive functioning is fundamentally important to tracking relevant stimuli, ignoring irrelevant stimuli, inhibiting unwanted responses, and correcting errors. Thus, the role of "difficulty identifying feelings" in executive functioning reinforces that alexithymia alters early stimulus processing, including attention and appraisal, which can produce downstream effects on cognition, such as memory and behaviour, even in neutral contexts. This is consistent with the expectations posed by both Panayiotou et al. (2021) and Luminet et al. (2021). Indeed, Correro et al. (2021) found "externally oriented thinking" was responsible for memory deficits, due to reduced meaningfulness or salience of important memoranda (i.e. "signal") relative to foils (i.e."noise"), and that poor executive functioning exacerbated this effect in older adults. Thus, the authors concluded that "externally oriented thinking" reduces the ability to use internal cognitive control processes that can facilitate effective memory storage and access (Dressaire et al., 2015). This poor internal monitoring results in risks for generally poorer cognitive functioning in older age.

Vermeulen (2021): Previous literature on memory and alexithymia has focused on long-term memory (LTM) abilities (albeit almost exclusively with short retention delays), showing that retrieval is hampered in high alexithymia when the to-be-remembered stimuli or the events are emotional (e.g. Vermeulen et al., 2018). While LTM also plays a central role in short-term memory (STM) performance, very few studies have examined STM (i.e. working memory) in alexithymia (DiStefano & Koven, 2012; Takahashi et al., 2015). In his paper for this special issue, Vermeulen (2021) extends prior investigations of STM for affective and neutral words by contrasting the effects of blocked- (Study 1; only positive, negative, or neutral stimuli) and mixed-valence memoranda (Study 2; positive frequent or rare, negative frequent or rare) in alexithymia.

The results showed that alexithymia was related to a deficit for short-term memory of words, but only in the blocked condition where lists included only one category of words (Study 1). Deficits were associated with "externally oriented thinking" for all word categories; for positive words, deficits were also associated with "difficulty describing feelings". It was suggested that the poorly integrated emotion schemas in alexithymia contribute to reducing access to emotion categories, and reducing the "richness" of emotion material in particular. The results fit well with the hypothesis that those with higher alexithymia have difficulty linking symbolic and sub-symbolic representations of their past (Bucci, 1997; Taylor & Bagby, 2004), as well as with the recent attention-appraisal model that attributes alexithymia specifically to deficits of attention ("externally oriented thinking") and appraisal ("difficulty identifying feelings, externally oriented thinking") in emotion processing (Preece et al., 2017).

Ridout et al. (2021). Nearly all memory studies in alexithymia have examined verbal memoranda. In contrast, Ridout et al. (2021) importantly extend the literature by examining the influence of alexithymia on memory for socially relevant non-verbal stimuli, including faces (Study 1) and social interactions

(Study 2). In Study 1, their findings showed that "difficulty describing feelings" contributed to poorer recognition memory for emotional faces. Moreover, the deficits were particularly strong when faces exhibited anger. This memory deficit, related to "difficulty describing feelings", was also apparent in a prior study with face stimuli (Donges & Suslow, 2015) and is consistent with other studies that highlight a specific deficit in alexithymia for detecting and attending to anger and, more generally, threat-related information (e.g. Fujiwara, 2018; Luminet et al., 2011; Vermeulen et al., 2006, 2008).

In Study 2, Ridout and colleagues (2021) found that "difficulty identifying feelings" was related to poorer memory for emotional social interactions, particularly for interactions featuring anger and happiness. However, "difficulty identifying feelings" was also related to *better* familiarity for neutral interactions. Similar results were shown with words by Dressaire et al. (2015). However, this finding differs from Correro et al. (2021), where neutral memory deficits attributed to "externally oriented thinking" were worsened in those with high "difficulty identifying feelings". Importantly, Correro and colleagues used an exclusively neutral context. In contrast, participants in Ridout et al. evaluated emotive and neutral social interactions; the neutral interactions were likely easier to appraise, relative to the emotive interactions. Thus, "difficulty identifying feelings" might *facilitate* processing, if the context, even a neutral context, allows for less difficult appraisal (Luminet et al., 2021; Preece et al., 2017).

Taken together, these three memory papers suggested that alexithymia impairs memory in both short-term and long-term forms, although attention and appraisal likely contribute significantly to the findings and to the facet responsible for those effects. Moreover, the three alexithymia factors were involved in memory deficits through different underlying processes. "Difficulty identifying feelings" was related to executive functions deficits that can be linked with decreased processing resources and greater difficulty mobilising them (Correro et al., 2021). It was also related to deficits in memory for social interactions, notably those involving anger. "Difficulty describing feelings" was also related to deficits in memory involving anger, but in relation to face processing (Ridout et al., 2021).

The implications of these results are important because an anger display is a central component of threat, which activates the search for urgent responses in order to avoid danger. Specific deficits for anger processing suggest that alexithymia leads to reduced attention and reactivity when situations require particularly fast responses (see Vermeulen et al., 2006 for an extended discussion of the role of anger deficits in alexithymia). "Difficulty describing feelings" was also related to decreased STM that was linked to poorly integrated cognitive schemata (Vermeulen, 2021). Finally, in addition to decreased STM, "externally oriented thinking" was related to decreased internal monitoring and awareness that reduces the ability to extract and prioritise meaningful or salient information from extraneous and inaccurate information (Correro et al., 2021).

Verbal and non-verbal language allows people to communicate inner thoughts and feelings and to understand the utterances of others, which is central to social life. Studies have explored language expression in alexithymia, finding consistent deficits in alexithymia, typified by reduced complexity, openness and emotional content (see Luminet et al., 2021; Welding & Samur, 2018), which are linked to deficits of empathy (Grynberg et al., 2018) and mentalizing affect (Fonagy et al., 2002). Such findings suggest that language comprehension would also suffer from deficits in alexithymia. However, there is a paucity of studies specifically examining language comprehension abilities in alexithymia, except as it pertains to attention (e.g. Stroop, priming; see Welding & Samur, 2018). Fortunately, two papers that contributed to this special issue have directly addressed language comprehension in alexithymia.

Samur et al. (2021): In their paper, Samur et al. (2021) conducted both a large-cohort online study and a smaller laboratory study to measure the influence of contextual support on language comprehension, as a function of narrative engagement in alexithymia. Participants read fictional narratives written from either first-person or a third-person perspective. First-person perspectives tend to better support and engage listeners, purportedly because they support "mental transportation", helping the person to better transcend the here and now and project themselves into distant times and places (Macrae et al., 2014), which contributes social-cognitive skills (Mar & Oatley, 2008). Their results showed poorer narrative engagement in alexithymia (both for the total score and for a poor fantasy life or fantasising facet[1]). Moreover, they found that only those scoring low on alexithymia were able to benefit from first-person narratives to enhance engagement; those scoring high on alexithymia via the fantasising facet had no difference in engagement based on the narrator perspective. These findings compellingly suggest a deficit of perspective-taking in alexithymia consistent with reduced narrative engagement, which is likely due to poorer mental imagery (van der Velde et al., 2013) and poor development of emotion schemas (Hoemann & Feldman Barrett, 2019) and empathy (Grynberg et al., 2018).

Jakobson and Pearson (2021): The paper by Jakobson and Pearson (2021) examined whether the mentalizing abilities required to understand the implicit intentions of a speaker are influenced by alexithymia. Participants watched video-taped vignettes of a speaker making sincere or insincere statements in response to a question posed by an interviewer. Participants were asked to judge whether the statements were meant to be taken literally or sarcastically (in jest) or as a "fib" (i.e. a trivial lie). These were either positive (e.g. compliments) or negative (e.g. criticisms). For each statement, viewers were given either no added context, where only non-verbal cues (e.g. facial expressions, voice, body language) could be used to discern the speaker's intentions, or they were given added verbal context cues. These verbal cues, which were provided in half the videos, were short vignette segments that preceded the exchange with the interviewer, where the speaker communicated their true intentions to a third person. Thus, when watching the vignette, the participant had insight into the speaker's true intention that did not have to be surmised from behavioural cues alone. The analyses controlled for verbal intelligence and sex. The results showed that alexithymia did not impair the accuracy of discerning the speaker's intent. Indeed, *better* accuracy was associated with "difficulty describing feelings", perhaps because thresholds for excitation and sensation are typically lower in alexithymia (Liss et al., 2008), which may have made these vignettes particularly engaging to those with alexithymia. The authors suggested that "difficulty describing feelings" would instead impair performance for emotionally charged vignettes. Importantly, "difficulty identifying feelings" resulted in slower decision-making about speaker intentions when relying on non-verbal cues, which could hamper everyday social functioning.

Taken together, the two language papers in this special issue uniquely and crucially show that socio-emotional interactions, including perspective-taking, emotional empathy, imagery, and language comprehension may be hampered by alexithymia. This is fitting with the suggestion that theory of mind, including making inferences about others' states of mind, is impaired in alexithymia (Grynberg et al., 2018). They furthermore highlight that analysis of the specific contributions of facets is important to revealing when and under what circumstances alexithymia might influence social interactions. Specifically, these two unique studies suggest different roles in language for each alexithymia facet.

"Difficulty identifying feelings" appears to hamper decision-making about others' communications (Jakobson & Pearson, 2021), which is consistent with reduced capacity for and mobilisation of executive function resources (e.g. Correro et al., 2021), which may be amplified in anger contexts (Ridout et al., 2021). "Difficulty describing feelings" may be helpful to understanding others' communications when the context is unemotional, though it may have the opposite effect under emotive conditions, perhaps particularly in anger or other threat contexts (e.g. Ridout et al., 2021). Finally, fantasising (closely linked to "externally oriented thinking") contributes to deficits in perspective-taking, perhaps due to poor empathy (Grynberg et al., 2018), emotion schemas (Hoemann & Feldman Barrett, 2019) and internal monitoring and extraction of meaningful information from the environment (Correro et al., 2021). Notably, the findings of these studies also strongly suggest the importance of the further study of language comprehension in social situations in alexithymia and point to the need for a more nuanced evaluation of fantasising and emotional reactivity to better interpret these effects (Jakobson & Pearson, 2021).

Gvirts and Dery (2021): The final paper, by Gvirts and Dery (2021), provides new perspectives on the impact of alexithymia on social alignment. Social alignment theory suggests that people create connectedness, closeness and likability by creating alliances with other members of a group through thoughts, emotions and behaviours (Shamay-Tsoory et al., 2019). Because of poor communication skills, those with higher alexithymia scores would exhibit reduced social alignment. To evaluate this hypothesis, participants were randomly assigned to play an online game with a group of seven other players. Unbeknownst to participants, these "players" were either other humans, or they were bots programmed to behave more rationally than humans. The game used five cards with animal images, each with a different point value. These specific values for each card differed between players and players only knew their own valuations. The goal of the game, involving 10 rounds, was to shift choices to reach a group consensus of card choice, before time expired. During the rounds, players could see the number of players who had chosen each card. Thus, to reach consensus, they had to actively shift their choice until a consensus was reached. If no consensus was reached prior to the deadline, zero points were earned, making consensus reaching valuable. It also required making choices that could reduce the individual points earned by prioritising the card preferred by others. This "opposing alignment" is indicative of rational decision-making.

Gvirts and Dery (2021) found that higher "externally oriented thinking" scores predicted irrational decisions, but for different underlying motives depending on the type of opponent. When playing with bots, those with high "externally oriented thinking" exhibited heightened opposing alignment, where players inhibited personally beneficial actions toward better promoting a consensus. It was suggested that this likely occurred because the drive to avoid conflict was higher due to high harmony amongst other players. In contrast, during games against humans, where consensus-building was less consistent, those with higher "externally oriented thinking" exhibited less opposing alignment, instead of tending to prioritise personal gain. Social alignment has been associated with reward (Shamay-Tsoory et al., 2019). As such, Gvirts and Dery suggested that those with higher "externally oriented thinking" are less reliant on reward sensations because they did not strive to prioritise group harmony when playing against other imperfect consensus-builders. They did so only when consensus was very high; not doing so would create high conflict and disrupt group harmony. Indeed "externally oriented thinking" has been linked to poor perspective-taking (Grynberg et al., 2010), social detachment (Vanheule et al., 2011) and various aspects of impaired cognitive processing (see Luminet et al., 2021). This study compellingly contributes to our understanding of the social difficulties that have been reported experimentally, and observed clinically, in those with high levels of alexithymia, such as impaired processing of the emotional states of others, deficits in empathy and compromised pro-sociality (Grynberg et al., 2018).

4. Conclusions and new perspectives

An important finding across the papers of this special issue is the repeated observation of a lack of correspondence amongst emotional responses in alexithymia. This lack of correspondence is first apparent between processes, as well as amongst the alexithymia facets. In the review by Luminet et al. (2021) and across multiple empirical papers in this special issue there was a strong dominance of emotion-related cognitive deficits, particularly in memory and language, contrasting with an over-responding to emotion or threat in behavioural responding. Impaired performance in the cognitive domain was associated with each of the alexithymia facets, but dominantly so with "externally oriented thinking". These effects have been linked to poor internal monitoring and avoidance behaviours (see Luminet et al., 2021; Preece et al., 2017). In contrast, "difficulty identifying feelings" was more often associated with an over-responding to emotion or threat (e.g. Teten et al., 2008; Velotti et al., 2016), and together with "difficulty describing feelings", was linked to the poor appraisal of stimuli, cognitive control and evaluation of salience (see Luminet et al., 2021; Preece et al., 2017). Thus, these studies collectively highlight that emotion processing is not homogeneous across processes. That is, it is not represented by a continuous dimension where "more is better". Instead, deviations in either direction from typical may reflect the influence of distinct underlying cognitive mechanisms. Alexithymia research exemplifies the opportunities available to better delineate and explain the foundations and mechanisms of these deviations.

The lack of correspondence between emotion processes found in the special issue corresponds to a small number of empirical studies that have simultaneously considered the three emotion components (physiological, behaviour-expressive and cognitive-experiential). These studies show that in low alexithymia the three components are positively associated, while in high alexithymia they are dissociated[2] (Constantinou et al., 2014; Pollatos & Gramann, 2011). Similarly, Peasley-Miklus et al. (2016) reported weaker physiological–cognitive/experiential and behavioural–cognitive/experiential associations in higher alexithymia participants. These responses contrast with a fuller, normal emotional experience that involves the activation of the three emotional components.

Studies that have examined combinations of the three components together (e.g. multi-component studies) show that in normative samples they are correlated, although not always strongly so (e.g. Bradley & Lang, 2000; Cacioppo et al., 1992; Mauss et al., 2005). A central outcome is that emotional awareness is generated through synchronisation amongst emotional components (Scherer, 2000, 2005; see also Grandjean et al., 2008), which fits with models suggesting that alexithymia is related to emotion awareness deficits (three-process model, Smith et al., 2018; see Luminet et al., 2021 for a discussion of the relevance of the model to account for cognitive–emotional impairments in alexithymia). Furthermore, dissociated emotional components have been demonstrated as a risk factor for long-term negative health outcomes (e.g. Myers, 2010; Schäflein et al., 2018), providing a process explanation for the ubiquitous negative mental and physical health outcomes in alexithymia (e.g. Morie & Ridout, 2018). Together, these findings illuminate the intersecting and situationally specific relationships amongst emotional components and emphasise the value of multi-component studies for a fuller understanding of the interface between cognition and emotion generally, and specifically in individual and personality differences.

The papers on the special issue also provide valuable insights for future research on the cognition–emotion interface. We briefly consider insights at three levels of analysis: extending the type of processes involved, considering systematically neutral and emotive contexts together, and improving methodological condition. At the process level, at least four papers in this special issue (Gvirts & Dery, 2021; Jakobson & Pearson, 2021; Ridout et al., 2021; Samur et al., 2021) illustrate the richness of systematical investigations into interpersonal and collective processes such as empathy, pro-social behaviours or norms adherence, clearly indicating these processes have important influences on cognitive-emotion interactions beyond the intra-individual level. Studies such as the one by Correro et al. (2021) furthermore highlight the importance of drawing better connections amongst multiple processes, toward disentangling the effects of early processes (e.g. attention) on later processes (e.g. memory and language). In addition, they suggest the value of better delineating relationships between cognitive processes, such as executive functions, and personality characteristics, including and beyond alexithymia.

At the context level, it is important to consider that the processing of neutral information is not simply a baseline measure to compare with emotional stimuli. While studies of the cognition–emotion interface tend to focus on processing during emotive contexts, the papers in this special issue show that neutral information is not immune to the influence of individual differences, resulting in both deficits (e.g. Correro et al., 2021; Vermeulen, 2021) and benefits (Ridout et al., 2021).

Finally, at the methodological level, the papers in this special issue demonstrate that the vast majority of studies of the cognition–emotion interface in alexithymia are done cross-sectionally and in normative samples. These papers highlight the need for a greater focus on longitudinal and experimental designs that allow for causal interpretations regarding influences on the cognition–emotion interface. Regarding normative samples, alexithymia is a stable personality trait, rather than simply a clinical categorisation (e.g. Luminet et al., 2001). Thus, it is important to consider that studies of the cognition–emotion interface in alexithymia, including all of the papers in this special issue, have almost exclusively employed normative rather than severe or clinical samples. Moreover, each paper demonstrated significant cognitive and behavioural implications of alexithymia without the aid of severe populations, and even extended beyond emotion processing into more general cognitive processing. It would therefore be expected for such effects to be more exaggerated, and even more important to address, in more severe alexithymia. This conclusion further implies that all studies of the cognitive-emotion interface would directly benefit from a greater consideration of the contributions of personality differences, alongside well-designed experimental methods, thereby allowing more thorough explanatory frameworks.

In conclusion, thea studies that compose this special issue highlight that alexithymia influences several aspects of how one perceives and responds to neutral and emotional situations and interacts with others in those situations. From the introductive vignette presented by Luminet et al. (2021), we can highlight that scoring high on alexithymia has multiple implications for daily life. A lack of variation in emotional responses, a scarcity of experiencing pleasant feelings, and an attribution of personal reactions to external rather than internal circumstances limits the extent and quality of their social network, increases the likelihood of somatic illnesses, and restricts their inner world to purely factual concerns. These outcomes are broad and consequential for their biological, psychological and social life. We expect that the findings presented in this special issue can help to advance the design and targeting of both future cognition–emotion research, and the development of effective interventions to improve emotion processing and reduce risk and manifestation of physical and emotional illness.

Notes

1. Poor fantasy life is assessed in some self-report scales such as the BVAQ (Bermond et al., 2015). It is closely related to externally oriented thinking.
2. Dissociation across emotional components can take different forms. Specifically, there can be simultaneous activation of one component while there is deactivation of another, or deactivation or activation of one component, with no activation of other components.

Disclosure statement

No potential conflict of interest was reported by the author(s).

Funding

This work was supported by Fund for Scientific Research – Belgium (FRS-FNRS).

ORCID

Olivier Luminet http://orcid.org/0000-0002-1519-2178
Kristy A. Nielson http://orcid.org/0000-0001-8977-3138
Nathan Ridout http://orcid.org/0000-0002-7111-2996

References

Aaron, R. V., Snodgress, M. A., Blain, S. D., & Park, S. (2018). Affect labeling and other aspects of emotional experiences in relation to alexithymia following standardized emotion inductions. *Psychiatry Research*, *262*, 115–123. https://doi.org/10.1016/j.psychres.2018.02.014

Alexander, F. (1950). *Psychosomatic medicine*. Norton & Company.

Bagby, R. M., Parker, J. D. A., & Taylor, G. J. (1994a). The twenty-item Toronto Alexithymia scale—I. Item selection and cross-validation of the factor structure. *Journal of Psychosomatic Research*, *38*(1), 23–32. https://doi.org/10.1016/0022-3999(94)90005-1

Bagby, R. M., Taylor, G. J., & Parker, J. D. A. (1994b). The twenty-item Toronto Alexithymia scale—II. Convergent, discriminant, and concurrent validity. *Journal of Psychosomatic Research*, *38*(1), 33–40. https://doi.org/10.1016/0022-3999(94)90006-X

Baumert, A., Schmitt, M., Perugini, M., Johnson, W., Blum, G., Borkenau, P., Costantini, G., Denissen, J. J. A., Fleeson, W., Grafton, B., Jayawickreme, E., Kurzius, E., MacLeod, C., Miller, L. C., Read, S. J., Roberts, B., Robinson, M. D., Wood, D., Wrzus, C., & Mõttus, R. (2017). Integrating personality structure, personality process, and personality development. *European Journal of Personality*, *31*(5), 503–528. https://doi.org/10.1002/per.2115

Bayot, M., Pleyers, G., Kotsou, I., Lefèvre, N., Sauter, D. A., & Vermeulen, N. (2014). Joint effect of alexithymia and mood on the categorization of nonverbal emotional vocalizations. *Psychiatry Research*, *216*(2), 242–247. https://doi.org/10.1016/j.psychres.2013.12.007

Beresnevaite, M. (2000). Exploring the benefits of group psychotherapy in reducing alexithymia in coronary heart disease patients: A preliminary study. *Psychotherapy and Psychosomatics*, *69*(3), 117–122. https://doi.org/10.1159/000012378

Bermond, B., Oosterveld, P., & Vorst, H. C. (2015). Measures of alexithymia. In G. J. Boyle, D. H. Saklofske, & G. Matthews (Eds.), *Measures of personality and social psychological constructs* (pp. 227–256). Elsevier.

Bradley, M. M., & Lang, P. J. (2000). Affective reactions to acoustic stimuli. *Psychophysiology*, *37*(2), 204–215. https://doi.org/10.1111/1469-8986.3720204

Bucci, W. (1997). *Psychoanalysis and cognitive science: A multiple code theory*. Guilford Press.

Cacioppo, J. T., Uchino, B. N., Crites, S. L., Snydersmith, M. A., Smith, G., Berntson, G. G., & Lang, P. J. (1992). Relationship between facial expressiveness and sympathetic activation in emotion: A critical review, with emphasis on modeling underlying mechanisms and individual differences. *Journal of Personality and Social Psychology*, *62*(1), 110–128. https://doi.org/10.1037/0022-3514.62.1.110

Constantinou, E., Panayiotou, G., & Theodorou, M. (2014). Emotion processing deficits in alexithymia and response to a depth of processing intervention. *Biological Psychology*, *103*, 212–222. https://doi.org/10.1016/j.biopsycho.2014.09.011

Correro IIA. N., Paitel, E. R., Byers, S. J., & Nielson, K. A. (2021). The role of alexithymia in memory and executive functioning across the lifespan. *Cognition and Emotion*, 1–16. https://doi.org/10.1080/02699931.2019.1659232

da Silva, A. N., Vasco, A. B., & Watson, J. C. (2017). Alexithymia and emotional processing: A mediation model. *Journal of Clinical Psychology*, *73*(9), 1196–1205. https://doi.org/10.1002/jclp.22422

DiStefano, R. A., & Koven, N. S. (2012). Dysfunctional emotion processing may explain visual memory deficits in alexithymia. *Personality and Individual Differences*, *52*(5), 611–615. https://doi.org/10.1016/j.paid.2011.12.007

Donges, U. S., & Suslow, T. (2015). Alexithymia and memory for facial emotions. *Universitas Psychologica*, *14*(1), 103–110. https://doi.org/10.11144/Javeriana.upsy14-1.amfe

Dressaire, D., Stone, C. B., Nielson, K. A., Guerdoux, E., Martin, S., Brouillet, D., & Luminet, O. (2015). Alexithymia impairs the cognitive control of negative material while facilitating the recall of neutral material in both younger and older adults. *Cognition and Emotion*, *29*(3), 442–459. https://doi.org/10.1080/02699931.2014.919898

Ellsworth, P. C., & Scherer, K. R. (2003). Appraisal processes in emotion. In R. J. Davidson, K. R. Scherer, & H. Goldsmith

(Eds.), *Handbook of affective sciences* (pp. 572–595). Oxford University Press.

Fonagy, P., Gergely, G., Jurist, E., & Target, M. (2002). *Mentalization, affective regulation and the development of the self*. Other Press.

Frijda, N. H. (1986). *The emotions*. Cambridge University Press.

Fujiwara, E. (2018). Looking at the eyes interferes with facial emotion recognition in alexithymia. *Journal of Abnormal Psychology*, *127*(6), 571–577. https://doi.org/10.1037/abn0000361

Grandjean, D., Sander, D., & Scherer, K. R. (2008). Conscious emotional experience emerges as a function of multilevel, appraisal-driven response synchronization. *Consciousness and Cognition*, *17*(2), 484–495. https://doi.org/10.1016/j.concog.2008.03.019

Groddeck, G. (1923). *Le livre du ça*. Gallimard.

Grynberg, D., Berthoz, S., & Bird, G. (2018). Social and interpersonal implications. In O. Luminet, G. J. Taylor, & R. M. Bagby (Eds.), *Alexithymia: Advances in research, theory, and clinical practice* (pp. 174–189). Cambridge University Press.

Grynberg, D., Luminet, O., Corneille, O., Grèzes, J., & Berthoz, S. (2010). Alexithymia in the interpersonal domain: A general deficit of empathy? *Personality and Individual Differences*, *49* (8), 845–850. https://doi.org/10.1016/j.paid.2010.07.013

Gvirts, H. Z., & Dery, L. (2021). Alexithymia and reaching group consensus. *Cognition & Emotion*, 1–14. https://doi.org/10.1080/02699931.2019.1675600.

Hoemann, K., & Feldman Barrett, L. (2019). Concepts dissolve artificial boundaries in the study of emotion and cognition, uniting body, brain, and mind. *Cognition and Emotion*, *33* (1), 67–76. https://doi.org/10.1080/02699931.2018.1535428

Hoppe, K. D., & Bogen, J. E. (1977). Alexithymia in twelve commissurotomized patients. *Psychotherapy and Psychosomatics*, *28*(1-4), 148–155. https://doi.org/10.1159/000287057

Horney, K. (1952). The paucity of inner experiences. *The American Journal of Psychoanalysis*, *12*(1), 3–9. https://doi.org/10.1007/BF01872367

Ihme, K., Sacher, J., Lichev, V., Rosenberg, N., Kugel, H., Rufer, M., Grabe, H.-J., Pampel, A., Lepsien, J., Kersting, A., Villringer, A., Lane, R. D., & Suslow, T. (2014b). Alexithymic features and the labeling of brief emotional facial expressions – An fMRI study. *Neuropsychologia*, *64*, 289–299. https://doi.org/10.1016/j.neuropsychologia.2014.09.044

Ihme, K., Sacher, J., Lichev, V., Rosenberg, N., Kugel, H., Rufer, M., Grabe, H.-J., Pampel, A., Lepsien, J., Kersting, A., Villringer, A., & Suslow, T. (2014a). Alexithymia and the labeling of facial emotions: Response slowing and increased motor and somatosensory processing. *BMC Neuroscience*, *15*(1), 40. https://doi.org/10.1186/1471-2202-15-40

Jakobson, L. S., & Pearson, P. M. (2021). Alexithymic traits predict the speed of classifying non-literal statements using nonverbal cues. *Cognition and Emotion*, 1–7. https://doi.org/10.1080/02699931.2020.1715346.

Joormann, J. (2019). Is the glass half empty or half full and does it even matter? Cognition, emotion, and psychopathology *Cognition and Emotion*, *33*(1), 133–138. https://doi.org/10.1080/02699931.2018.1502656

Kätsyri, J., Saalasti, S., Tiippana, K., von Wendt, L., & Sams, M. (2008). Impaired recognition of facial emotions from low-spatial frequencies in asperger syndrome. *Neuropsychologia*, *46*(7), 1888–1897. https://doi.org/10.1016/j.neuropsychologia.2008.01.005

Kelman, N. (1952). Clinical aspects of externalized living. *The American Journal of Psychoanalysis*, *12*(1), 15–23. https://doi.org/10.1007/BF01872369

Koole, S. L., & Rothermund, K. (2019). Revisiting the past and back to the future: Horizons of cognition and emotion research. *Cognition and Emotion*, *33*(1), 1–7. https://doi.org/10.1080/02699931.2019.1574398

Koven, N. S. (2014). Abnormal valence differentiation in alexithymia. *Personality and Individual Differences*, *68*, 102–106. https://doi.org/10.1016/j.paid.2014.04.007

Krystal, H. (1988). *Integration and self-healing: Affect, trauma, alexithymia*. Analytic Press.

Kuppens, P., Stouten, J., & Mesquita, B. (2009). Individual differences in emotion components and dynamics: Introduction to the special issue. *Cognition and Emotion*, *23*(7), 1249–1258. https://doi.org/10.1080/02699930902985605

Lane, R. D., Reiman, E. M., Axelrod, B., Yun, L. S., Holmes, A., & Schwartz, G. E. (1998). Neural correlates of levels of emotional awareness: Evidence of an interaction between emotion and attention in the anterior cingulate cortex. *Journal of Cognitive Neuroscience*, *10*(4), 525–535. https://doi.org/10.1162/089892998562924

Larwood, J. L., Vanman, E. J., & Dingle, G. A. (2021). Negative valence specific deficits in judgements of musical affective quality in alexithymia. *Cognition and Emotion*, 1–10. https://doi.org/10.1080/02699931.2019.1707514.

Liss, M., Mailloux, J., & Erchull, M. J. (2008). The relationships between sensory processing sensitivity, alexithymia, autism, depression, and anxiety. *Personality and Individual Differences*, *45*(3), 255–259. https://doi.org/10.1016/j.paid.2008.04.009

Luminet, O., Bagby, R. M., & Taylor, G. J. (2001). An evaluation of the absolute and relative stability of alexithymia in patients with major depression. *Psychotherapy and Psychosomatics*, *70*(5), 254–260. https://doi.org/10.1159/000056263

Luminet, O., Grynberg, D., Ruzette, N., & Mikolajczak, M. (2011). Personality-dependent effects of oxytocin: Greater social benefits for high alexithymia scorers. *Biological Psychology*, *87* (3), 401–406. https://doi.org/10.1016/j.biopsycho.2011.05.005

Luminet, O., Nielson, K. A., & Ridout, N. (2021). Alexithymia as a fundamental dimension of emotional life: An integrative review. *Cognition and Emotion*. https://doi.org/10.1080/02699931.2021.1908231

Luminet, O., Rimé, B., Bagby, R. M., & Taylor, G. J. (2004). A multimodal investigation of emotional responding in alexithymia. *Cognition and Emotion*, *18*(6), 741–766. https://doi.org/10.1080/02699930341000275

Luminet, O., Vermeulen, N., Demaret, C., Taylor, G. J., & Bagby, R. M. (2006). Alexithymia and levels of processing: Evidence for an overall deficit in remembering emotion words. *Journal of Research in Personality*, *40*(5), 713–733. https://doi.org/10.1016/j.jrp.2005.09.001

Luminet, O., & Zamariola, G. (2018). Emotion knowledge and emotion regulation in alexithymia. In O. Luminet, R. M. Bagby, & G. J. Taylor (Eds.), *Alexithymia: Advances in research, theory, and clinical practice* (pp. 49–77). Cambridge University Press.

Luminet, O., Zech, E., Rimé, B., & Wagner, H. L. (2000). Predicting cognitive and social consequences of emotional episodes:

The contribution of emotional intensity, the five factor model and alexithymia. *Journal of Research in Personality*, *34*(4), 471–497. https://doi.org/10.1006/jrpe.2000.2286

Lundh, L. G., Johnsson, A., Sundqvist, K., & Olsson, H. (2002). Alexithymia, memory of emotion, emotional awareness, and perfectionism. *Emotion*, *2*(4), 361–379. https://doi.org/10.1037/1528-3542.2.4.361

MacLean, P. D. (1949). Psychosomatic disease and the « visceral brain » – recent developments bearing on the papez theory of emotion. *Psychosomatic Medicine*, *11*(6), 338–353. https://doi.org/10.1097/00006842-194911000-00003

Macrae, C. N., Christian, B. M., & Miles, L. K. (2014). Imagination and behavioral control. In J. P. Forgas & E. Harmon-Jones (Eds.), *Motivation and its regulation: The control within* (pp. 79–94). Taylor & Francis.

Mann, L. S., Wise, T. N., Trinidad, A., & Kohanski, R. (1994). Alexithymia, affect recognition, and the five-factor model of personality in normal subjects. *Psychological Reports*, *74*(2), 563–567. https://doi.org/10.2466/pr0.1994.74.2.563

Mar, R. A., & Oatley, K. (2008). The function of fiction is the abstraction and simulation of social experience. *Perspectives on Psychological Science*, *3*(3), 173–192. https://doi.org/10.1111/j.1745-6924.2008.00073.x

Marty, P., & de M'Uzan, M. (1963). La pensée opératoire. *Revue Française de Psychanalyse*, *27*(suppl.), 345–356.

Mather, M., & Sutherland, M. R. (2011). Arousal-biased competition in perception and memory. *Perspectives on Psychological Science*, *6*(2), 114–133. https://doi.org/10.1177/1745691611400234

Mauss, I. B., Levenson, R. W., McCarter, L., Wilhelm, F. H., & Gross, J. J. (2005). The tie that binds? Coherence among emotion experience, behavior, and physiology. *Emotion*, *5*(2), 175. https://doi.org/10.1037/1528-3542.5.2.175

McEwen, B. S. (1998). Stress, adaptation, and disease: Allostasis and allostatic load. *Annals of the New York Academy of Sciences*, *840*(1), 33–44. https://doi.org/10.1111/j.1749-6632.1998.tb09546.x

Mischel, W., & Shoda, Y. (1998). Reconciling processing dynamics and personality dispositions. *Annual Review of Psychology*, *49* (1), 229–258. https://doi.org/10.1146/annurev.psych.49.1.229

Morie, K. P., & Ridout, N. (2018). Alexithymia and maladaptive regulatory behaviors in substance use disorders and eating disorders. In O. Luminet, G. J. Taylor, & R. M. Bagby (Eds.), *Alexithymia: Advances in research, theory, and clinical practice* (pp. 158–174). Cambridge University Press.

Myers, L. B. (2010). The importance of the repressive coping style: Findings from 30 years of research *Anxiety, Stress, & Coping*, *23*(1), 3–17. https://doi.org/10.1080/10615800903366945

Nemiah, J. C., & Sifneos, P. E. (1970). Psychosomatic illness: A problem in communication. *Psychotherapy and Psychosomatics*, *18*(1-6), 154–160. https://doi.org/10.1159/000286074

Nielson, K. A., & Correro IIA. N. (2017). Post-learning arousal enhances veridical memory and reduces false memory in the Deese–Roediger–McDermott paradigm. *Neurobiology of Learning and Memory*, *144*, 198–207. https://doi.org/10.1016/j.nlm.2017.07.009

Oatley, K., Parrott, W. G., Smith, C., & Watts, F. (2011). Cognition and emotion over twenty-five years. *Cognition and Emotion*, *25*(8), 1341–1348. https://doi.org/10.1080/02699931.2011.622949

Panayiotou, G., Panteli, M., & Vlemincx, E. (2021). Adaptive and maladaptive emotion processing and regulation, and the case for alexithymia. *Cognition and Emotion*, 1–19. https://doi.org/10.1080/02699931.2019.1671322.

Papciak, A. S., Feuerstein, M., & Spiegel, J. A. (1985). Stress reactivity in alexithymia: Decoupling of physiological and cognitive responses. *Journal of Human Stress*, *11*(3), 135–142. https://doi.org/10.1080/0097840X.1985.9936750

Parker, J., Taylor, G. J., & Bagby, R. M. (1993b). Alexithymia and the processing of emotional stimuli: An experimental study. *New Trends Experimental and Clinical Psychiatry*, *9*(1/2), 9–14.

Parker, J. D. A., Taylor, G. J., & Bagby, R. M. (1993a). Alexithymia and the recognition of facial expressions of emotion. *Psychotherapy and Psychosomatics*, *59*(3-4), 197–202. https://doi.org/10.1159/000288664

Peasley-Miklus, C. E., Panayiotou, G., & Vrana, S. R. (2016). Alexithymia predicts arousal-based processing deficits and discordance between emotion response systems during emotional imagery. *Emotion*, *16*(2), 164–174. https://doi.org/10.1037/emo0000086

Pollatos, O., & Gramann, K. (2011). Electrophysiological evidence of early processing deficits in alexithymia. *Biological Psychology*, *87*(1), 113–121. https://doi.org/10.1016/j.biopsycho.2011.02.016

Preece, D., Becerra, R., Allan, A., Robinson, K., & Dandy, J. (2017). Establishing the theoretical components of alexithymia via factor analysis: Introduction and validation of the attention-appraisal model of alexithymia. *Personality and Individual Differences*, *119*, 341–352. https://doi.org/10.1016/j.paid.2017.08.003

Prkachin, G. C., Casey, C., & Prkachin, K. M. (2009). Alexithymia and perception of facial expressions of emotion. *Personality and Individual Differences*, *46*(4), 412–417. https://doi.org/10.1016/j.paid.2008.11.010

Quirin, M., Robinson, M. D., Rauthmann, J. F., Kuhl, J., Read, S. J., Tops, M., & DeYoung, C. G. (2020). The dynamics of personality approach (DPA): 20 tenets for uncovering the causal mechanisms of personality. *European Journal of Personality*, https://doi.org/10.1002/per.2295

Reise, S. P., Bonifay, W. E., & Haviland, M. G. (2013). Scoring and modeling psychological measures in the presence of multidimensionality. *Journal of Personality Assessment*, *95*(2), 129–140. https://doi.org/10.1080/00223891.2012.725437

Ridout, N., Smith, J., & Hawkins, H. (2021). The influence of alexithymia on memory for emotional faces and realistic social interactions. *Cognition and Emotion*, 1–19. https://doi.org/10.1080/02699931.2020.1747991

Robinson, M. D., Klein, R. J., & Persich, M. R. (2019). Personality traits in action: A cognitive behavioral version of the social cognitive paradigm. *Personality and Individual Differences*, *147*, 214–222. https://doi.org/10.1016/j.paid.2019.04.041

Ruesch, J. (1948). The infantile personality. *Psychosomatic Medicine*, *10*(3), 134–144. https://doi.org/10.1097/00006842-194805000-00002

Samur, D., Tops, M., Slapšinskaitė, R., & Koole, S. L. (2021). Getting lost in a story: How narrative engagement emerges from narrative perspective and individual differences in alexithymia. *Cognition and Emotion*, 1–13. https://doi.org/10.1080/02699931.2020.1732876.

Schäflein, E., Sattel, H. C., Pollatos, O., & Sack, M. (2018). Disconnected – impaired interoceptive accuracy and Its association with self-perception and cardiac vagal tone in patients with dissociative disorder. *Frontiers in Psychology*, *9*, 897. https://doi.org/10.3389/fpsyg.2018.00897

Scherer, K. R. (2000). Emotions as episodes of subsystem synchronization driven by nonlinear appraisal processes. In M. D. Lewis & I. Granic (Eds.), *Emotion, development, and selforganization: Dynamic systems approaches to emotional development* (pp. 70–99). Cambridge University Press.

Scherer, K. R. (2005). What are emotions? And how can they be measured? *Social Science Information*, *44*(4), 695–729. https://doi.org/10.1177/0539018405058216

Schmidt, U., Jiwany, A., & Treasure, J. (1993). A controlled study of alexithymia in eating disorders. *Comprehensive Psychiatry*, *34*(1), 54–58. https://doi.org/10.1016/0010-440X(93)90036-4

Shamay-Tsoory, S. G., Saporta, N., Marton-Alper, I. Z., & Gvirts, H. Z. (2019). Herding brains: A core neural mechanism for social alignment. *Trends in Cognitive Sciences*, *23*(3), 174–186. https://doi.org/10.1016/j.tics.2019.01.002

Shoda, Y., & Mischel, W. (2000). Reconciling contextualism with the core assumptions of personality psychology. *European Journal of Personality*, *14*(5), 407–428. https://doi.org/10.1002/1099-0984(200009/10)14:5<407::AID-PER391>3.0.CO;2-3

Sifneos, P. E. (1973). The prevalence of 'alexithymic' characteristics in psychosomatic patients. *Psychotherapy and Psychosomatics*, *22*(2-6), 255–262. https://doi.org/10.1159/000286529

Sifneos, P. E., Apfel-Savitz, R., & Frankel, F. H. (1977). The phenomenon of « alexithymia ». observations in neurotic and psychosomatic patients. *Psychotherapy and Psychosomatics*, *28*(1-4), 47–57. https://doi.org/10.1159/000287043

Smith, R., Killgore, W. D., & Lane, R. D. (2018). The structure of emotional experience and its relation to trait emotional awareness: A theoretical review. *Emotion*, *18*, 670–692.

Takahashi, J., Hirano, T., & Gyoba, J. (2015). Effects of facial expressions on visual short-term memory in relation to alexithymia traits. *Personality and Individual Differences*, *83*, 128–135. https://doi.org/10.1016/j.paid.2015.04.010

Taylor, G. J. (2000). Recent developments in alexithymia theory and research. *The Canadian Journal of Psychiatry*, *45*(2), 134–142. https://doi.org/10.1177/070674370004500203

Taylor, G. J., & Bagby, R. M. (2004). New trends in alexithymia research. *Psychotherapy and Psychosomatics*, *73*(2), 68–77. https://doi.org/10.1159/000075537

Taylor, G. J., Bagby, R. M., & Parker, J. D. A. (1997). *Disorders of affect regulation: Alexithymia in medical and psychiatric illness*. Cambridge University Press.

Taylor, G. J., Bagby, R. M., & Parker, J. D. A. (2016). What's in the name 'alexithymia'? A commentary on "affective agnosia: Expansion of the alexithymia construct and a new opportunity to integrate and extend Freud's legacy.". *Neuroscience and Biobehavioral Reviews*, *68*, 1006–1020. https://doi.org/10.1016/j.neubiorev.2016.05.025

Teten, A. L., Miller, L. A., Bailey, S. D., Dunn, N. J., & Kent, T. A. (2008). Empathic deficits and alexithymia in trauma-related impulsive aggression. *Behavior Sciences and the Law*, *26*(6), 823–832. https://doi.org/10.1002/bsl.843

van der Velde, J., Servaas, M. N., Goerlich, K. S., Bruggeman, R., Horton, P., Costafreda, S. G., & Aleman, A. (2013). Neural correlates of alexithymia: A meta-analysis of emotion processing studies. *Neuroscience & Biobehavioral Reviews*, *37*(8), 1774–1785. https://doi.org/10.1016/j.neubiorev.2013.07.008

Vanheule, S., Meganck, R., & Desmet, M. (2011). Alexithymia, social detachment and cognitive processing. *Psychiatry Research*, *190*(1), 49–51. https://doi.org/10.1016/j.psychres.2010.06.032

Velotti, P., Garofalo, C., Petrocchi, C., Cavallo, F., Popolo, R., & Dimaggio, G. (2016). Alexithymia, emotion dysregulation, impulsivity and aggression: A multiple mediation model. *Psychiatry Research*, *237*, 296–303. https://doi.org/10.1016/j.psychres.2016.01.025

Vermeulen, N. (2021). Alexithymia disrupts verbal short-term memory. *Cognition and Emotion*, 1–10. https://doi.org/10.1080/02699931.2019.1701418

Vermeulen, N., Domachowska, I., & Nielson, K. A. (2018). Memory and executive functions in alexithymia. In O. Luminet, G. J. Taylor, & R. M. Bagby (Eds.), *Alexithymia: Advances in research, theory, and clinical practice* (pp. 49–77). Cambridge University Press.

Vermeulen, N., Luminet, O., & Corneille, O. (2006). Alexithymia and the automatic processing of affective information: Evidence from the affective priming paradigm. *Cognition and Emotion*, *20*(1), 64–91. https://doi.org/10.1080/02699930500304654

Vermeulen, N., Luminet, O., De Sousa, M. C., & Campanella, S. (2008). Categorical perception of anger is disrupted in alexithymia: Evidence from a visual ERP study. *Cognition and Emotion*, *22*(6), 1052–1067. https://doi.org/10.1080/02699930701597635

Welding, C., & Samur, D. (2018). Language processing in alexithymia. In O. Luminet, G. J. Taylor, & R. M. Bagby (Eds.), *Alexithymia: Advances in research, theory, and clinical practice* (pp. 90–104). Cambridge University Press. https://doi.org/10.1017/9781108241595.

Wittkower, E. (1938). Ulcerative colitis: Studies of personality. *British Medical Journal*, *2*(4069), 1356–1360. https://doi.org/10.1136/bmj.2.4069.1356

Yiend, J. (2010). The effects of emotion on attention: A review of attentional processing of emotional information. *Cognition and Emotion*, *24*(1), 3–47. https://doi.org/10.1080/02699930903205698

Cognitive-emotional processing in alexithymia: an integrative review

Olivier Luminet, Kristy A. Nielson and Nathan Ridout

ABSTRACT

Alexithymia is a multifaceted personality construct characterised by difficulties identifying one's feelings and distinguishing them from bodily sensations, difficulties describing one's feelings to others, and an externally oriented cognitive style. Over the past 25 years, a burgeoning body of research has examined how alexithymia moderates processing at the cognition–emotion interface. We review the findings in five domains: attention, appraisals, memory, language, and behaviours. The preponderance of studies linked alexithymia with deficits in emotion processing, which was apparent across all domains, except behaviours. All studies on behaviours and a proportion of studies in other domains demonstrated emotional over-responding. Analysis at the facet level revealed deficits in memory and language that are primarily associated with externally oriented thinking, while over-responding was most often linked to difficulty identifying feelings and difficulty describing feelings. The review also found evidence for contextual modulation: The pattern of deficits and over-responding was not restricted to emotional contexts but also occurred in neutral contexts, and in some circumstances, emotional over-responding in alexithymia was beneficial. Taken together, this review highlights alexithymia as a central personality dimension in the interplay between cognition and emotion.

Chris is fifty years old, divorced, has two adult children, and works as a civil engineer in a large technology company. Chris displays little emotion other than mild irritability. They have hypertension and has suffered from irritable bowel syndrome for over ten years. They show little insight into their feelings or inner life, and focus primarily on impersonal factors like the weather, their diet, or their job as potential causes of their physical problems. Chris sometimes reports a sense of inner emptiness and finds that they are about to cry, but cannot explain these behaviours. Chris mentions that they never experience pleasant emotions other than mild enjoyment when meeting with their children each week. They report having no noticeable feelings during their divorce four years earlier or after their brother's suicide the following year. Chris has only weak emotional connections with their few friends. They rarely recall their dreams and seldom experiences fantasies.

The above vignette describes a typical profile of the men and women who score high on alexithymia. Alexithymia is a multifaceted personality construct targeting socio-emotional competencies. Individuals scoring high on this construct have (a) difficulty identifying feelings and distinguishing feelings from bodily sensations of emotional arousal; (b) difficulty describing their feelings to others; (c) a restricted fantasy life; and (d) a cognitive style in which the focus of attention is external, with little interest for introspection or insight (e.g. Taylor et al., 2016). People scoring high on alexithymia can experience emotions and do get distressed by their emotions. Nevertheless, they lack adequate mental representations to experience them as identifiable and describable feelings (Taylor et al., 2016). Alexithymia therefore constitutes a vulnerability factor for both mental and somatic illnesses (e.g. Baudic et al., 2016; Porcelli et al., 2007; Tolmunen et al., 2010).

Over the last twenty-five years, many papers have examined the role of alexithymia in various aspects in the cognitive processing of emotion. Our goal in this article is to unlock this line of research for emotion researchers, by conducting a theoretically oriented review of alexithymia research. In what follows, we start by describing two different models of alexithymia: The first model regards alexithymia as a deficit in emotional processing, whereas the second model regards alexithymia as emotional over-responding. Next, we provide background on the early foci of research and its measurement. In the main section of the paper, we review evidence for the deficit and over-responding models of alexithymia in research on attention, appraisals, memory, language, and behaviour. Our review includes both a general assessment and an analysis at the level of alexithymia facets, a critical assessment of methodological factors and the role of context, the clinical significance of the results, and neuro-imaging findings. We finish with the implications of our findings for major emotion theories (attentional bias and control, appraisal, and emotion awareness).

1. Introduction

1.1. Deficit and "Over-responding" models

A fundamental unanswered question is under which circumstances alexithymia involves a deficit or an excess of emotional processing (i.e. "over-responding"). Since its inception, alexithymia has been viewed as a deficit in emotion identification and communication (Sifneos et al., 1977), and cognitive processing and regulation of emotions (Taylor, 2000). This view corresponds to the ability/ deficit hypothesis of alexithymia developed by Preece et al. (2017) in which they highlight that people with higher alexithymia scores have poorly organised, differentiated, and integrated emotional schemas, which means they are unable to focus on the most relevant aspects of their emotional responses or to make accurate interpretations of input information about emotions. In parallel, alexithymia has sometimes been conceptualised as a defensive reaction to overly intense feelings that we will refer to as over-responding (OR) for the remainder of this paper (e.g. Knapp, 1983; Marchesi et al., 2014). Preece et al. (2017) proposed that avoidance in alexithymia causes the individual to regress to operating at an earlier developmental level of information processing. These models are not mutually exclusive, with some authors adopting both the deficit and the defensive approaches (Krystal, 1982, 1988; McDougall, 1982–83; Nemiah, 1977; Preece et al., 2017). However, to date, no systematic efforts have been made to integrate these models and delineate the conditions that would produce deficits vs. over-responding. This is a major goal of this review. We further distinguish between over-responding that is detrimental to functioning and over-responding that is beneficial to functioning. To effectively draw these delineations, as well as contribute to their potential clinical applications, considering situational context is essential, such as whether effects occur under neutral and/or under emotional activation, and/or under pleasant or unpleasant conditions.

Another key focus of this paper is to examine the distinct role of alexithymia facets, rather than total alexithymia scores. Identifying the unique processes (e.g. attention, appraisals, memory, language, behaviours) that are particularly related to specific facet of alexithymia allows identification of which factors are the most related to individual vulnerabilities for mental and somatic outcomes. For the purposes of this paper, we consider the primary facets described in the literature, which are (a) difficulty identifying feelings (DIF), (b) difficulty describing feelings (DDF), and externally oriented thinking (EOT). Fantasising is sometimes included but is less emphasised in this review. Thus, if we take the example of mental and somatic outcomes, many studies evidence a positive association with DIF and DDF, but not with EOT (e.g. Hund & Espelage, 2006; Nowakowski et al., 2013). In contrast, higher EOT scores have been related to fewer intrusive thoughts (Luminet et al., 2004), reduced physiological reactivity after being exposed to films inducing sadness (Davydov et al., 2013), and reduced craving for alcohol (Luminet et al., 2016). These consequences could decrease mental and somatic vulnerabilities. We therefore predict that specific alexithymia facets affect some processes more than others, and might distinguish deficits vs. over-responding. DIF, reflecting deficits in emotion perception, is expected to mainly impact early emotion processing (e.g. attention) and emotion intensity. DDF, reflecting deficits in expressing and communicating emotion to others, is expected to impact later processing of emotion (e.g. memory, language) and interpersonal relationships. Finally, EOT is expected to reduce interpretation and elaboration of emotional information, leading mainly to deficits.

1.2. Early alexithymia research

1.2.1. Early foci of alexithymia studies prior to the validated assessment

Early studies examined the relationship of HA with somatic illness (e.g. Parker et al., 1993a; Schmidt et al., 1993), suggesting vulnerability to illness in alexithymia through deficits in the cognitive processing of emotions (Taylor, 2000; Taylor et al., 1997) and the arrested development of affective regulation and interpersonal outcomes (e.g. Krystal, 1988). Other studies examined discordance (i.e. "decoupling") of physiological from cognitive-experiential components of emotional responses (e.g. Papciak et al., 1985), neurobiological bases of alexithymia (e.g. Hoppe & Bogen, 1977; Lane et al., 1998), and interventions aimed at reducing alexithymia (e.g. Beresnevaite, 2000). However, these studies, along with studies that attempted to address the cognition–emotion interface (Mann et al., 1994; Parker et al., 1993a, 1993b) had notable methodological weaknesses due to the lack of a valid instrument for measuring alexithymia.

1.2.3. The TAS-20 as a valid instrument to measure alexithymia

The Toronto Alexithymia Scale 20-item (TAS-20) was developed in the early 1990s in response to the limitations of existing alexithymia measures, including the earlier 26-item TAS (Taylor et al., 1985) and the Revised TAS (TAS-R, Taylor et al., 1992). The TAS-20, rated on five-point Likert scales, assesses three central components of the alexithymia construct: DIF, a difficulty identifying feelings and distinguishing between feelings and the bodily sensations of emotional arousal; DDF, a difficulty describing feelings to others; and EOT, an externally oriented style of thinking (see Figure 1). The threefold factor structure has good construct validity in clinical and nonclinical samples (Parker et al., 2003), which includes factorial validity; strong convergent/concurrent validity (e.g. negative correlations with psychological mindedness, need for cognition, and emotional intelligence (see Sekely et al., 2018a) and discriminant validity (e.g. no or low associations with Agreeableness or Conscientiousness); see Taylor, Bagby, & Luminet, 2000); good test-retest reliability for short (3 weeks) or long (6 months) intervals (Bagby et al., 1994a; Kojima et al., 2001); and good internal reliability for the total score, DIF and DDF, although somewhat lower for EOT. Measurement invariance was also demonstrated, including factorial invariance across clinical and nonclinical samples, and across different modes of administration of the scale (e.g. internet and pencil and paper) (e.g. Preece et al., 2018). Taxometric investigations indicate that the TAS-20 yields continuous scores rather than categorical scores, which supports the preference for considering alexithymia as a continuous dimension (Bagby et al., 2020).

To some readers, it might seem paradoxical to assess alexithymia with self-reports given that HA have difficulties accessing their internal world and can thus be unable to accurately report their emotional difficulties and evaluate their low awareness for emotional feelings (e.g. Muller et al., 2008). This is an important consideration, which has led to the recent development of a complementary multimethod approach to assess alexithymia, the Toronto Structured Interview for Alexithymia (TSIA) (e.g. Bagby et al., 2006; Sekely et al., 2018b). Studies using the TSIA have not yet been applied in the contexts we examine for this paper. Moreover, and importantly, studies have found a high overlap between the TAS-20 and the TSIA, despite their differences, both when considering the total and the factor scores (e.g. Bagby et al., 2006; Montebarocci & Surcinelli, 2018). Finally, concerns about using self-report measures are most relevant in very severe alexithymia. As such, the problem seems less relevant for the current review, in which the preponderance of the studies had moderate score ranges and most studies include normative samples, making the issue unlikely.

The TAS-20 further demonstrates independence from negative affect (e.g. psychological distress, medical/psychiatric symptoms), with relative stability over time despite score reductions associated with symptom reduction (e.g. Luminet et al., 2001; Luminet et al., 2007). Yet, due to shared variance of negative affect and alexithymia, covarying negative affect is valuable to discerning clear alexithymia effects (see the general discussion for a full development of the issue of overlap with negative and positive affect). Thus, the advent of the TAS-20 importantly allowed systematic study of the

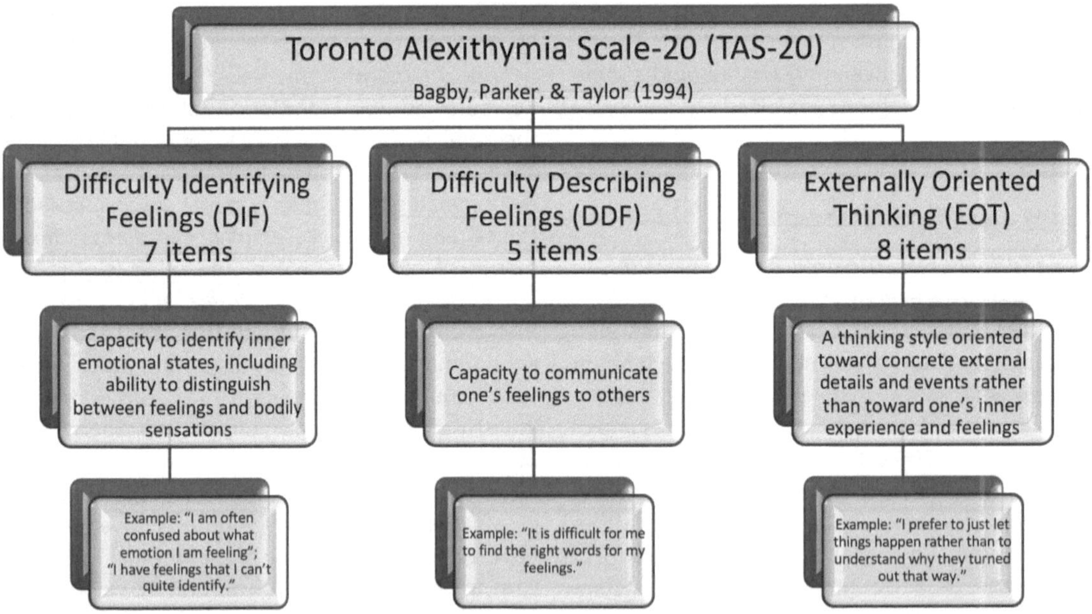

Figure 1. Overview of the three facet scores, with example items, from the Toronto Alexithymia Scale-20 (TAS-20; Bagby et al., 1994).

cognition–emotion interface in alexithymia. Although the overwhelming majority of studies included in this review report results based on the TAS-20, some used a different validated instrument, the BVAQ (Bermond et al., 2015). The BVAQ measures the three similar facets DIF, DDF, and EOT, as well as a difficulty with fantasising facet. Fantasising ability has often been considered a core aspect of the alexithymia construct. Yet, it is absent from the TAS-20 because the items designed to measure fantasising lacked clear validation due to their persistent correlation with social desirability and ability to experience emotion (Sekely et al., 2018a). In addition, the fantasising facet of the BVAQ tends to correlate highly with the EOT facet (Zech et al., 1999). The fantasising facet is hence less frequently investigated than DIF, DDF, and EOT. As such, it is not well represented in the studies evaluated in this review.

2. Alexithymia and the cognition–emotion interface: a review of 25 years of behavioural research

In this review, we adopt a framework that is loosely inspired by the modal model of emotion (e.g. Gross, 2014) toward examining evidence that alexithymia may have a moderating impact on five major processes of the cognition–emotion interface: (1) attention, (2) appraisals, (3) memory, (4) language, and (5) action tendencies and behaviours. For each section, we searched as comprehensively as possible, without setting the needed criteria for a systematic review, as that was not the goal of this paper. Specifically, we used major primary search engines (e.g. Google Scholar, Scopus, Web of Science) and prior review papers that included (a) empirical studies, (b) of these specific topics (including using major paradigms as search terms, such as "Stroop" for attention, etc.), (c) in the context of alexithymia. We do not claim to have exhaustively included all possible papers, but we endeavoured to be comprehensive and included every study found that fit this description.

We have limited the scope of the review primarily to behavioural outcomes, particularly response time and accuracy measures for conscious and automatic information processing, adding other outcomes where they help to clarify or interpret behavioural findings (e.g. psychophysiology, Panayiotou et al., 2018, 2021, this issue). For each section, we give a definition of the process under study. We then indicate why this process is critical for understanding the deficit vs. over-responding nature of HA responses. When necessary, we distinguish between sub-dimensions in the process under study and we hypothesise how it may be associated with total alexithymia scores and specific alexithymia factors. We conclude with a sub-section that (a) summarises the characteristics of the studies (such as their clinical/non-clinical nature or the type of emotion induction), (b) reports the proportion of studies that support deficits or OR (dysfunctional or functional), and (c) gives the proportion of studies that included control variables. We also complement the text with tables that give more detailed information about sample size and characteristics, alexithymia assessment and control, paradigms involved, results (with facet level findings when provided) and study implications (see Tables 1–5).

Early research in personality employed a primarily categorical approach, comparing mean differences between groups based on clinical cutoffs or median splits. There has since been a shift toward a continuous/dimensional approach, using correlations and regression to test the moderating impact of alexithymia. We view a continuous approach as preferred as it more accurately and sensitively considers behavioural and cognitive differences across individuals. We endeavour to report the approach used (see tables), but for synthesis, have used "HA" to refer to those with high(er) alexithymia scores, and "LA" to refer to those with low(er) scores, regardless of approach.

2.1. Attention

Attention involves alerting, orienting, and executive control that manages the focus, selection, and direction of one's limited pool of cognitive resources (Petersen & Posner, 2012). It involves orienting towards stimuli in the environment and the selection of certain stimuli, over others, for further processing or action. It includes both early processes (e.g. orienting, priming) that occur automatically and without awareness or intention, and later processes that require conscious and intentional effort (e.g. selecting and maintaining information in awareness). Emotional events capture attention more readily than do non-emotional stimuli, even when task irrelevant. They can also interrupt ongoing non-emotional processing, leading to slower responding or poorer accuracy. The influence of alexithymia on attention is of central importance, because biases during the early stage of processing can influence subsequent processing, such as appraisal and memory (see sections 2.2 and 2.3). Specifically, emotional stimuli are thought to bias competition for attentional priority through heightened salience, exhibiting influence across the continuum from early automatic processing to later controlled processing (Yiend, 2010).

To the extent that alexithymia is a deficit in emotion processing (Taylor, 2000), where emotion is thought to be a less salient aspect of alexithymic individuals' mental life, we would expect HA to show impaired attentional processing of affective stimuli. Moreover, although emotional reactions occur, high EOT has been conceptualised as a deficit in the ability to attend to such emotional reactions (Preece et al., 2017). As such, we would specifically predict under-responding to emotional stimuli linked to the EOT facet. We found 16 papers (19 studies) that examined the influence of alexithymia on attention (see Table 1). Most of these (n=16) examined early, automatic processing of emotional stimuli, though work has begun to investigate later, controlled attentional processing.

Attentional processing in alexithymia has focused primarily on early, automatic orienting and priming. Emotional Stroop tasks have been common, where emotional and non-emotional words are presented, with participants asked to report the ink colour of the words, but to ignore their meaning. One emotional Stroop study found no relationship between alexithymia and colour-naming times (Galderisi et al., 2008) and another found no bias toward threat stimuli (i.e. pain) in a dot-probe paradigm (Liossi et al., 2009). Yet, others have demonstrated slowed colour-naming of threat words (Pandey, 1995; Parker et al., 1993b) and illness words (Lundh & Simonsson-Sarnecki, 2002), indicative of an attention bias for threat in HA. Similarly, attention was biased in HA toward distracting negative faces on a face-word variant of the emotional Stroop task (Hsing et al., 2013). However, these studies did not control for negative affect (NA), which has been linked to an attention bias towards threat (MacLeod, 2019). Studies that incorporated such controls showed reduced emotion interference in those with HA (Coffey et al., 2003; Mueller et al., 2006), suggesting that individuals with higher alexithymia scores have a deficit in the automatic processing of affect.

Affective priming tasks provide an alternative way to examine early attention processes. They do so by asking subjects to respond to a target stimulus that is briefly preceded by another stimulus, known as the "prime". Prime-target pairs either have congruent valence, which facilitates accuracy and response speed, or incongruent valence, which slows response

Table 1. Alexithymia and attention.

Study	Sample size & characteristics	Alexithymia measures/ controls	Attention measures	Results (Total/Facets (if specified))	Implications
Brandt et al. (2015)	89; 60% F M_{age}=32; M_{TAS} =42; M_{OAS}=41	TAS-20 (C, OAS) Controls(**1**): depression (BDI), positive/negative affect (PANAS), symptoms (SOMS)	**Affective priming** Faces (angry, happy, & neutral) and words (positive, negative, neutral & illness) as both primes and targets	HA<LA: TAS-20 related to faster RTs for illness words primed with positive and negative faces.	HA = Deficit [↓] in automatic attention to affect.
Coffey et al. (2003)	129; 58%F M_{age} = 19; M_{TAS} = 46	TAS-20 (C) w/facets Controls (**2**): emotional intelligence (TMMS); mood (MAS); extraversion, neuroticism (NEO; likened to positive/negative affect)	**Emotional Stroop** Positive, negative, and neutral words	HA<LA: Stroop interference positively related to 'attention to emotion' factor, which was negatively associated with EOT.	HA (EOT)= Deficit [↓] in attention to emotion.
Fujiwara (2018)	76 LA (M_{TAS}=42), 62% F, M_{age}=20; 73 HA (M_{TAS}=67), 52% F, M_{age}=19	TAS-20 (D) Controls(**1**): depression, anxiety (DASS-21)	**Eye-tracking** Eye movements recorded whilst participants judged the ratio of emotions in a set of blended faces	HA=LA: accuracy, face task. HA<LA: dwell time, eyes. HA<LA: HA fewer errors related to eye dwell time.	HA= Deficit [↑] in attention to eyes, but this led to more accurate performance.
Galderisi et al. (2008)	28 PD, 68% F, M_{age}=31, M_{TAS}=57; 32 HC, 59% F, M_{age}=28, M_{TAS}=39	TAS-20 (C) Controls(**1**): depression (HRSD), anxiety (HRSA, SCRAS), IQ (WAIS-R)	**Emotional Stroop** Positive, neutral, panic-related and threat words	No association between TAS scores and Stroop RTs.	*No alexithymia effect* on attention to words.
Grynberg et al. (2014)	Study 1: 41, 73% F, M_{age}=22; M_{TAS}=46 Study 2: 68, 79% F, M_{age}=22, M_{TAS}=44	TAS-20 (C) w/facets Controls(**2**): positive/ negative affect (PANAS)	**Rapid Serial Visual presentation (RSVP)** Study 1: T1 targets: faces (fear, pain, happy, neutral). T2 targets: neutral scenes. Distractors: neutral faces. Study 2: T1 targets: faces (fear, anger, neutral); T2: as study 1.	HA>LA: (DDF, Study 1[#]; EOT, Study 2) associated with increased delay following T1 before T2 targets can be accurately detected, but only when T1=faces of negative affect.	HA (DDF & EOT) = OR [↓] to threat. HA associated with prolonged processing of negative affect.
Hsing et al. (2013)	115, 57% F, M_{age}=19, Mdn_{TAS} =47 56 HA 59 LA	TAS-20 (D) Controls(**2**): depression (BDI), anxiety (STAI), verbal IQ (ERVT)	**Emotional Stroop** Task required classifying adjectives as angry or sad; images of sad, angry or neutral faces were superimposed, varying in display time (primes)	HA=LA: classification of adjectives and faces (presented alone). HA>LA: slower responding overall, and to sad words with sad (congruent) and angry (incongruent) primes. HA>LA (trend): when affect controlled, lower IQ HA had greater Stroop interference.	HA = OR [↓] greater distraction from negative faces with sad target words. HA: *no deficit* in overall Stroop interference, or categorising isolated verbal, nonverbal stimuli.
Liossi et al. (2009)	15 CH, 60% F, M_{age}=33, M_{TAS}=50 18 HC, 72% F M_{age}=30, M_{TAS}=41	TAS-20 (C) Controls: none	**Visual Probe Task** Pain words paired with neutral words, presented for short (500ms) or long (1250ms) durations before probe onset	TAS-20 not associated with probe RTs under any condition.	*No alexithymia effect* on attention to pain words.
Lundh and Simonsson-Sarnecki (2002)	120, 52% F, M_{age}=37, M_{TAS}=39 20 HA (>49) 20 LA (<31)	TAS-20 (C, D) Controls(**2**): somatic anxiety (KSP), health (HQL-I)	**Emotional Stroop** Illness-related, negative, and neutral words	HA=LA, no alexithymia correlations in total sample. HA>LA, HA had greater Stroop interference to	HA= OR [↓] to illness words.

(*Continued*)

Table 1. Continued.

Study	Sample size & characteristics	Alexithymia measures/ controls	Attention measures	Results (Total/Facets (if specified))	Implications
				unmasked illness words than masked negative words[#].	
Mueller et al. (2006)	45, 67% F, M_{age}=45, M_{TAS}=54 Psychiatric inpatient sample	TAS-20 (D), OAS Controls(**2**): depression (BDI), anxiety (STAI, ASI), traits (NEO) symptoms (SCL-90)	**Emotional Stroop** Positive, negative, neutral, and body-related words	HA<LA: HA had reduced interference from negative and body words[#].	HA=Deficit [↓] in responding to negative and body words.
Pandey (1995)	12 HA (M_{TAS}=66) 12 LA (M_{TAS}=36) 0% F, M_{age}=NR (undergraduates)	TAS-20 (D) Controls: None	**Emotional Stroop** Baseline (nonword, OOOOO), neutral and emotionally arousing (sexual) words	HA>LA: HA exhibited greater Stroop interference for arousing words.	HA= OR [↓] to arousing words.
Sharpe et al. (2016)	52, 100% F M_{age}=22, M_{TAS}=45 Eating disorder sample	TAS-20 (C) Controls(**2**): depression (BDI), anxiety (STAI), symptoms (EDI)	**Eye-tracking** Free viewing of happy and angry faces paired with neutral faces	HA=LA; TAS-20 not related to attention bias metrics.	*No alexithymia effect* on attention to faces.
Suslow (1998)	32, 59% F, M_{age}=27, M_{TAS}=39	TAS-20 (C) w/facets Controls: none	**Affective Priming** Positive and negative words primed with positive, negative, or neutral words	HA (DDF): greater priming facilitation, negative prime-targets. HA (EOT): greater priming facilitation, positive prime-targets.	HA (DDF & EOT) =OR [↑] in automatic attention to affective primes.
Suslow and Junghanns (2002)	31, 52% F, M_{age}=26, Mdn_{TAS}=39 15 HA (M_{TAS}=51) 16 LA (M_{TAS}=30)	TAS-20 (C, D) w/facets Controls: none positive/ negative affect measured (DES) but did not analyse because no group difference	**Affective Priming** Neutral, emotional, and non-words primed with congruent or incongruent situational scenarios	Lexical decision times for emotional words: HA: congruent > incongruent LA: congruent < incongruent DIF associated with reduced situation priming	HA (DIF)=Deficit [↓] in automatic attention towards the emotional primes
Vermeulen et al. (2006)	Study 1: 64, 61% F, M_{age}=20, M_{TAS}=50 Study 2: 58, 84% F, M_{age}19, M_{TAS}=49 Study 3: 60, 75% F, M_{age}=21, M_{TAS}=47	TAS-20 (C) Controls(**1**): Negative affect (NAS; Study 1,3), anxiety (STAI, Study 2,3), depression (ZDS; Study 2,3)	**Affective Priming** Study 1: Targets: words (positive, negative, neutral). Primes: words (positive, negative, neutral) and faces (happy, threat, neutral) Study 2: As Study 1 plus sad faces and words Study 3: As Study 2, plus face targets (happy, sad, angry, disgusted)	HA<LA; HA correlated with reduced priming from angry schematic faces (Study 1, 2, 3). HA=LA; face priming by verbal stimuli did not correlate with alexithymia.	HA=Deficit [↓] in automatic attention to angry faces. *No alexithymia effect* in attention to emotional words.
Vermeulen et al. (2019)	55, NR % F, M_{age}=22, Mdn_{TAS}=45 27 HA (M_{TAS} =53) 28 LA (M_{TAS} =38)	TAS-20 (D) Controls: None	**Rapid Serial Visual presentation (RSVP)** Task with relaxation and exercise conditions T1 targets: neutral words T2 targets: neutral and low or high arousal words Distractors: random symbols	HA<LA. For T2 target accuracy, HA exercise= relaxation and no difference by target category, while LA exercise>relaxation, with high arousal>low arousal or neutral targets.	HA=Deficit [↓] in attention to arousing stimuli. HA= Deficit [↓] in attentional benefit of situational arousal.

(*Continued*)

Table 1. Continued.

Study	Sample size & characteristics	Alexithymia measures/ controls	Attention measures	Results (Total/Facets (if specified))	Implications
Wiebe et al. (2017)	99, 63% F, M_{age}=24, M_{TAS}=41	TAS-20 (C) w/facets Controls(**1**): depression (BDI), anxiety (STAI), IQ (WAIS-R), sex	**Eye-tracking** Free viewing of pictures (positive, neutral, threat-relevant, depression-relevant) presented in a 2x2 grid.	HA<LA (EOT). HA had reduced dwell time on depression-relevant images.	HA (EOT)= Deficit [↓] in strategic attentional processing of negative images.

Notes**.** All studies used non-clinical samples (unless otherwise stated); TAS-20: Toronto Alexithymia Scale 20 Items (C-continuous, D-dichotomous, OAS- Observer Alexithymia Scale); DIF: Difficulty Identifying Feelings subscale of the TAS-20; DDF: Difficulty Describing Feelings subscale from the TAS-20; EOT: Externally Oriented Thinking subscale of the TAS-20; LA: Low Alexithymia Scorers; HA High Alexithymia Scorers; F=Female; CH=chronic headache; HC=healthy controls; PD=panic disorder; M_{TAS}= mean (Mdn=median) TAS-20 total score; M_{age}=mean (Mdn=median) age (years); NR=not reported; ns=not significant; OR=over-responding; [↓]=detrimental effect of HA; [↑]=potentially beneficial effect of HA; (**1**)results reported effects after affect variables controlled; (**2**)results reported indicating separable or unique effect of controls; (**3**)negative affect control reduced alexithymia effect.

Instruments: ASI = Anxiety Sensitivity Index; BDI=Beck Depression Inventory; BVAQ = Bermond-Vorst Alexithymia Questionnaire; ERVT=The Extended Range Vocabulary Test; DAS-21=Depression, Anxiety and Stress Scale; DES = Differential Emotions Scale; HQL-I= Health and Quality of Life Interview; EDI=Eating Disorders Inventory; HRSA=Hamilton Anxiety Rating Scale; HRSD =Hamilton Rating Scale for Depression; KSP = Karolinska Scales of Personality; MAS=Mood Awareness Scale; NAS = Negative Affectivity Schedule; NEO = The NEO Five-Factor Inventory (60 items); PANAS=-positive and negative affect scale; SCRAS =Sheehan Clinician Rated Anxiety Scale; SCL-90=90-item Symptom Checklist Revised; SOMS=Screening for Somatoform Symptoms; STAI=State Trait anxiety Inventory; TMMS= Trait Meta Mood Scale; WAIS-R= Wechsler Adult Intelligence Scale (verbal); ZDS=Zung Depression scale.

times and reduces target accuracy. In HA, Suslow (1998) reported greater facilitation of congruent prime-target pairs with greater DIF (positive pairs) and EOT (negative pairs), suggesting enhanced automatic processing of emotion in HA. However, when negative affect was controlled, other studies instead showed reduced emotional priming in HA. For example, Suslow and Junghanns (2002) found HA had reduced priming (interference) from incongruent verbal primes. Over three experiments, Vermeulen et al. (2006) reported reduced priming (both facilitation and interference) from angry face primes in HA. Finally, Brandt et al. (2015) reported that when categorising illness words, HA exhibited reduced interference from positive and negative primes. Taken together, when negative affect is controlled, the findings in early attention processing support the deficit model of alexithymia (Taylor, 2000), with also some evidence supporting the role of EOT in this deficit (Coffey et al., 2003), in line with the attention-appraisal model (Preece et al., 2017).

Another way to examine early attentional processing that allows for processing both early and later aspects of attention is the so-called "attentional blink" (AB). The AB is the phenomenon that one fails to detect, or identify, the second of two targets when it occurs close in time to the first target. The Rapid Serial Visual Presentation (RSVP) task used to assess AB therefore presents a stream of rapidly presented stimuli, requiring participants to detect two targets (T1, T2) within that stream. Longer ABs indicate prolonged T1 processing, while shorter ABs indicate enhanced T2 detection. Grynberg et al. (2014) reported that DDF (study 1) and EOT (study 2) were linked to longer ABs when negative faces were presented at T1. In contrast, Vermeulen et al. (2019) reported that arousing T2 stimuli produced shorter ABs, and that T2 detection was enhanced if arousal was induced through exercise prior to the task. Yet, this effect only occurred in LA, suggesting that HA have a deficit in attention to arousing stimuli. Together, these findings suggest a different profile for HA depending on the phase of attention processing. Specifically, HA exhibit a deficit in automatically orienting towards threat, but prolonged processing of threat (over-responding) during the conscious maintenance phase of attention.

An additional approach to examining both early and later influences on attention is through eye-tracking. Using tracking technology, variations in eye movements, such as speed of movement, duration

Table 2. Alexithymia and appraisals.

Study	Sample Size & Characteristics	Alexithymia Measures/ Controls	Appraisal Measures	Results (Total/Facets (if specified))	Implications
Aaron et al. (2018)	108, 67% F, M_{age}=19, M_{TAS}=46	TAS-20(C); w/facets Controls: none	**Valence** Presented 14 video clips eliciting discrete emotion states (anger, amusement, contentment, disgust, fear, sadness, surprise). Primary, secondary emotions (open-ended) assessed: emotional granularity (fine-grained emotional distinctions) and dialecticism (recognising concurrent pleasant and unpleasant states)	HA<LA (DDF): reduced emotional granularity, only for negative videos. HA<LA (EOT): reduced dialecticism, only for negative videos.	HA (DDF, EOT): <u>Deficit</u> [↓]. HA had reduced ability to for fine and gross distinctions of negative situations. Unpleasantness reduced in negative context. *No effect*: pleasantness in positive context.
de Timary et al. (2008)	28, 0% F, M_{age}=21, M_{TAS}=48	TAS-20(C); w/facets Controls: none	**Stress anticipation, response** Ps exposed to stressful task (TSST), measured effects of anticipatory appraisals on cortisol response	HA>LA (DDF): cortisol response, stress anticipation. HA=LA: stress exposure and recovery.	HA (DDF): <u>OR</u> [↓] Stronger stress response when appraising potential threat.
Fantini-Hauwel et al. (2015)	225, 69% F M_{age}=21, M_{TAS}=49	TAS-20(C); w/facets Controls(**1**): sex; negative, positive frequency (when predicting intensity; vice versa)	**Valence** Measured overall affect intensity (AIM; positive, negative subscales) and affect frequency (PANAS) without manipulation or reference to emotional events	(1) HA>LA (DIF): higher positive intensity. (2) HA<LA (DDF): lower positive intensity. (3) HA>LA (DIF): higher negative frequency.	HA (DDF): <u>Deficit</u> [↓] positive intensity. HA (DIF): <u>OR</u> [↓] higher positive intensity and greater negative frequency.
Koven (2014)	96, 59% F, M_{age}=19, M_{TAS}=46	TAS-20(D) Controls(**2**): negative affect (POMS), anhedonia (CRSPAS)	**Valence** Ps viewed appetitive and aversive words and pictures	HA<LA: appetitive words and pictures rated less positively. HA=LA: aversive word and picture ratings.	HA: <u>Deficit</u> [↓] Pleasantness decreased in positive contexts. *No effect*: unpleasantness in negative context.
Larwood et al. (2021) (this issue)	162, 56% F, M_{age}=21, M_{TAS}=54	TAS-20(C) Controls(**2**): depression (DASS).	**Valence** Ps listened to ten 15 sec musical pieces (happy, sad, tender, angry, fearful), listed emotion word conveyed by music.	HA=LA: number of emotion words generated. HA<LA: sad, angry, fearful music judged more neutral. HA=LA: happy, tender.	HA: <u>Deficit</u> [↓] negative stimuli. Unpleasantness reduced, negative context. *No effect*: pleasantness, positive context.
Luminet et al. (2000)	<u>Study 1</u>: 99, 86% F, M_{age}=20, M_{DDF}=23, M_F=16 <u>Study 2</u>: 101, 74% F, M_{age}=22, M_{DDF}=22, M_F=17	BVAQ(C); w/facets Controls(**1**): Emotional intensity event; Neuroticism and Extraversion (NEO PI-R)	**Valence** Measured rumination and social sharing for recent (3 months, Study 1; 6 months Study 2) negative and positive autobiographical events	HA<LA (DF): less rumination about positive, but not negative events. HA<LA (DDF): less sharing with others, lower emotional involvement in sharing for negative, but not positive events.	HA (DF, DDF): <u>Deficit</u> [↓] Decreased unpleasantness in negative context (DDF) Decreased pleasantness in positive context (DF)
Luminet et al. (2004)	50, 44% F, M_{age}=64, M_{BVAQ}:NR	BVAQ(C); w/facets Controls: gender, age, health status	**Valence, familiarity, importance** Measured familiarity, importance, emotional reactions to sad movie	HA<LA (EOT): lower unpleasantness. HA<LA (DDF): lower familiarity. HA<LA (EOT): lower importance.	HA (DDF, EOT): <u>Deficit</u> [↓] potentially due to avoidance. Decreased unpleasantness in negative contexts (EOT, DDF).

Notes. All studies used non-clinical samples. TAS-20=Toronto Alexithymia Scale 20; BVAQ=Bermond Vorst Alexithymia Questionnaire (DF=difficulty fantasising); C=continuous, D=dichotomous; DDF=difficulty describing feelings; DIF=difficulty identifying feelings; EOT=externally oriented thinking; F=Female; M_{TAS}= mean TAS-20 total score; M_{DIF}= mean DIF factor; M_{DDF} = mean DDF factor; M_{EOT}= mean EOT factor; M_F= mean difficulty fantasising factor; M_{age}=mean (Mdn=median) age (years); Ps=participants; OR=over-responding; [↓]=detrimental effect of HA; [↑]=potentially beneficial effect of HA; NR=not reported; (**1**)results reported effects after affect variables controlled; (**2**)results reported indicating separable or unique effect of controls; (**3**)negative affect control reduced alexithymia effect.

Instruments: AIM= Affect Intensity Measure; CRSPAS= Chapman Revised Social and Physical Anhedonia Scales; DASS= Depression, Anxiety and Stress Scale; NEO PI-R = NEO Personality Inventory-Revised; PANAS= Positive Affectivity Negative Affectivity Schedule; POMS= Profile of Mood States; STAI= State-Trait Anxiety Inventory (S=State; T=Trait); TSST= Trier Social Stress Test; Zung= Zung depression questionnaire.

of fixations, pattern of visual search and even frequency or pattern of blinking can be assessed to understand the individual's attention to the environment. Few studies have yet been done in alexithymia, but the existing results focus on later attentional processes and amplify findings with other approaches. One study reported no contribution of alexithymia to eye-tracking metrics during free-viewing of emotional and neutral faces (Sharpe et al., 2016). In contrast, Fujiwara (2018) reported that HA spent less time looking (i.e. dwell time) at the eye-region of faces that had blended emotions, particularly those with faces featuring anger. Interestingly, attending to the eyes improved emotion recognition judgments in LA, but it impaired in HA (i.e. deficit). Wiebe et al. (2017) included a facet-level analysis, reporting that dwell time was reduced for depression-relevant images in those with higher EOT, suggesting a specific EOT-related deficit in attention processing for such images. Thus, as with early attention studies focused on orientation and priming, these studies examining the later maintenance phase of attention are also consistent with an alexithymia deficit model (Taylor, 2000) and the attention-appraisal model (Preece et al., 2017).

2.1.1. Summary

We found 19 studies in 16 papers examining the influence of alexithymia on attention were reviewed. Only two studies used clinical samples; 17 of 19 (90%) employed normative (*n*=5) and student samples (*n*=12), thereby focusing findings on young subjects (mean age range=19-45 yrs, median of means=25 yrs). Most studies investigated attention for words (*n*=10, 53%) or faces (*n*=6, 32%), while one (5%) examined affective images. The majority (12/19, 63%) controlled for negative affect, with two of these studies also controlling for positive affect. Eight studies (42%) examined the results before and after controlling for mood and the majority of these (5/8, 63%) reported no change in results following control for affect.

The weight of the evidence (10/19 studies, 53%; Table 1) suggests alexithymia is linked to deficits in early, automatic attention to affect, as well as later, controlled attention. These findings are consistent with Taylor's (2000) deficit view of alexithymia. Furthermore, although most studies examined the total TAS-20 score or dichotomous groups, evidence is emerging linking attentional deficits to specific facets of alexithymia. Consistent with the attention-appraisal model of alexithymia (Preece et al., 2017), EOT was most frequently reported (Coffey et al., 2003; Wiebe et al., 2017).

Four of the six studies that reported over-responding to emotional stimuli in alexithymia (67%) did not control for negative affect. However, Grynberg et al. (2014) did so and reported prolonged attentional processing of threatening faces linked to EOT (study 1) and DDF (study 2), which was inconsistent with either the deficit (Taylor, 2000) or attention-appraisal models (Preece et al., 2017). However, the rapid serial visual presentation task might be better characterised as measuring stimulus appraisal (T1, emotional faces) rather than prolonged processing of threat. Thus, their findings could be interpreted as due to slowed appraisal, thereby consistent with the appraisal element of the attention-appraisal model (Preece et al., 2017; see also section 2.2.).

2.2. Appraisals

Appraisals are a person's subjective evaluation of the personal significance of a situation, object, or event (Scherer, 1999). Experienced feelings are continually modified because appraisals may change in relevance and intensity over time depending on personal meaning, such as values, beliefs, goals, and experiences (Ellsworth & Scherer, 2003). Different models have been proposed, including the following dimensions: valence, importance, familiarity, novelty/expectedness, agency/intentionality, coping potential/power, goal conduciveness, fairness, and compatibility with social standards and norms (for a review, see Scherer, 2019). In their recent model, Preece et al. (2017) suggested that difficulties in the appraisal stage of emotion processing might be a central feature of alexithymia. HA have under-developed emotion schemas (e.g. Luminet et al., 2006; Lundh et al., 2002; Suslow & Junghanns, 2002; Vermeulen et al., 2006) leading to increased difficulty interpreting patterns of input in a sufficiently differentiated way. Thus, they evaluate their emotional states in a diffuse manner ("I am feeling bad") rather than in a specific manner ("I am feeling angry").

Among the various appraisal dimensions, alexithymia research has only substantively examined valence. Valence is the degree to which a situation is evaluated as potentially agreeable/pleasant or disagreeable/unpleasant. Importantly, although alexithymia scores are moderately inflated by negative affect, alexithymia is largely independent of it, as

Table 3. Alexithymia and memory.

Study	Sample Size & characteristics	Alexithymia measures/ controls	Memory measures	Results (Total/Facets (if specified))	Implications
Correro et al. (2021) (this issue)	Exp. 1: 296, 73% F, M_{age}=20, M_{TAS}=45 Exp. 2: 139, 67% F, 18–89 yrs, M_{TAS}=43 Exp. 3: 121, 67% F, 18–92 yrs, M_{TAS}=41	TAS-20(C), w/facets Screened: intact cognition Controls (all exp.)(**4**): age, sex, anxiety (BSI.BAI), depression (BSI/BDI)	**Neutral Words, Narratives** Exp. 1: neutral word list (*d′*, 60 min delay). Exp. 2: EF battery. Exp. 3: EF; memory: WMS-III (neutral story; 30-min delay).	Exp. 1: HA<LA; EOT and DIF predicted memory, but EOT fully mediated DIF. Exp. 2: HA<LA: DIF predicted EF. Exp. 3: HA<LA: DIF predicted EF; EOT predicted memory; moderation: poor EF + EOT = poor memory.	HA: Deficit [↓], poorer memory (EOT) and executive function (cognitive control) (DIF) in *neutral context*. Executive function interacts with EOT [↓] to influence memory.
DiStefano and Koven (2012)	12 LA (M_{TAS}=46), 12 HA (M_{TAS}=63) 18–22 yrs 75% F	TAS-20(D) Controls: none	**Neutral Words, Faces, Narratives, Scenes** WMS-III (neutral), immediate, 30-min delay; verbal: words, story; visual: faces, social scenes.	HA=LA verbal, immediate and delayed; HA<LA visual, immediate and delayed	HA: Deficit [↓], visual memory (not verbal) in *neutral* context.
Donges and Suslow (2015)	40, 100% F, M_{age}=23, M_{TAS}=35	TAS-20(C), w/facets Controls(**2**): vocab (MVT), anxiety (STAI-T), depression (BDI) Correlational analysis.	**Emotive Faces** Intentional encoding of faces (angry, fearful, happy, neutral). 30 min delayed recognition.	HA<LA (DDF): DDF inversely correlated with angry, fearful hits; HA=LA: happy, neutral	HA (DDF): Deficit [↓] emotive face memory (anger, fear).
Dressaire et al. (2015)	Exp. 1 (negative words): 60, 50% F, 35–99 yrs, M_{TAS}=52 Exp. 2 (neutral words): 60, 50% F, 35–98 yrs, M_{TAS}= 51	TAS-20(C), w/facets Controls(**1**): age, anxiety and depression (HADS)	**Neutral, Emotive Words** Directed forgetting (list method); 1 min retrieval delay. Exp. 1: negative words Exp. 2: neutral words	Exp. 1 (negative): HA<LA (EOT); HA predicted poorer recall, greater false memory; Exp. 2 (neutral): HA<LA (EOT); EOT correlated with poorer retrieval; HA>LA (DIF); DIF predicted *better* recall.	HA (EOT): Deficit [↓] *negative*; *neutral* (ns); HA (EOT): OR [↓] false negative memory (cognitive control *deficit*); HA (DIF): OR [↑] *neutral*.
Jacob and Hautekeete (1998)	21 LA (TAS-26<62) 24 HA (TAS-26>74) ~90% F, 18–22 yrs	TAS-26 (French; D) Controls(**1**): anxiety (non-standard), depression (BDI)	**Neutral, Emotive Words** Incidental learning, sentence game (phrase substitution, w/tone (negative, positive, neutral)). Immediate recognition (old/new).	HA>LA: slower response time HA<LA: errors (*more* correct rejections, not more hits). HA=LA: positive>negative >>neutral.	HA: Deficit [↓] in decision time only, not memory; HA: OR [↑]; fewer errors (rigorous decision criterion, greater need for cues).
Luminet et al. (2006)	42 HA (TAS>56), 40 LA (TAS<40) 56% F, age NR (undergraduates)	TAS-20(D), w/facets Controls(**2**): positive/ negative affect (PANAS), optimism (LOT-R), depression (ZSDS)	**Neutral, Emotive Words** Incidental word learning (positive, negative, neutral), R/K paradigm, retrieval delay, 1-min w/distraction.	HA<LA: R (confident), poorer positive (total, all facets) and negative (DIF), whether shallow or deep processing. HA=LA for recall, K (familiarity), Neutral.	HA: Deficit [↓], conscious access to emotional words (*positive*: DIF, DDF, EOT; *negative*: DIF).
Lundh et al. (2002)	Exp. 1: 88, 76% F, M_{age}=29, M_{TAS}=40	TAS-20(C), w/facets Controls: none	**AMT** (positive, negative prompts).	HA=LA; No correlation of TAS-20 (total or facets) with latency or retrieval of positive or negative memories.	Alexithymia *did not contribute to* retrieval time or memory.
Meltzer and Nielson (2010)	42 LA (TAS<43) 43 HA (TAS>42) 69% F, M_{age}=19	TAS-20(D) Controls: none	**Neutral, Emotive Words** Incidental learning (word rating); positive, negative, neutral, illness words. Recall delay, 45 min.	HA<LA: negative recall HA>LA: illness recall, HA>LA: neutral recall (trend).	HA: Deficit [↓], *negative*; HA: OR [↓], *illness*, possibly pre-occupation, salience of illness

(*Continued*)

Table 3. Continued.

Study	Sample Size & characteristics	Alexithymia measures/ controls	Memory measures	Results (Total/Facets (if specified))	Implications
Muir et al. (2017)	185, 92% F, 18–36 yrs, M_{TAS}=49	TAS-20(C), w/facets Controls: none	**AMT** (negative, positive, neutral memory probes); Fading of Affect Bias (FAB, over time, negative> positive fading).	HA<LA (total score only) FAB; HA: greater positive fading, less negative fading. No effects were significant with TAS subscales.	HA: OR [↓] less affect fading; due to greater positive fading, negative persistence (*negative* salience).
Nielson and Meltzer (2009)	30 LA (TAS<38), 67% F 30 HA (TAS>53), 57% F Age NR (undergraduates)	TAS-20(D) Controls(**4**): vocab. (WAIS-R), stress (PSS), depression (BDI), anxiety (BAI)	**Neutral Words** Intentional learning, word list (neutral) followed by arousing or neutral video. Retrieval delay 24-hrs (surprise).	HA<LA: immediate recall HA<LA subjective arousal HA=LA physiological arousal HA=LA 24 hr recall, arousal condition (deficit direction).	HA: Deficit [↓] of arousal appraisal and immediate memory of *neutral* stimuli; *No effect*: delayed memory.
Ridout et al. (2021) (this issue)	Exp. 1: 39, 100% F, M_{age}=20, M_{TAS}=40 Exp. 2: 38, 100% F, M_{age}=20, M_{TAS}=42	TAS-20(C), w/facets Controls(**1**): age, depression (HADS), anxiety (HADS)	**Neutral, Emotive Faces, Scenes** Emotion identification (angry, sad, happy, neutral), intentional learning. R/K paradigm, retrieval delay: 5 min. Exp. 1: faces. Exp. 2: social videos.	Exp. 1: HA=LA emotion identification; HA<LA (DDF): *d'*, angry; HA>LA (DIF): *d'*, sad; Exp. 2: HA<LA (DIF, EOT); HA predicted poorer emotive memory (DIF, EOT: hits; DIF: R, anger and happy); HA>LA (DIF); HA predicted better neutral familiarity (K).	HA: Deficit [↓], *anger* (faces, DDF; videos, DIF, EOT) and *happy* videos (DIF, EOT); HA: OR (DIF) [↓], *better* retrieval of *sad* faces; HA: OR (DIF) [↑], greater familiarity of *neutral* videos.
Senior et al. (2020)	83, 87% F, M_{age}=20, M_{TAS}=46	TAS-20 (C), w/facets Controls(**2**): depression (HADS), anxiety (HADS) Correlational analysis.	**Emotive Faces** Affect matching, short-term memory (faces; anger, disgust, fear, happy, sad, surprise, neutral), with RM (25% increased / decreased expression intensity) during match decisions.	HA<LA (Total), accuracy; HA<LA (DIF), errors, forward cond. HA>LA (DIF), response time, forward cond. HA<LA (EOT): RM effect (forward > backward; fear, happy), except reduced in HA trend, *p*=.07. (Note accuracy >95%).	HA (total): Deficit [↓], accuracy; HA (DIF): Deficit [↓], slower RT; HA (EOT): Deficit [↓], RM effect HA (DIF): OR [↑], *reduced* errors to forward trials, possible benefit RM perception.
Suslow et al. (2003)	30, 50% F, M_{age}=36, M_{TAS}=38	TAS-20 (C), w/facets Controls(**2**): depression (BDI), vocab. (WAIS-R) Correlational analysis	**Neutral, Emotive Words** Incidental memory, pair evaluation (positive, negative adjective targets; positive, negative, neutral noun distractors). Immediate free recall.	HA>LA (DIF): DIF positively correlated with intrusions to positive distractors. HA=LA, positive, negative targets, and neutral distractors.	HA (DIF): OR [↓], more intrusion errors in recall, positive stimuli. HA: Emotional valence less salient, poorer memory organization.
Takahashi et al. (2015)	Exp. 1: 15 LA (TAS<52), 53% F, M_{age}=21; 15 HA (TAS>60), 73% F, M_{age}=20 Exp. 2: 8 LA (TAS<52), 63% F, M_{age}=21; 8 HA (TAS>60), 63% F, M_{age}=20	TAS-20(D) Controls: none	**Neutral, Emotive Faces** Visual STM; search and change detection of abstract faces. Exp 1: montage, encoding v. storage; happy, angry. Exp. 2: probed single item (storage v. retrieval); happy, angry, neutral.	Exp. 1: HA=LA in search and change detection response time; HA<LA in change accuracy (*d'*) for happy, and within HA, happy<angry; storage effect, not encoding. Exp. 2: HA=LA (happy, angry; neutral presented but not probed); no effect on retrieval.	HA Deficit [↓], *happy* accuracy only, via immediate memory storage. No effect on response speed. Note: face stimuli were not realistic.
Terock et al. (2019)	Exp. 1: 1980, 53% F, M_{age}=55, M_{TAS}=45 Exp. 2: 3799, 51% F, M_{age}=51, M_{TAS}=42	TAS-20(C), w/facets Controls(**1**): age, sex, education, lifetime major depression (MCIDI)	**Neutral Words** Intentional neutral word list learning, multiple trials; Delay interval: immediate, 20-min;	Exp. 1: HA<LA (EOT, DIF): poorer immediate, delayed recall predicted by EOT, with DIF to lesser degree. Exp. 2: HA<LA (EOT): replicated Exp. 1, trend only at delayed recall.	HA (EOT) Deficit [↓], immediate, delayed word memory for *neutral* words in neutral context.

(*Continued*)

Table 3. Continued.

Study	Sample Size & characteristics	Alexithymia measures/ controls	Memory measures	Results (Total/Facets (if specified))	Implications
Vermeulen (2021) (this issue)	Exp. 1: 44, 66% F, M_{age}=21, M_{TAS}=45 Exp. 2: 44, 75% F, M_{age}=21, M_{TAS}=48	TAS-20(C), w/facets Controls(**1**): age, sex, positive/negative affect (PANAS)	**Neutral, Emotive Words** Verbal STM (auditory); 20 6-item lists; positive, negative, neutral. Exp. 1: pure lists (one word valence type/ list) Exp 2: mixed lists	Exp. 1 (pure): HA< LA (TAS-total, EOT); EOT predicted poorer positive, negative recall (neutral-trend); HA<LA (DDF); DDF predicted poorer positive recall. Exp. 2 (mixed): HA=LA;.	HA: Deficit [↓] (EOT *negative, positive,* and *neutral* (trend) stims; DDF *positive* stims) when contextually cohesive. No effect in mixed context.
Vermeulen and Luminet (2009)	65, 83% F, M_{age}=19, M_{TAS}=48	TAS-20(C), w/facets Controls(**1**): anxiety (STAI-S); positive/ negative affect (PANAS)	**Neutral, Emotive Words** Incidental learning; word evaluation task of neutral, joy, disgust, and anger words (shallow or deep processing). Surprise immediate (Remember/ Know) retrieval.	HA<LA (DIF); DIF associated with poorer emotion word memory (R); HA>LA (EOT) *better* memory, all categories, via emotional introspection EOT items, not external thinking items.	HA (DIF): Deficit [↓], emotive words; emotion regulation difficulty, lack of motivation for emotion processing; HA (EOT): OR [↑], improved all categories.
Vermeulen et al. (2010)	55 LA (TAS<47), 73% F, M_{age}=22 52 HA (TAS>48), 67% F, M_{age}=21	TAS-20(D) Controls(**1**): positive/ negative affect (PANAS)	**Neutral, Emotive Words** Incidental learning; word evaluation task of neutral, joy, disgust, and anger words (shallow or deep processing) with happy or sad background music. Surprise immediate (Remember/ Know) retrieval.	HA>LA: Congruent music facilitated word processing, deep condition. HA<LA anger word retrieval, overall memory w/ angry music. HA>LA congruence effect (happy music: joy>anger; angry music: anger>joy). HA=LA: processing time.	HA Deficit [↓], anger. HA OR [↑], *congruence effect;* matching context provided support for memorising, retrieving anger and joy words.

Notes. All studies used non-clinical samples; TAS-26: Toronto Alexithymia Scale 26 Items; TAS-20: Toronto Alexithymia Scale 20 Items (C-continuous, D-dichotomous); DIF: Difficulty Identifying Feelings subscale of the TAS-20; DDF: Difficulty Describing Feelings subscale from the TAS-20; EOT: Externally Oriented Thinking subscale of the TAS-20; LA: Low Alexithymia Scorers; HA High Alexithymia Scorers; F=Female; *d′*= d-prime, recognition sensitivity (accuracy); EF=executive functioning; K= 'know' response (familiarity in recognition); M_{TAS}= mean TAS-20 total score; M_{age}=mean age (years); NR=not reported; ns=not significant; OR=over-responding; R= 'remember' response (confident retrieval in recognition); RM= representational momentum, perceptual extrapolation in direction of an implied trajectory; STM=short-term memory; [↓]=detrimental effect of HA; [↑]=potentially beneficial effect of HA; (**1**)results reported effects after affect variables controlled; (**2**)results reported indicating separable or unique effect of controls; (**3**)negative affect control reduced alexithymia effect; (**4**)affect variables left out of analysis as they did not correlate with DV.
Instruments: AMT=Autobiographical Memory Test; BAI=Beck Anxiety Inventory; BDI= Beck Depression Inventory; BSI=Brief Symptom Inventory; HADS=Hospital Anxiety and Depression Scale; *KSP*=Karolinska Scales of Personality (Trait); LOT-R=Life Orientation Test-Revised; MCIDI=Munich Composite International Diagnostic Interview; MVT=Multiple-choice Vocabulary Test; PANAS=-Positive Affectivity Negative Affectivity Schedule; PSS=Perceived Stress Scale; SPM=Raven's Standard Progressive Matrices; STAI=State-Trait Anxiety Inventory (S=State; T=Trait); WAIS-R=Wechsler Adult Intelligence Scale-Revised (vocabulary subtest); WMS-III=Wechsler Memory Scale-III; ZSDS=Zung Self-rating Depression Scale.

Table 4. Alexithymia and language.

Study	Sample Size & Characteristics	Alexithymia Measures/ Controls	Language Measures	Results (Total/Facets (if specified))	Implications
Camia et al. (2020)	4 LA, 75% F, M_{age}=50, M_{TAS}=44; 4 HA, 25% F, M_{age}=43, M_{TAS}=64 Chronic alcoholism sample	TAS-20 (D) Controls: none	**Expressive: Autobiographical Narratives** Qualitative narrative analysis (LIWC) of personal events (TSIA); 6 yes/no questions per TAS-20 facet, with elaboration using personal examples.	HA=LA: specificity HA>LA: personalisation, concreteness, avoidance. HA<LA: coherence, affect ratio (HA: positive> negative), elaboration (context, feelings, interpretation).	HA Deficit [↓] in language expression, particularly negative processing; reflected personalised but low quality, unelaborated, concrete, avoidant approach.
Edwards et al. (2020)	96; 76% F, M_{age}=21, M_{TAS}=44	TAS-20(C) w/facets Controls(**1**): positive/ negative affect (PANAS)	**Expressive: Autobiographical Narratives** Narrative analysis of 6 probed personal events (5 min; 3 negative and 3 neutral or positive). Linguistic analysis (LIWC). Uncorrected correlations.	HA<LA (DIF, DDF): less positive language. HA>LA (DIF, DDF): more negative language, more self-focus, and stronger emotion-situation correspondence.	HA (DIF, DDF) Deficit [↓] in positive expression. HA (DIF, DDF) OR [↓] More negative language and perseveration on self-relevance (salience) in emotive context.
Jakobson and Pearson (2021) (this issue)	70, 51% F, M_{age}=21, M_{TAS}=47	TAS-20(C) w/facets Controls: sex, verbal IQ (WASI)	**Receptive: Social Inference** Social video vignettes (neutral), infer speaker intentions (literal, sarcastic, jocular, white lies) with or w/o verbal context.	HA>LA (DDF): *better* accuracy when no context. HA>LA (DIF): *slower* on non-literal exchanges when no context.	HA (DIF) Deficit [↓], via response time and when no context available. HA (DDF) OR [↑], *better* accuracy when no context.
Jelinek et al. (2010)	N_{PTSD}= 25, 64% F M_{age}=41, M_{TAS}=54; $N_{nonPTSD}$= 54, 48% F M_{age}=39, M_{TAS}=44 Trauma sample	TAS-20 (C) Controls: none	**Expressive: Autobiographical Narratives** Interview about trauma experience, analysed with LIWC.	HA=LA: no correlation with affect word use in full sample or non-PTSD. HA<LA: negative correlation in those with PTSD.	HA Deficit [↓] in language expression. Reduced emotional expression discussing trauma in HA with PTSD.
Kreitler (2002)	100, 50% F, M_{age}=23, M_{TAS}=55	TAS-20 (C) w/facets Controls: none	**Expressive: Autobiographical Narratives (neutral)** The Meaning Test; Communicate personal meaning of a 11 probe words (e.g. "telephone") to another person (i.e. neutral context).	HA>LA: concrete, simple, visual, externalized. (DIF: concreteness; DDF: avoidance of emotion (perceived, experienced); EOT: concrete, externalized).	HA (DIF, DDF, EOT) Deficit [↓] in *general* language expression qualitatively poorer (*neutral* context).
Luminet et al. (2004)‡	50, 44% F, M_{age}= 64, M_{BVAQ}= NR	BVAQ (C) w/facets (independent, as TAS-20) Controls: age, sex, health status	**Expressive: Emotional Narrative** Emotional video (sad), re-exposure 2d later, recount most emotional part; lexical task (bird names, emotion words). Scored emotion word content/frequency.	HA=LA: no correlation with emotion or neutral word frequency HA<LA (DDF): negatively correlated with emotion word frequency about film.	HA (DDF) Deficit [↓] in language expression. HA have sufficient emotion vocabulary, access, but use it less in emotional situations.
Meganck et al. (2009)	50, 62% F, M_{age}= 42 M_{TAS}= 60 Psychiatric inpatient sample	TAS-20 (C) w/facets Controls(**1**): positive/ negative affect (PANAS)	**Expressive: Autobiographical Narratives** Interview using CDI (2 hr; covering complaints, relationships, work/school, symptoms, etc. and follow-up probes). Used LIWC analysis of communication word frequency, complexity.	HA=LA: word frequency HA<LA (DIF, EOT) lower complexity HA>LA (EOT) more references to others v. self.	HA (DIF, EOT) Deficit [↓] in language expression. HA (EOT) OR [↓] more other-focused. HA discussions had reduced vividness, differentiation and self-disclosure.

(*Continued*)

Table 4. Continued.

Study	Sample Size & Characteristics	Alexithymia Measures/ Controls	Language Measures	Results (Total/Facets (if specified))	Implications
Paez et al. (1999)	Exp. 3: 70 (via Exp. 1, 2); ≈65% F; M_{age}≈19; Md_{DDF}=12	TAS-20 (D)-DDF, median split. Controls: none PPSS, positive/ negative affect (PANAS) measured but did not analyse because no group difference	**Expressive: Autobiographical Narratives** Expressive writing about traumatic or social event.	HA<LA: emotion words, esp. positive; introspection, self-reference. HA>LA: inhibition.	HA (DDF) Deficit [↓] in language expression. Intensive writing was *beneficial* relative to brief writing.
Parker et al. (2000)	8 LA, 50% F, M_{TAS}=31; 8 HA, 50% F, M_{TAS}=66; Age: NR (undergraduates)	TAS-20 (D) Controls: none	**Expressive: Autobiographical Narratives** Sleep study; dream recounting upon awakening from REM (dream) sleep.	HA=LA: valence of dreams, number of words. HA<LA: fantasy content	HA Deficit [↓] in language expression, specifically in elaboration and imagination.
Roedema and Simons (1999)	31 LA, 48% F, M_{TAS}<52; 34 HA; 56%; M_{TAS}>72; Age: NR (undergraduates)	TAS-26 (D) Controls: none	**Expressive: Autobiographical Narratives** Emotional slides; ratings, psychophysiological measures. Subjects wrote adjectives to describe how the slide made them feel.	HA<LA emotion words.	HA Deficit [↓] in language expression.
Samur et al. (2021) (this issue)	Online: 541, 55% F, M_{age}=36, M_{BVAQ}=100; Lab: 55, 55% F, M_{age}=22, M_{BVAQ}=100	BVAQ/subscores (Cognitive, aka TAS-20 total; Affective (DF)= emotionalising, fantasising) Controls: none	**Receptive: Narrative Engagement** Ss read fictional narrative, with either 1st- or 3rd-person perspective. Narrative engagement measured using TS.	HA<LA: (Total, DF): negatively correlated with narrative engagement. HA<LA (DF): effect of perspective (engagement 1st > 3rd) in LA, not in HA.	HA (Total, DF) Deficit [↓] in narrative processing, even w/ 1st person perspective. Developmental role in empathy, perspective-taking.
Smyth et al. (2002)	39_{asthma}, 73% F, M_{age}≈41 32_{RA}, 71%F, M_{age}≈51 Overall, M_{TAS}=44	TAS-20 (C) Controls: none	**Expressive: Autobiographical Narratives** Writing on 3 consecutive days (20 min ea.) about traumatic experience, coded for personal, emotional content and narrative structure.	HA=LA: No correlation with personal, emotional expression, change in positive or negative affect after writing; or narrative structure.	HA: no effect.
Tull et al. (2005)	541; 67% F, M_{age}=27, M_{TAS}=46	TAS-20 (C) w/facets Controls(**1**): negative affect (PANAS)	**Expressive: Autobiographical Narratives** 5-min interview about distressing past event, linguistic analysis with LIWC.	HA<LA (DIF): negative correlation with frequency, variety of positive words. HA>LA (DIF): *positive* correlation with frequency of negative words.	HA (DIF) Deficit [↓] in positive expression; may reflect reduced positive vocabulary store/access. HA (DIF): OR [↓] negative expression; may reflect mood and emotion regulation ability.
Vanheule et al. (2011)	32, 63% F, M_{age}=43, M_{TAS}=56 Mental health outpatient sample	TAS-20 (C) w/facets Controls(**1**): depression (BDI)	**Expressive: Autobiographical Narratives** Clinical interview (2hr); narrative analysis (LIWC) for frequency, complexity (diversity) of cognitive and social word use.	HA>LA (DIF): *more* cognitive words (CI incl. 0). HA<LA (EOT): *fewer* cognitive words (CI incl. 0), *fewer, less complex* social words, *less complex* cognitive words.	HA (EOT) Deficit [↓] in language expression. Reduced social word use, diversity of expression (i.e. social detachment, impaired cognitive processing).
Wagner and Lee (2008)	Exp. 1: 55, 100% F, M_{age}=20, M_{TAS}=47 Exp. 2: 54, 100% F, M_{age}=21, M_{TAS}=50	TAS-20 (C) w/facets Controls: none	**Expressive: Autobiographical Narratives** Oral narrative of a personal positive and negative event (w/ or w/o female experimenter present). Correlational analysis.	Exp. 1: HA<LA (DIF): less positive expression in positive context. HA< LA (DIF, EOT): less negative expression in negative context.	HA (DIF, EOT) Deficit [↓] in language expression congruent with context (DIF both positive, negative; EOT negative, may be mediated by DIF).

(*Continued*)

Table 4. Continued.

Study	Sample Size & Characteristics	Alexithymia Measures/ Controls	Language Measures	Results (Total/Facets (if specified))	Implications
				Exp. 2: HA<LA; Replicated Exp. 1; social context, ns.	
Wotschack and Klann-Delius (2013)	52 LA, 42% F, M_{age}=34; M_{TAS}=38; 50 HA; 42%; M_{age}=36; M_{TAS}=68	TAS-20 (D) Controls: none	**Expressive: Autobiographical Narratives** Interviews on positive, negative personal experiences (emotion word cues, autobiographical narratives, pictures, LEAS).	HA<LA: types of emotion words, emotion synonyms, fewer symptomatic and physiological words.	HA Deficit in [↓] language expression. Suggested reduced, less diverse semantic and conceptual vocabulary for emotion.

Notes. All studies used non-clinical samples except as noted; BVAQ: Bermond-Vorst Alexithymia Questionnaire (DF=difficulty fantasising); TAS-26: Toronto Alexithymia Scale 26 Items; TAS-20: Toronto Alexithymia Scale 20 Items (C-continuous, D-dichotomous); DIF: Difficulty Identifying Feelings subscale of the TAS-20; DDF: Difficulty Describing Feelings subscale from the TAS-20; EOT: Externally Oriented Thinking subscale of the TAS-20; LA: Low Alexithymia Scorers; HA High Alexithymia Scorers; ‡=study appears in more than one table and section of the paper; F=Female; M_{TAS}= mean TAS-20 total score; M_{age}=mean age (years); *d'*= d-prime, recognition sensitivity (accuracy); PTSD=post-traumatic stress disorder; RA=rheumatoid arthritis; NR=not reported; ns=not significant; OR=over-responding; CI=Confidence Interval (contains 0=low confidence of true significance); [↓]=detrimental effect of HA; [↑]=potentially beneficial effect of HA; (**1**)results reported effects after affect variables controlled; (**2**)results reported indicating separable or unique effect of controls; (**3**)negative affect control reduced alexithymia effect.
Instruments: BDI= Beck Depression Inventory; CDI=Clinical Diagnostic Interview; LEAS= Levels of Emotional Awareness Scale; LIWC= Linguistic Inquiry Word Count; PANAS=Positive Affectivity Negative Affectivity Schedule; PPSS=Pennebaker Physical Symptoms Scale; TSIA=Toronto Structured Interviews for Alexithymia; TS=Transportation Scale; WASI= Wechsler Abbreviated Scale of Intelligence-2nd Ed. (vocabulary, similarities subtests).

demonstrated by the relative stability of alexithymia scores even in situations of strong psychological distress (e.g. Luminet et al., 2001, 2007; see section 1.2.3.). Although HA may be impaired in their ability to experience, elaborate, and express subjective feelings, they are still able to feel pleasantness or unpleasantness. However, their distress may not be expressed through language, but by other channels such as somatic sensations or symptoms, or impulsive behaviours (see section 2.5).

Our first prediction was that individuals with high alexithymia scores would experience negative events as more unpleasant, especially as HA is linked to difficulties in differentiating somatic arousal and experienced feelings. We also predicted that HA scorers would appraise positive events as being less pleasant, given the association between alexithymia and anhedonia, which suggests individuals with HA have a limited capacity to experience positive emotions (Krystal, 1988). Because alexithymia correlates with other personality dimensions (e.g. positively with neuroticism, negatively with extraversion and openness; Luminet et al., 1999), control over NA and PA is important. This was accomplished by six out of eight (75%) of the valence studies (see Table 2). Because of the lack of literature on types and intensity of appraisals and alexithymia, we also considered how initial valence of events can affect long-term emotional reactions such as social sharing of emotion and rumination.

We found a total of seven papers (eight studies) addressing appraisal. Two papers examined the early processing of emotion. One showed that high alexithymia scores were linked to reduced unpleasantness ratings in response to negative stimuli (Luminet et al., 2004), whereas the other reported that alexithymia was not linked to appraisals of aversive stimuli but was associated with diminished responsivity to appetitive words and pictures (Koven, 2014). Regarding later processing of emotion, individuals with poorer fantasy scores[1] ruminated less after positive events, and those with higher DDF scorers had deficits in sharing emotions in a negative context (Luminet et al., 2000). Deficits of emotional responding in HA would appear to occur only under specific valence conditions. These results have important implications for psychological adaptation. Thinking about positive events from the past can increase the availability of positive memories, which then increases positive mood. By not benefitting from the protective effect of positive rumination,

Table 5. Alexithymia, action tendencies and behaviours.

Study	Sample size & characteristics	Alexithymia measures/controls	Action tendencies/ behaviours measures	Results (Total/Facets (if specified))	Implications
Edwards and Wupperman (2017)	96, 76% F, Mdn_{age}=20, M_{TAS}=44	TAS-20(C) Controls: none	**Aggression** Self-reported impulsive aggression (IPAS), emotion regulation (DERS)	HA>LA: HA positively correlated wtih agression, which was mediated by emotion dysregulation.	HA: OR [↓] Poor access to emotion information produces emotion dysregulation in HA, predisposing them to acts of impulsive aggression.
Gvirts and Dery (2021) (this issue)	116, 65% F, M_{age}=24, M_{TAS-20}=46	TAS-20(C, D), w/ facets Controls: none	**Social agreement** Videogame where Ps unaware whether playing with a bot (who acts rationally, always seeks consensus), or with other Ps.	HA<LA (EOT): HA had impaired ability to reach social agreement; evident when group harmony is low but not when group harmony is high.	HA (EOT): Deficit [↓] for interpersonal functions. Possibly due to low reliance on reward from social interactions.
Laloyaux et al. (2015)	Study 1: 255, 69% F, M_{age}=20; M_{TAS-20}=49 Study 2: 1111, 50% F, M_{age} = 41, M_{BVAQ}=106	Study 1: TAS-20(C); w/facets Study 2: BVAQ(C); w/ facets Controls: age, education	**Emotion regulation** Used the ERQ; with reappraisal and suppression dimensions.	HA>LA (DDF): greater use of emotional suppression in HA; HA=LA: reappraisal	HA (DDF): OR [↓] excessive use of emotional suppression.
Panayiotou et al. (2015)	Study 1 (HC): 205, 79% F, M_{age}=21, M_{TAS}=53 Study 2 (anxiety sample): 163, 37% F, M_{age}=30; M_{TAS}=56	TAS-20(C), w/facets Controls: none	**Experiential avoidance** Self-report measures of psychosomatic symptoms (PHQ-15), depression (BDI), and experiential avoidance (AAQ)	HA>LA (DIF,DDF): positive correlation w/ symptoms (Study 1), depression (Study 2); mediated by experiential avoidance. DIF reduced with depression treatment (Study 2); mediated by reduced experiential avoidance.	HA (DIF, DDF): OR [↓] (somatic symptoms, depression); mediated by experiential avoidance. Alexithymia change (DIF) with treatment due to change in experiential avoidance.
Teten et al. (2008)	38, 8% F, M_{age}=59, M_{TAS}=63 Trauma sample	TAS-20(C) Controls: none	**Aggression** Measured impulsive aggression (IPAS), verbal/physical aggression (BPAQ), empathic concern (IRI)	HA>LA: HA predicted higher impulsive agression (R^2 = .10)	HA: OR [↓] HA results in greates impulsive aggression, but not general aggression.
Velotti et al. (2016)	HC: 617, 46% F, M_{age}=37, M_{TAS}=43 Inpatient psychiatric sample: 257, 50% F, M_{age}=44, M_{TAS}=55	TAS-20(C) Controls(**2**): age, sex depression (BSI)	**Aggression** Measured aggression (AQ), emotion dysregulation (DERS), impulsivity (BIS-11)	HA>LA: HA positively correlated with aggression (both samples), which was mediated by emotion dysregulation (both samples), and impulsivity (only HC).	HA: OR [↓] emotion dysregulation responsible for the role of HA in aggression.

(*Continued*)

Table 5. Continued.

Study	Sample size & characteristics	Alexithymia measures/controls	Action tendencies/ behaviours measures	Results (Total/Facets (if specified))	Implications
Venta et al. (2013)	64, 59% F, M_{age}=16, HA: M_{TAS}=71, LA: M_{TAS}=45 Psychiatric inpatient sample	TAS-20(D) Controls: none (age, sex, verbal IQ were comparable)	**Experiential avoidance** Examined self-reported emotion regulation (DERS), experiential avoidance (AFQ-Y)	HA>LA: HA positively associated with emotion dysregulation, which was mediated by experiential avoidance in this adolescent inpatient sample.	HA: OR [↓] HA exhbit emotion dysregulation, due to experiential avoidance.

Notes. All studies used non-clinical samples except as noted. TAS-20: Toronto Alexithymia Scale 20 Items (C-continuous, D-dichotomous); DIF: Difficulty Identifying Feelings subscale of the TAS-20; DDF: Difficulty Describing Feelings subscale from the TAS-20; EOT: Externally Oriented Thinking subscale of the TAS-20; BVAQ: Bermond Vorst Alexithymia Questionnaire (C-continuous, D-dichotomous); LA: Low Alexithymia Scorers; HA High Alexithymia Scorers; F=Female; M = Male; M_{TAS}= mean TAS-20 total score; M_{age}=mean age (years; Mdn=median); HC=healthy controls (community sample); OR=over-responding; Ps = Participants; [↓]=detrimental effect of HA; [↑]=potentially beneficial effect of HA; (**1**)results reported effects after affect variables controlled; (**2**)results reported indicating separable or unique effect of controls; (**3**)negative affect control reduced alexithymia effect.

Instruments: AAQ= Acceptance and Action Questionnaire (II); AFQ-Y= Questionnaire for Youth; AQ= Aggression Questionnaire; BIS-11=Barratt Impulsiveness Scale-11; BDI= Beck Depression Inventory(II); BPAQ= verbal and physical aggression, Buss–Perry Aggression Questionnaire; BSI=Brief Symptom Inventory; DERS= Difficulties in Emotion Regulation Scale; ERQ= Emotion Regulation Questionnaire; IPAS= Impulsive-Premeditated Aggression Scale (Impulsive Aggression Subscale); IRI= Interpersonal Reactivity Index; PHQ-15= Patient Health Questionnaire-15.

HA may be more impacted by thoughts generated after a negative event. Furthermore, as verbal disclosure of negative events is related to positive health outcomes (e.g. Pennebaker & Smyth, 2016), it is possible that individuals with HA experience less mitigation of health impacts through disclosure.

The distinction between affect intensity (i.e. magnitude of individuals' experiences of emotional responses; Larsen, 1985) and affect frequency (i.e. how often mood states are experienced in a particular period) is another dimension to consider. Regarding positive emotion intensity, Fantini-Hauwel et al. (2015) found a dissociation, with DDF linked to lower intensity and DIF with higher intensity. This highlights the importance of considering the alexithymia facets separately. Furthermore, while high positive frequency is considered healthy, high positive intensity is related to psychological dysfunctions, such as bipolar disorders (Diener et al., 1985a, 1985b). DIF was also related to a higher frequency of experiencing negative affect, which is likely to have deleterious effects on mood regulation.

Aaron et al. (2018) used a more refined method to examine how alexithymia moderates the appraisal process, distinguishing emotional granularity, the ability to make fine-grained distinctions between emotional experiences (Barrett et al., 2001), and emotional dialecticism, one's tendency to simultaneously recognise pleasant and unpleasant states (Bagozzi et al., 1999). High alexithymia was linked to reduced emotional granularity (DDF) and dialecticism (EOT) in response to negative videos. Specifically, individuals with higher DDF used a smaller set of adjectives to describe their emotional reactions and those with higher EOT experienced fewer pleasant states concurrently with unpleasant ones. Reduced granularity of negative emotions in HA was previously suggested by Erbas et al. (2014). Finally, Larwood et al. (2021, this issue) examined the influence of alexithymia on the appraisal of emotions in musical extracts, and reported that HA assessed negative musical emotions (sad, angry, fearful) as more neutral than LA, but appraisal of positive musical emotions (happy, tender) was not linked to alexithymia, highlighting again that HA is related to a mitigation of the valence of stimuli.

Regarding other appraisals, Luminet et al. (2004) found deficits for importance (EOT) and familiarity (DDF). The first result suggests that HA is related to reduced interest and concern for emotional topics, but reduced familiarity indicates a greater discomfort in dealing with affective themes in those with HA. The latter finding supports the hypothesis that HA would also result in avoidance of negative situations. Early clinical evidence indicated that HA experience elevated discomfort during social interaction, thereby avoiding social relationships (Nemiah & Sifneos, 1970; Sifneos et al., 1977). Finally, anticipatory appraisals, which are measured before people are exposed to stressful situations were considered in one study (de Timary et al., 2008). Higher DDF was related to elevated cortisol at baseline, but no alexithymia factor was related to cortisol secretion during stress exposure or during recovery, suggesting that alexithymia modulates anticipation of stress rather than the stress response.

2.2.1. Summary

Most of the literature on appraisal and alexithymia has examined valence. After unpleasant situations, almost all studies showed a deficit in emotional responding rather than the predicted over-responding. Importantly, the results were not modified when controlling for negative affect. The driving factors were consistently DDF and EOT, while the only finding for greater reactivity towards negative situations was found with DIF. Regarding the moderating impact of alexithymia in pleasant situations, fewer studies are available, which corresponds to the general lack of attention to positive context in the emotion research domain. Two studies, which controlled for positive affect, found decreased ratings of positivity. HA also involved alterations in importance and familiarity appraisals, and stress anticipation. In their model, Preece et al. (2017) predicted that DIF and DDF are the main driving factors of the appraisal stage, which is only partially supported in our data where DDF and EOT were the significant factors associated to appraisals.

Among the seven papers reviewed, all (100%) involved non-clinical samples, with six (86%) of them with a student population and one examining older adults. Five of the papers (71%) used controls for negative affect. Participants were primarily exposed to emotional materials (i.e. emotive video, pictures, music; four papers, 57%), with other approaches characterising one paper each (social stress task, autobiographical rumination task, affect intensity ratings with no manipulation). Six (86%) found evidence for deficits, one (14%) found dysfunctional over-responding, and one found both, strongly suggesting an overall pattern of deficit in HA. DDF and EOT seem to be the driving factors, although the number of studies that examined how alexithymia factors are related to appraisals dimensions is very limited. This is a clear priority for future research.

2.3. Memory

Just as emotion perception and responses are influenced by people's appraisals of the experience, memory is influenced by individual differences in how events are experienced (Kensinger, 2009). Memory is the encoding of our experiences, which we retrieve to guide our future thoughts, decisions and actions. Encoding, which is the formation of initial memory traces, is assessed by short-term testing and is influenced by stimulus perception and attention (Levine & Edelstein, 2009). Encoding processes in turn influence memory storage and what is later retrieved. Emotion evokes physiological and subjective experiences that can both contribute to a memory advantage for emotive memoranda and contexts (e.g. LaBar & Cabeza, 2006). Ultimately, emotion influences memory priority by triggering salience or top-down goals (Mather & Sutherland, 2011). However, what constitutes "priority" is influenced by individual differences in the appraisal of and response to emotion. At the facet-level, EOT is associated with both inhibited arousal responding (Davydov et al., 2013) and impaired emotional appraisal (section 2.2). Thus, we would predict deficits of both short-term and delayed emotive memory in HA, particularly associated with EOT.

We found 18 papers with 24 studies that specifically examined memory performance in alexithymia (Table 3). The earliest study, examining incidental learning of emotion words, found longer decision times and *fewer* recognition errors in HA, but no difference in memory accuracy (Jacob & Hautekeete, 1998). Superficially, fewer errors appeared beneficial, but the effect was due to better *distractor rejection*, while acceptance of targets was actually poorer in HA. Thus, HA had a more conservative style, rejecting both targets and distractors, thereby hinting at a memory deficit in HA. Furthermore, although few studies have examined processing time, others have not replicated longer memory processing time in HA (Lundh et al., 2002; Vermeulen et al., 2010).

Since 1998, all but one paper (Lundh et al., 2002) has reported some form of memory deficits in HA (94%); only half also examined TAS-20 facets (Table 3). When the context is emotive (most papers), memory deficits in alexithymia at immediate testing have been typically shown for emotive but not neutral memoranda. This finding is apparent across intentional and incidental learning paradigms, nearly all of which used verbal stimuli. For example, poorer memory was found in HA for emotive words (e.g. negative, positive), with no effect for neutral words (Luminet et al., 2006; Meltzer & Nielson, 2010; Vermeulen & Luminet, 2009). One paper instead reported elevated intrusion errors (over-responding to positive distractors; Suslow et al., 2003). These effects were isolated to confident "remember" responses versus familiarity (Luminet et al., 2006), and specifically to DIF (Suslow et al., 2003; Vermeulen & Luminet, 2009). In contrast, other papers have isolated emotive memory deficits in HA to EOT. Directed forgetting, where subjects learn certain lists or items while forgetting others, showed greater EOT associated with deficits in memory for negative wanted items and over-responding via greater intrusion of negative unwanted items (i.e. false memory; Dressaire et al., 2015). Another paper showed memory deficits with EOT for negative and positive items in "pure" (single valence) but not mixed-valence lists (Vermeulen, 2021, this issue). These papers suggest pervasive interference with emotive links to conscious memory in alexithymia (Bucci, 1997; Taylor, 2000), thereby interfering with internal cognitive control and producing a more conservative acceptance criterion, perhaps due to difficulty managing uncertainty and motivation to process emotion (Vermeulen & Luminet, 2009).

Papers examining non-verbal emotive memory in alexithymia have typically been consistent with verbal studies, including deficits in immediate and delayed memory for faces and social scenes or interactions (DiStefano & Koven, 2012; Donges & Suslow, 2015; Ridout et al., 2021, this issue) and memory for change of facial expression (happy; Takahashi et al., 2015). Some face memory effects were specific to anger and/or fear rather than happy or neutral (Donges & Suslow, 2015; Ridout et al., 2021, this issue); these were notably attributable to DDF. In contrast, deficits for social interactions in video stimuli were associated with DIF and EOT (Ridout et al., 2021, this issue). One paper produced a paradoxical *benefit*: increasing the intensity of facial expressions should produce greater errors in subsequent matching comparisons than for reduced intensity (i.e. representational momentum). However, fewer errors (over-responding) resulted in HA (total score) due to reduced intensity sensitivity (Senior et al., 2020).

Some instances of better memory in HA have appeared alongside deficits, though not all these effects were beneficial. Specific findings include fewer errors in HA (Jacob & Hautekeete, 1998), which Senior et al. (2020) link to DIF; and better memory for emotive or neutral memoranda associated with DIF (sad, Ridout et al., 2021; neutral, Dressaire et al., 2015; Ridout et al., 2021) or EOT (Vermeulen & Luminet, 2009). It is possible that negative affect contributed to better sad face memory through salience (context congruency), though depression covariance analysis decreased this likelihood. Yet, in support of the salience explanation and indicating detrimental over-responding, HA had better memory for illness words (via preoccupation), despite poorer memory for other negative words (Meltzer & Nielson, 2010). Similarly, while Fading Affect Bias predicts that negative memories fade more over time than positive memories, the effect was opposite in HA, with positive memories fading more and negative memories fading less (Muir et al., 2017). Thus, HA experiencing negative emotion as more negative, along with reduced intensity of positive emotion (Krystal, 1988), may inadvertently protect negative memory salience over time as positive memories fade. Finally, despite generally reduced emotive memory, Vermeulen et al. (2010) found HA-specific context effects with improved joy word retrieval when encoding was accompanied by happy background music, and anger word retrieval with angry music. These results implicate a role for cognitive control in alexithymia, showing that setting a congruent context can be beneficial in helping HA better process and later retrieve emotive information.

Although memory studies in alexithymia typically reported no effects on neutral stimuli, most employed an emotionally charged context. However, as learning context critically influences memory (e.g. Smith, 1994), we must also ask whether alexithymia influences genuinely neutral memory. Seven papers have addressed this question. Two of them (29%) reported *better* immediate memory (beneficial over-responding) for neutral stimuli via DIF (Dressaire et al., 2015; Ridout et al., 2021), although one also reported a negative correlation with EOT (Dressaire et al., 2015). The other five papers (71%) reported a neutral memory deficit attributable to EOT for immediate memory (DiStefano & Koven, 2012; Nielson & Meltzer, 2009; Terock et al., 2019; Vermeulen, 2021) and delayed memory (Correro et al., 2021; DiStefano

& Koven, 2012; Terock et al., 2019). Correro et al. (2021, this issue) further found DIF contributed to poorer executive functioning, which interacted with EOT to impair memory. Importantly, emotion typically triggers physiological reactivity, rumination, and attentional shifts from external to internal thoughts (Luminet et al., 2004). However, EOT reduces translation of these external cues to internal cues in all contexts. We suspect that, because EOT impairs emotional appraisal (see section 2.2. on Appraisal) and inhibits arousal responses and processing concomitant with internally directed cognition (Davydov et al., 2013), the fundamental processes for establishing priority in memory (Mather & Sutherland, 2011) are disadvantaged by EOT even in neutral contexts.

The majority of memory studies tested retention within one minute after encoding (67%; see Table 3). Testing was delayed five minutes in one study (5%; Ridout et al., 2021), and 20 min to 24 h in five studies (28%; Correro et al., 2021; DiStefano & Koven, 2012; Meltzer & Nielson, 2010; Nielson & Meltzer, 2009; Terock et al., 2019). Arguably, nuanced long-term memory assessment requires a sufficient delay to allow for some consolidation to occur. Indeed, all neutral memoranda studies with 20–60 min delays showed an HA deficit (EOT; Correro et al., 2021; DiStefano & Koven, 2012; Terock et al., 2019), while one study showed no effect after 24 hrs despite an immediate retrieval deficit (Nielson & Meltzer, 2009). Long-term retrieval with mixed stimuli instead saw a deficit for negative words, but over-responding to illness words and neutral words (Meltzer & Nielson, 2010). Alongside an immediate memory deficit in neutral but not mixed contexts (EOT; Vermeulen, 2021), and enhanced happy or angry memory within matching musical backgrounds (Vermeulen et al., 2010), these studies suggest context dependency, likely interacting with appraisal tendencies, are impactful on encoding and retrieval in HA. However, not enough is yet known about storage influences in alexithymia (see Takahashi et al., 2015).

2.3.1. Summary

All the 18 memory papers (including 24 studies; Table 3) reviewed examined normative samples, mostly using young adults (typically college students). Six out of these 18 papers (33%) examined middle aged to older adults or compared older adults with young adults (range=18-99 yrs). The vast majority of papers (12/18, 67%) used emotional and/or neutral words or narratives as memoranda, while five (28%) used emotional and/or neutral faces or scenes, and two (11%) used autobiographical memory tests. Twelve of the 18 papers (67%) controlled for negative affect (four also controlled positive affect); none reported that affect contributed to prediction of memory outcomes, though results were not commonly compared with and without inclusion. However, it should be noted that in most of these studies, affect correlated with alexithymia, but not necessarily with the memory metrics. Importantly, affect control is of no value if it does not correlate with the outcome measures (see discussion section for a detailed elaboration on the conditions for affect control).

Taken together, 15 of 18 papers (83%) demonstrated that memory is poorer in HA, particularly for emotional stimuli and even for neutral stimuli in neutral contexts. Of the seven studies (39%) examining only the TAS-total score, *all* (100%) showed memory deficits, while three (43%) reported in addition over-responding to salient content, including one showing context congruence effects can be beneficial (i.e. functional over-responding). Eleven of the 18 papers (61%) examined TAS-20 facets. DIF contributed to memory or cognitive control deficits in five papers (45%) and over-responding in five papers; OR was dysfunctional (more intrusion of affective memories) in two papers (18%), and OR was beneficial in three papers (memory was better for neutral stimuli or fewer errors in HA; 27%). DDF was linked to memory deficits in four papers (36%), two for positive stimuli and two for anger or fear; it was not associated with over-responding. Overall, differences were isolated to specific retrieval (e.g. recall, "remember") rather than familiarity (e.g. "know") and were associated with poorer cognitive control and greater influences of salience and context on HA, suggesting the influence of early appraisal tendencies on later memory processes. Finally, EOT was the primary contributor to memory deficits (7/11 studies, 64%), with also dysfunctional over-responding in one study (i.e. increased false memory; 9%) and functional over-responding in one study (9%); the stimulus type that was influenced differed across paradigms. Thus, an externally oriented thinking style seems particularly detrimental to memory across paradigms, likely due to reduced cues that are needed to establish priority in memory. Studies that use a facet level analysis while specifically interrogating cognitive control within memory paradigms, as well as studies manipulating of memory priority, are particularly important future directions.

2.4. Language

Language, verbal and non-verbal, is a structured form of communication that allows people to share inner thoughts and feelings and to understand the utterances of others. These are central aspects of social life. Language furthermore reveals much about cognition, as it relies on the integrity of the range of cognitive processes and in turn, influences and shows how we feel, remember and think. Many emotion theories, from nativist to constructionist, attribute some role for language in emotion processing (Hobson et al., 2019) and include its role in the development and adaptation of emotion concepts and schemas and emotion regulation (Hoemann & Feldman Barrett, 2019). These schemas then afford the ability to identify emotion when it occurs, and to communicate it to others. Language also pervades most aspects of cognition. Certainly, any task using verbal stimuli and/or requiring a verbal response is founded in language. That said, herein we examine "language" only in its receptive and expressive capacities, without consideration of non-verbal cues, influences of verbal tasks (e.g. appraisal, attention, memory), or emotion schemas (i.e. concept formation), because empirical alexithymia research has not yet addressed these areas.

The importance of language to alexithymia is evident in its very definition. For example, difficulty identifying feelings suggests difficulty translating sensations (i.e. sub-symbolic representations) into concepts (i.e. symbolic representations), which can then limit ability to describe feelings due to poor symbolic representations. Indeed, other reviews have addressed these concepts about language disturbances in alexithymia (see Welding & Samur, 2018), with one review further postulating "the language hypothesis of alexithymia" (Hobson et al., 2019). Given the important relationship between language development and emotional-social development (e.g. Izard et al., 2011), and the under-development of emotion schemas evident in HA through attention, memory (e.g. Luminet et al., 2006; Vermeulen et al., 2006) and appraisal (see section 2.2. on Appraisal and Preece et al., 2017), we would predict significant deficits in language expression and reception for emotive contexts in HA, particularly related to DDF and DIF.

There is a good deal of overall consistency across studies that examine language expression and reception in alexithymia, showing a general pattern of deficits (Table 4). We found 16 papers; all but one (Smyth et al., 2002) evidence some form of language deficit in alexithymia. All but two of these asked subjects to write or speak about their emotional experiences. Consistently, they report HA have reduced emotional expression, including fantasy content of dreams (Parker et al., 2000), frequency of emotion words and descriptions used in speech or writing (Jelinek et al., 2010; Luminet et al., 2004 (DDF); Paez et al., 1999; Roedema & Simons, 1999; Tull et al., 2005 (DIF); Vanheule et al., 2011; Wotschack & Klann-Delius, 2013), reduced complexity of emotion vocabulary or expression (Meganck et al., 2009 (DIF, EOT); Vanheule et al., 2011 (EOT; DIF (only positive)); Wotschack & Klann-Delius, 2013), and a less open communication style (Kreitler, 2002; Wagner & Lee, 2008). This was most evident when people were trying to verbalise intense or traumatic experiences (Paez et al., 1999 (DDF); Jelinek et al., 2010; though see Smyth et al., 2002). The samples for these papers ranged from normative to clinical. Notably, although few employed controls for comorbidities such as affect or depression (25%), those that did so still found language deficits in alexithymia.

No clear pattern emerged about which facet(s) of alexithymia are most relevant to language. Only 8 papers examined facets rather than the total score; one examined only DDF. All three facets were associated with deficits: DIF in six studies (75%) (Edwards et al., 2020; Jakobson & Pearson, 2021; Kreitler, 2002; Meganck et al., 2009; Tull et al., 2005; Wagner & Lee, 2008), DDF in four studies (50%) (Edwards et al., 2020; Kreitler, 2002; Luminet et al., 2004; Paez et al., 1999), and EOT in five studies (62.5%) (Kreitler, 2002; Meganck et al., 2009; Samur et al., 2021, this issue; Vanheule et al., 2011; Wagner & Lee, 2008). DDF was associated with *better* performance in one study (Jakobson & Pearson, 2021, this issue), as was DIF in another, but the confidence interval included zero suggesting an unreliable effect (Vanheule et al., 2011). Indeed, a large study that examined writing about a distressing past event while controlling for negative affect showed that DIF was associated with a deficit of positive expression, but greater negative expression (Tull et al., 2005). This finding fits with appraisal and memory studies associating DIF with over-responding to negative material, even after controlling for negative affect (see sections 2.2. on Appraisal, and 2.3. on Memory). The only language expression study to examine neutral, everyday topics, found all three facets significantly predicted general deficits in language expression (Kreitler, 2002). This finding too is consistent with recent studies showing alexithymia deficits (typically EOT) in memory for neutral material (section 2.3. on Memory). These findings support our predictions, suggesting that the under-developed emotion schemas that influence attention, memory, and appraisal further influence language expression, resulting in deficits (Preece et al., 2017; Taylor, 2000). This was apparent in emotive contexts and may be most associated with DIF, but limited work suggested deficits in neutral contexts as well.

Studies of language reception (i.e. comprehension) per se in alexithymia are scarce. Two new papers, however, both in this issue, do explicitly examine it. Jakobson and Pearson (2021, this issue) presented videos of neutral vignettes with subjects required to infer speaker intentions as literal or non-literal; half provided contextual assistance while half did not. No alexithymia effects were apparent when context was included. Without context, HA had slower decision time (DIF), but *better* accuracy (DDF). As DDF and DIF are associated with ease of excitation and lowered sensory thresholds, it was concluded that heightened engagement in HA when context is lacking could improve performance (DDF), but retard decision-making (DIF). Paradoxically, this could impair performance in more emotionally charged displays. Similarly, fictional first – or third-person narratives showed impaired language comprehension in HA (emotionalising/fantasising) through low narrative engagement (Samur et al., 2021; this issue). Specifically, HA were unable to benefit from the "support" of first-person narratives, perhaps due to difficulty with perspective-taking, or mentally simulating another's world. These findings correspond with HA having poorer mental imagery ability (e.g. Davydov et al., 2013; Luminet et al., 2004) and difficulty with empathy (e.g. Grynberg et al., 2018). These context effects also reinforce a difficulty processing non-verbal and abstract cues in HA, highlighting the importance of providing concrete, verbal cues and context during interactions.

2.4.1. Summary

Of the 16 language papers reviewed, nine (56%) had samples with average ages from 30s to 60s; samples were older than typical college-aged samples. Four studies (25%, all with samples older than college age) included clinical samples. Fourteen of 16 papers (87.5%) involved language expression and 100% of these used a narrative approach, with all but one (93%) employing an autobiographical emotive paradigm; the other was neutral. Two papers (12.5%) measured receptive language, which examined social inference and engagement.

The literature is quite consistent in showing a deficit in language expression, and in two new papers, reception, in alexithymia. All but one of 16 papers (94%) showed a deficit characterised by reduced complexity, a less open style, and reduced emotional content in HA. Control over mood or affect was rare four studies controlled NA (25%), two also controlled PA (12.5%), but deficits were not mitigated by such controls. Furthermore, the effects were strongest under higher intensity conditions. Three papers (19%) also evidenced dysfunctional over-responding with more negative language (DIF, DDF) or more outward focus (EOT). Few studies have directly examined language comprehension (reception; only two papers herein (12.5%)), but these also are indicative of HA deficits, particularly when no context is available, although one of them showed functional over-responding to inferences when no context was available (DDF). Specific facet distinctions, however were not forthcoming in this review. Despite ten papers (63%) investigating the TAS-20 facets, the findings were relatively equivocal. DIF was associated with deficits most frequently, in six papers (60%), and also with over-responding in two papers (20%). By comparison, DDF was linked to deficits in four papers (40%) and over-responding in two papers (20%), while EOT was associated with deficits in five papers (50%) and over-responding in one paper (10%)

2.5. Action tendencies and behaviours

Emotions are connected with actions and behaviours. Due to socialisation and normative constraints, emotions rarely lead to observable behaviours (e.g. verbal or physical aggression while experiencing anger), but the potential exists and is captured by action tendencies or action readiness (e.g. antagonism; Frijda et al., 1989). Action tendencies represent urges to carry out certain behaviours when experiencing emotion. For example, when experiencing intense anger, a will toward physical or psychological aggression is automatically activated. Action tendencies therefore involve inhibition capacities to prevent external behaviours from occurring.

Emotions provide individuals with necessary information to guide, control, and regulate their behaviours. Any restricted access to emotional information is likely to result not only in dysregulated emotional responses, but also in behavioural responses. Clinical studies showed that HA manifest their emotions more often in actual behaviours, while not necessarily feeling them mentally (e.g. MacLean, 1949; Vanheule, 2008), which led many to suggest that HA may attempt to regulate emotional states behaviourally, rather than cognitively, resulting in impulsive behaviours such as substance abuse or eating disorders (Morie & Ridout, 2018; Taylor et al., 1997). Examining behavioural reactions in contrast with cognitive processes could therefore highlight some important dissociations. That is, we might expect dominance of dysfunctional over-responding for behaviours, in contrast with the dominance of deficits that was found across the four cognitive processes we investigated in the previous sections. One caveat is that this section does not address the domain of facial expressions and emotional expressivity. This was thoroughly reviewed by Grynberg et al. (2012), showing that alexithymia was associated with impaired perceptual abilities and deficits in labelling emotional facial expressions, but only among those with clinical disorders.

Surprisingly, no studies yet directly examined whether and how alexithymia may moderate the type and intensity of action tendencies (see Table 5). We can therefore only focus on actual behaviours, with a set of seven (with nine studies) coherent papers examining actual behaviours. Of these seven papers, six (86%) demonstrated over-responding, indicative of elevated rates of behaviours such as aggression. HA was related to higher scores for impulsive aggression (Edwards & Wupperman, 2017; Teten et al., 2008; Velotti et al., 2016), with emotion dysregulation being a potential explanatory factor (Edwards & Wupperman, 2017; Velotti et al., 2016). Alexithymia characteristics may facilitate aggressive behaviours by limiting the cognitive and affective resources that are necessary to turn down distressing emotions and to inhibit impulsive action, suggesting deficient emotion regulation abilities. Unfortunately, none of these studies controlled for NA or examined the role of alexithymia facets.

One potential explanation for these findings is the tendency of HA to avoid linking available input information about the stimulus (i.e. the emotion) to their emotion schemas Preece et al. (2017). One specific aspect of avoidance, experiential avoidance, might be as a central process involved in HA. Experiential avoidance, encompassing both avoidance and escape behaviours, consists of two related aspects: (a) desire to disconnect from aversive private experiences, and (b) actions taken to alter aversive experiences or their eliciting sources (Hayes et al., 1996). Experiential avoidance is associated with a wide range of psychopathologies (e.g. Kashdan & Rottenberg, 2010; Kingston et al., 2010); in contrast engaging fully in one's current activity, is linked to well-being and psychological adjustment (Ciarrochi et al., 2011). An initial paper supported the mediating role of experiential avoidance in the association between alexithymia and difficulties regulating one's emotions (Venta et al., 2013). Two other studies supported the assumption that experiential avoidance mediates the association between alexithymia and psychosomatic and depressive symptoms (Panayiotou et al., 2015).

Experiential avoidance overlaps with other pathogenic constructs such as avoidant coping, thought suppression, stress intolerance and anxiety sensitivity; these constructs are close to the emotion regulation strategy of suppression. In two studies, Laloyaux et al. (2015) found a strong positive association between alexithymia total scores (and its facets) and suppression, while for reappraisal, there was a negative correlation of smaller magnitude. Notably, during suppression a person attempts to down-regulate emotion-expressive behaviours and change the behavioural response to the event (John & Gross, 2004), which results in decreased positive, but not negative, emotion experience (Gross & John, 2003). In contrast, reappraisal modifies emotional responding by altering one's way of thinking during an experience (Webb et al., 2012), which effectively reduces negative emotions and increases positive emotions (Gross & John, 2003). The strong tendency for HA to use suppression as an emotion regulation strategy could thus be an explanatory process for the decreased level of pleasantness observed for positive events (see section 2.2 on Appraisal).

One limitation of these studies is their rather static approach to the role of avoidance by using cross-sectional designs. Studies adopting a more dynamic view, such as assessing flexibility to switch between confrontation and avoidance across situations, have suggested HA lack flexibility in response to threat. The reduced priming effects for HA after exposure to threatening information (Vermeulen et al., 2006, see attention section) suggest that avoidance responses can occur at a very early stage of information processing. This early avoidance orientation can later have deleterious effects for interpersonal relations. For instance, Luminet et al. (2011) found HA had reduced ability to recognise threatening stimuli, which can then increase the risk of responding inappropriately or without due caution in interpersonal situations.

Another promising approach to examine behavioural tendencies in more dynamic situations is the one developed by Gvirts and Dery (2021, this issue), who considered social alignment, the tendency to align with other members of the group in terms of thoughts, emotions, and behaviours. They examined consensus-reaching as a cognitive dimension of social alignment, and found that EOT was associated with an impaired ability to reach agreements, in some cases to minimise conflicts, and in others because of lower reliance on the rewarding sensation associated with social alignment.

2.5.1. Summary

We could not find studies investigating how alexithymia can moderate action tendencies, despite the importance of this construct in the cognitive processing of emotions. When turning to actual behaviours, seven papers describing nine studies were evaluated; four with clinical samples (44%) and five with normative samples (56%) (all but one used college students), some as controls for clinical samples. Only one paper, using a psychiatric inpatient sample, controlled for negative affect (14%). The findings converged showing across six papers (8/9 studies, 89%) that HA is related to a higher proneness for aggression, and particularly its impulsive dimension, which points to detrimental over-responding to emotion. Regarding explanatory processes, several studies showed that HA use more dysfunctional strategies (suppression, experiential avoidance, emotion dysregulation) when exposed to emotion that can explain this higher propensity for aggression. When a facet level analysis was available, DIF and DDF were the factors involved in over-responding, while EOT was the factor involved for the only study suggesting deficits.

3. Discussion

Alexithymia is a multi-faceted personality trait that involves difficulties in emotion processing that elevates risk for mental and somatic disorders. In this paper, we considered how, since the 1990s, alexithymia can be validly measured, and that over the last 25 years, the number of studies examining the cognitive processing of emotional information has rapidly grown. We reviewed the results of these studies across five major domains (attention, appraisals, memory, language, and behaviour). Using this process-oriented framework, we considered whether alexithymia, and more specifically the different alexithymia facets, can modulate emotion processing in the direction of deficits or over-responding across these domains.

In the discussion, we first summarise the main results for each domain. We then take a more general perspective, examining how alexithymia and the three specific facets are related to the deficit vs. over-responding models. We then turn to the issue of covariates, in particular negative and positive affect, and review current approaches to alexithymia, offering concrete recommendations for improvement through a process-oriented approach. Finally, we integrate our findings briefly with existing neuro-imaging research and clinical implications, and finally position them with respect to several major emotion theories (attention bias and control, appraisal, awareness) to consider important future directions.

3.1. Overview of the results using total alexithymia scores

Nearly half of the papers we reviewed examined only the total alexithymia score, although the proportion varied by domain, with more papers using only the total score to examine attention (69%) and behaviours (57%), than language (38%), memory (33%), or appraisal (29%). Regarding attention, only half of the studies supported the deficit hypothesis, which occurred to affect at both the early attention stage and in the later, controlled attention stage (see Table 6).

Among the studies that supported the over-responding model, greater distraction from negative faces when processing emotion words and greater interference when processing illness or arousing words were identified. Further investigations need to clarify whether this is due to prolonged attentional processing of threat, or to a longer processing time needed to appraise emotional stimuli. For appraisals, the studies (2/2) pointed to a deficit in valence in both negative and positive contexts, suggesting that both negative and positive stimuli are evaluated as less intense in HA. The few studies looking at other types of appraisals also support the deficit hypothesis. Caution is needed, however, because of the small number of studies examining this domain. Memory has been more extensively examined. Within this larger sample of studies, all of them (6/6; 100%) support the deficit hypothesis.

Two studies also demonstrated functional over-responding, one in which there were fewer errors in alexithymia, and one particularly important that showed context congruence effects can be beneficial for HA, leading to facilitated retrieval for positive information (see section 3.4, clinical significance). The dominance is even more striking when examining language, with 100% (6/6) of studies supporting deficits, while none supporting over-responding. The findings include mainly language expression with evidences for reduced complexity, a less open style, and reduced emotional content. Yet, two new studies that examined language comprehension also supported the deficit hypothesis. In contrast, studies examining behaviours in response to emotional situations show exclusively dysfunctional over-responding (4/4), with a tendency for HA to display impulsive aggression. The few studies that examined mediation processes suggest that suppression, experiential avoidance, and emotion dysregulation might play a role in the link between alexithymia and aggressive behaviours. To conclude, when examining only total alexithymia score, 19 of 25 (76%) papers examining the four cognitive processes found support for the deficit model. Conversely, all four papers (100%) examining behaviour supported dysfunctional over-responding.

3.2. Overview of the results regarding alexithymia facets

Studies considering total alexithymia scores supported a broad pattern of deficits. Is the same pattern observed when examining alexithymia facets? A glance at Table 6 suggests a different pattern. While EOT offers a pattern similar to the total alexithymia score, with the majority of papers supporting deficits, results for DIF and DDF indicate a much smaller prevalence of deficits and greater representation of over-responding. To gain a better appreciation of these patterns, we will briefly overview the results obtained for each process, distinguishing by alexithymia facet and deficits vs. over-responding.

For attention, the facets have been too little studied and the results fail to convey a clear pattern upon which to draw conclusions. In appraisal, most studies observed deficits under negative valence due to DDF and EOT. Yet, one study related DIF to over-responding, which could suggest some dissociations between facets. Furthermore, this possibility supports the value of facet level analysis, as total alexithymia scores do not reveal such patterns. In memory, all three facets contributed to deficits, but EOT was the primary contributor, with memory deficits for both emotive and neutral stimuli. This was explained by a reduced need for cues to establish priority in memory. Memory deficits were also associated with DDF in four studies, half for positive and half for negative stimuli, and with DIF specifically for retrieval ("remember"), rather than familiarity of emotive stimuli, reflective of cognitive control failures, as well as for over-responding, both functional (reduced errors, better neutral memory) and dysfunctional (intrusion of affective memories). For language, the findings did not implicate a particular facet; DIF, DDF and EOT were all associated with deficits in emotional expression; DIF was particularly linked to reduced positive expression, and EOT to reduced self-reference and linguistic complexity. Two papers also associated DIF and DDF with over-responding in use of negative language.

This brief overview highlights that EOT is a central facet involved in emotion deficits, as we had hypothesised in the introduction. However, contrary to our expectations, DIF was not particularly related to early emotion processing such as attention or appraisal, nor was DDF the facet most associated with later processing, such as memory or language. The number of available studies using a facet approach is small, which precludes strong conclusions. We can, however, conclude that analysis at the facet level provides a finer-tuned process-oriented approach that is crucial to understanding the nature of dysregulated processing of information related to personality traits (Quirin et al., 2020; Robinson et al., 2019). Disentangling specific deficit effects from detrimental over-responding at the facet level is also particularly important for designing future interventions toward reducing alexithymia. This disentanglement might also contribute to work toward further refinements of the TAS-20 itself.

The influence of the EOT facet seems distinct from the influence of DIF and DDF. As such, incorporating all facets into a total score may mask more complex relationships of alexithymia facets with cognition and emotion, leading to overly simplistic conclusions and false negative findings. It is also important to

Table 6. Frequencies of primary findings from the papers reviewed tallied across domains, for alexithymia total vs. facet scores, supporting deficits vs. over-responding.

	TAS-20		Facet-Level Analysis					
	Total Only		DIF		DDF		EOT	
	Deficit	OR+/-	Deficit	OR+/-	Deficit	OR+/-	Deficit	OR+/-
Cognitive								
Attention (n=16*)	5/11	3/11	1/5	0/5	0/5	2/5	2/5	2/5
Appraisal (n=7*)	2/2	0/2	0/5	1/5	4/5	1/5	3/5	0/5
Memory (n=18)	6/6	4/6	5/12	5/12	4/12	0/12	7/12	2/12
Language (n=16)	6/6	0/6	6/10	2/10	4/10	2/10	5/10	1/10
Total (n=57*)	19/25 (76%)	7/25 (28%)	12/32 (38%)	8/32 (25%)	12/32 (38%)	5/32 (16%)	17/32 (53%)	5/32 (16%)
Behavioural (n=7)	0/4 (0%)	4/4 (100%)	0/3 (0%)	1/3 (33%)	0/3 (0%)	2/3 (67%)	1/3 (33%)	0/3 (0%)

Notes. OR -: over-responding with detrimental effect of HA. OR+: over-responding with beneficial effect of HA. *One paper (Luminet et al., 2004) appears in two domains and is counted twice. Percentage is not absolute; some studies produced no findings, others produced more than one primary finding, resulting in final percentages that may not tally to 100%.

consider the risk of false positive findings. Analyses using the TAS-20 total score involve only one measure, while a facet analysis involves three measures. Three measures increase the opportunity to find effects, but could do so at the expense of more false positives. It is therefore crucial to prevent this issue by avoiding multiple separate analyses.

The three alexithymia facets are best incorporated into the same model (e.g. regression) to examine the effect of each while holding the others constant. Several studies in this review, including some in this issue (e.g. Correro et al., 2021; Ridout et al., 2021; Vermeulen, 2021) used this approach, showing important differences between the facets. Indeed, intercorrelations amongst the facets were not high enough to surpass the 0.80 threshold for serious concern about multicollinearity (Field, 2009). Thus, facet effects are robust enough to survive this conservative analytic approach.

Although the question of total alexithymia vs. factor scores remains undecided, psychometric analyses can further evaluate whether factor scores provide unique information over the total score (e.g. bifactor modelling, which tests the commonality among and unique contributions of the facets, Reise, 2012). Indeed, Bagby et al. (2019) found a majority of the TAS-20 variance was reflective of a single construct, concluding that total scores are little influenced by unknown admixtures of subscale multidimensionality. Yet, EOT was acknowledged as a somewhat separate construct from what the total scores assesses. Thus, for clinical assessment, the TAS-20 total scores are likely best, but for research purposes, the facet approach seems more advisable.

One challenge for future studies will be to use more dynamic analyses, toward determining when and under which circumstances deficits (particularly via EOT) switches to increased dysfunctional over-responding in handling particularly negative emotions (especially via DIF). It is unknown how these facet-level contributions correspond across processing levels, such as feed-forward effects resulting from priority to salient material. Studies have not yet tracked such effects across the processing domains or over time.

Another challenge will be to disentangle amongst deficit explanations those related to salience (mainly DIF/DDF) and those related to avoidance (mainly EOT). Importantly, results at the facet level diverged by valence type. For deficit effects, DIF was notable for negative emotion, DDF for positive emotion, and EOT for neutral stimuli. For functional over-responding, DIF was related to better processing of neutral information, but no facet was specific for emotional material. A valence-by-facet analysis is therefore also required in future studies, including a systematic assessment for the processing of neutral information. This approach might be facilitated by a recently developed alexithymia scale, the Perth Alexithymia Questionnaire, which simultaneously assesses impairments in emotion processing for both positive and negative affect, while existing instruments only consider impairments of negative affect perception and experience (Preece et al., 2018). The latter analyses could provide needed evaluation of the attention-appraisal model (Preece et al., 2017), which postulates that higher EOT scores would contribute to difficulties focusing attention on emotions, while higher DIF and DDF scores would contribute to difficulties at the appraisal stage of emotion processing. There are insufficient data to currently evaluate these assumptions, although its predictions for the involvement of EOT in attention and DDF in appraisal (though not DIF), appear supported by our review.

3.3. Critical assessment of alexithymia research and directions for improvement

3.3.1. The role of affect in alexithymia research

Those with higher alexithymia often exhibit elevated negative affect, including mood (e.g. depression, anxiety) and trait (e.g. neuroticism, depression and anxiety), along with reduced positive affect (e.g. Luminet et al., 1999; Taylor & Bagby, 2013). Thus, alexithymia is not related to overall decreased affective responses, but rather to a dissociation between elevated distress and reduced experience of positive affect. Negative and positive affect instead represent distinct dimensions that can result from alexithymia (e.g. confusion about feelings increasing negative affect) or contribute to it (e.g. frequent negative mood might increase difficulty identifying precise feelings). As such, is control over affect necessary to accurately measure the specific contribution of alexithymia (total score or facets) to outcome variables? If so, how would this be best accomplished?

Covarying negative and positive affect can importantly reveal the effects of alexithymia on dependent variables after isolating the influence of affect. Yet, this approach is typically undertaken when affect correlates with alexithymia or to ostensibly control group differences. However, covariance analysis is only effective when the covariate correlates with an outcome; otherwise it would remove variance shared with alexithymia without achieving control of "background noise" (Miller & Chapman, 2001). We therefore recommend reporting negative and positive affect ratings and their correlations with alexithymia and outcome variables. Analyses should be shown with and without covariates (when appropriate), which would reveal whether alexithymia results are or are not changed. If the results are unchanged, confident conclusions could be drawn. If instead the results are altered, more cautious conclusions or nuanced follow-up analyses are indicated. Mediation models, particularly with bootstrapping (see Hayes, 2013; Preacher & Hayes, 2008), and structural equation modelling in such cases can better isolate the contributions of both predictors and covariates. Thus, multiple hypothesis-driven models and paths can be tested (e.g. from affect to alexithymia facets, with separate paths from affect to/from alexithymia to outcome(s)), with clarity about which path(s) best fit the data.

Our review revealed considerable variability in analytic approaches used to address positive and negative affect. This prevents firm conclusions from the current literature about the role of NA/PA in alexithymia. Considering only the 63 unique papers reviewed (76 experiments), 26 (41%) lacked controls and 4 (6%) only controlled for non-emotional variables such as IQ. Of the 33 that controlled for affect, 11 papers (33%) controlled for both NA and PA, while 22 (67%) controlled only for NA. Furthermore, 17 of these papers (51%) only reported the final results after controls were applied, while 14 (42%) reported results with and without control, or reported whether controls altered the results (see Tables 1–5). Notably, two papers (6%) specifically documented that affect correlated only with alexithymia but not with the dependent measures and thus, left these variables out of the analyses (e.g. Correro et al., 2021, this issue; Nielson & Meltzer, 2009). Moreover, of the 33 papers examining affective controls, 29 (87.9%) showed that controls had no meaningful effect on alexithymia in the analysis, as they explained very little variance (see Correro et al., 2021; Grynberg et al., 2014; see also, Suslow & Donges, 2017). Only four papers found reduced alexithymia effects after controlling affect ratings (Grynberg et al., 2014; Lundh & Simonsson-Sarnecki, 2002; Mueller et al., 2006; Suslow et al., 2003); three were in the domain of attention, suggesting attention is most vulnerable or perhaps most sensitive to such effects. However, all four studies had small samples, leaving some question about remaining power to detect effects after controls. Indeed, despite moderate inflation of TAS-20 by anxiety or depression, the available evidence supports alexithymia as a stable personality trait, rather than simply a reflection of distress or illness severity (e.g. Luminet et al., 2001, 2007). Thus, while statistically controlling for negative and positive affect may be important in some cases, it is unlikely to greatly influence study outcomes.

3.3.2. Moving from correlational to causal interpretations

One major domain of improvement would be to move alexithymia research from predominantly correlational designs to designs that permit interpretation regarding the causal direction of relationships. Firstly, given that alexithymia has been explained as resulting from arrested emotional development (e.g. Lane & Schwartz, 1987; Taylor, 2000; Taylor et al., 2016), longitudinal studies are needed to evaluate emotional abilities from very early childhood to adulthood. Yet, these critically important studies do not yet exist. Indeed, longitudinal studies in alexithymia are scarce, with only two primary sets existing. The first study examined vulnerability for somatic diseases, showing that alexithymia predicts long-term health risks independently from other risk factors (Kauhanen et al., 1996; Tolmunen et al., 2010). The second study examined the course of chronic or acute stress, concluding that although alexithymia increases with distress, it also has relative stability over time (e.g. de Timary et al., 2008; Luminet et al., 2001; Luminet et al., 2007). These sets of studies further highlight the need to better discern how and under what circumstances deficits dominate, versus when over-responding occurs (see Preece et al., 2017).

In addition to longitudinal studies of emotional development, investigations of early emotion processing is needed to capture precisely how early deficits in processes such as attention and appraisal might lead to or trigger later processes, such as over-responding behaviours (e.g. aggression). Although memory deficits are noted for negative emotion stimuli in alexithymia, salience effects on early processing are thought to underlie the over-responding to meaningful stimuli such as illness words (e.g. Meltzer & Nielson, 2010), but few studies have disentangled these effects. Isolating early triggers would allow systematic study of the underlying mechanisms that lead to such downstream effects.

Causal interpretations of alexithymia also require the incorporation of experimental manipulations of emotional context and emotional intensity. Such study designs are still rare in alexithymia research, but highly insightful. One study showed the irrelevance of level of processing at encoding (i.e. perceptual vs. semantic) in HA; memory for emotive stimuli was equally deficient in both conditions (Luminet et al., 2006). Another study highlighted a difficulty of inhibiting irrelevant information in HA by manipulating task demands (remember vs. forget); HA exhibited deficits of remembering when processing negative information, but over-responding when required to forget (Dressaire et al., 2015). Similarly, physiological reactivity is often measured in alexithymia, but rarely is this manipulated along with measuring cognitive outcome variables. One such study found HA and LA had comparable physiological response and long-term memory enhancement when arousal was induced after learning, despite the lack of subjective arousal response and poorer immediate recall in HA (Nielson & Meltzer, 2009). This finding suggests that memory deficits in high alexithymia may occur at the encoding stage, rather than consolidation stage, fitting with the idea that early processing influences are responsible for downstream effects. Across all domains we examined, context and affect manipulations would greatly enrich our understanding of the conditions under which alexithymia produces deficits, over-responding, or nil effects.

In the studies that we reviewed, normative samples with moderate TAS-20 scores predominated. Few clinical studies examining the cognition–emotion interface is detrimental to a full understanding of alexithymia. Yet, more important perhaps is the clear indication of dysfunction in higher alexithymia even in normative samples. We would expect greater degrees of alexithymia severity would further amplify these dysfunctions. This highlights the importance of considering alexithymia when studying precisely how emotion and cognition interface, and further invites the longitudinal study of origins and outcomes in clinical cases.

3.4. The clinical significance of emotion and its impact on emotion regulation

In this review, alexithymia was linked to deficits of emotion processing in multiple domains, but it was also linked to over-responding to emotion. In most cases, over-responding was maladaptive. These findings are consistent with evidence that alexithymia predicts reduced effectiveness of psychotherapies based on insight, self-awareness, and client-therapist rapport (Ogrodniczuk et al., 2018), with DIF (Terock et al., 2015) and DDF (Leweke et al., 2009) in particular predicting poorer outcomes. Alexithymia also predicts reduced benefits of emotion rehearsal, including disclosure of emotion (Pennebaker & Smyth, 2016), via DDF (Paez et al., 1999). Thus, reducing emotion dysfunction in HA, even in those with modest alexithymia severity seems of paramount importance.

Cognition may be an important target in the therapeutic process in alexithymia as alexithymia has been shown to mediate treatment success among those with poor emotion processing (Sugiura, 2007). Because emotion processing biases in HA occur during early automatic processing, addressing them will be challenging. Fortunately, directed interventions have been found successful in reducing early attention biases to threat in anxiety disorders (MacLeod, 2019). Thus, it might be useful as an intervention to focus HA on the emotional aspects of their environment, as well as to elucidate the role of attention deficits in alexithymia.

Problems with emotion regulation are central to many forms of psychopathology (Sheppes et al., 2015). HA is linked to maladaptive emotion regulation strategies, such as suppression (e.g. Laloyaux et al., 2015), specifically via the DDF facet. Given the strong links between alexithymia and psychopathology (Honkalampi et al., 2018; Morie & Ridout, 2018), it is plausible that alexithymia might underpin, or at least contribute to, emotion dysregulation in psychiatric patients. Indeed, Clyne et al. (2010) demonstrated that alexithymia-specific training toward improving emotion recognition and attention to emotional reactions was more effective for binge eating disorder than cognitive–behavioural therapy or antidepressants alone. Alexithymia, particularly DIF, is linked to experiential avoidance, which mediates the link between alexithymia and difficulties regulating emotion (e.g. Venta et al., 2013), depression, and somatic symptoms (Panayiotou et al., 2015). Thus, interventions targeting experiential acceptance, improving affect labelling, and linking labels to visceral sensations might improve emotion regulation and reduce psychopathology in HA (Preece et al., 2017). Finally, effective methods are needed to assist HA to effectively process, encode, and retrieve autobiographical memories, particularly for positive events, which one study suggested might be achieved through inducing emotionally positive non-verbal contexts, such as using music (Vermeulen et al., 2010).

3.5. Neural correlates of the foundations of alexithymia

This review illuminated appraisal and attention deficits in emotion processing that may contribute to memory, language and behaviour effects in HA. These conclusions are complemented by neuroimaging findings. Specifically, impaired automatic processing of emotive stimuli in HA, particularly for threat-related and negative stimuli, have been reported corresponding to reduced activity in the amygdala, insula, precuneus, anterior cingulate, posterior cingulate, and prefrontal cortex (see Goerlich, 2018; Goerlich & Aleman, 2018). Given that reduced awareness of emotion occurs at the most fundamental perceptual levels, this may generate multiple downstream effects on physiological responding, emotional appraisal, decision-making, actions, memory, and language (Goerlich, 2018). Furthermore, this review illuminated deficits of cognitive control (e.g. executive functioning) in HA (see in particular Correro et al., 2021, this issue) that are consistent with dysfunction particularly in the prefrontal cortices (Hogeveen et al., 2016; Williams & Wood, 2010). A small but notable literature reinforces dysfunction of cognitive control, linking HA to excessive perseverative errors, impaired switching of task demands, and difficulty inhibiting irrelevant information (see Vermeulen et al., 2018).

Dysfunction of cognitive control and prefrontal regions is consistent with the difficulty HA have in linking concrete bodily experiences of emotions with symbolic and sub-symbolic representations (Bucci, 1997), which impairs using those experiences to form images and use words to reflect upon and communicate subjective experience (Taylor & Bagby, 2013). These effects, and more atypical findings of over-responding in HA (e.g. Meltzer & Nielson, 2010; Ridout et al., 2021; Vermeulen et al., 2010), are furthermore consistent with HA dysfunctions in self-referential processes and perhaps hyperactive salience effects, not restricted to emotion processing. Similar effects are evident in studies tapping the salience network (anterior insula, dorsal anterior cingulate cortex), default-mode network connectivity (a broad network most active during rest (Raichle, 2015), semantic processing (Binder & Desai, 2011)), and inter-hemispheric information transfer (see Goerlich & Aleman, 2018). Indeed, EOT may be particularly relevant as it appears to reduce the ability to detect and utilise necessary cues for establishing cognitive priority, even in neutral contexts. Systematic studies that integrate these approaches, use sensitivity and response bias metrics in analysis and seek to tease apart encoding from later memory stages will help characterise downstream effects of attention and appraisal in HA.

3.6. Integration between alexithymia research and emotion science

There are several emotion-theoretical frameworks that can help to contextualise the findings of this alexithymia review and the facet-specific effects. We discuss three general frameworks: (1) attentional bias and control; (2) appraisal; and (3) awareness. For each framework, we underscore important interpretations of the current findings in alexithymia, provide guidance for the issues, and directions to be addressed in future research.

3.6.1. Attentional bias and control

Emotion influences attentional processing across the continuum from early automatic (orientation) to later controlled processing (maintenance, avoidance) by biasing competition for attentional priority through heightened salience (Yiend, 2010). Attentional bias theory, indeed has shown salience effects can reduce or enhance processing. In anxiety disorders, salient threat-relevant stimuli are given preference in early and late processing phases (MacLeod, 2019), but they are also used to strategically avoid threat during later processing to regulate mood (Cisler & Koster, 2010). In alexithymia, elevated negative affect and reduced positive affect (e.g. Luminet et al., 1999; Taylor & Bagby, 2013) suggests that attention would be biased towards negative stimuli and/or away from positive stimuli. Several studies did report an attention bias to threat, such as to illness-related stimuli. This may be related to anxiety, but only one study controlled for negative affect (Grynberg et al., 2014). Indeed, the primary finding was instead reduced attentional processing of emotional stimuli during early and late processing, which might be due to emotion having reduced salience in alexithymia; thus, it does not capture attention.

Neuroimaging studies in HA are consistent with this explanation, demonstrating reduced amygdala activation to masked emotional faces (Recker et al., 2010) and reduced early visual evoked responses (P1) to emotional pictures (Pollatos & Gramann, 2011). Yet, some of these findings, particularly those associated with later attentional processing, might instead represent strategic avoidance of emotion. As HA exhibit poorly differentiated interpretations of emotion stimuli due to under-developed emotion schemas (e.g. Luminet et al., 2006), they experience diffuse and ambiguous emotional states and might strategically avoid processing emotional stimuli to avoid activating these states.

Attentional control theory (Eysenck et al., 2007) can also be related to alexithymia findings. It proposes that anxiety impairs executive function, resulting in more stimulus-driven ("bottom-up") processing and reduced "top-down" cognitive control of attention. There is evidence of deficient cognitive control in HA (see Correro et al., 2021, in this issue; Vermeulen et al., 2018), which could account for salience-related biases, while EOT might explain the predominant findings of attention deficits. Although a minority of studies took a facet-level approach, those that did so most often implicated EOT in attentional deficits in HA, supporting the importance of attentional control in alexithymia.

3.6.2. Appraisal

The emotion process approach of Scherer and Moors (2019) examines how the appraisal process produces differential outcomes for action tendencies, facial and vocal expressions, or bodily reactions, which then influence how feelings are categorised and labelled. This is a particularly valuable framework for clearly needed future alexithymia research evaluating appraisal during experimental emotion manipulations, particularly because HA are prone to aggression – and avoidance-related action tendencies during emotional situations.

To more closely link appraisals and action tendencies, Scherer and Moors (2019) indicate that inducing novel/unexpected situations increase approach action tendencies (orientation/exploration), together with immediate shift in attention (Brosch et al., 2013). Within negative stimuli, those that cause goal conflict instigate behavioural adjustments to increase effort to overcome conflict, as well as to avoid subsequent conflict. Finally, while other agency can increase the tendency to aggress, mitigating information providing evidences for circumstances-agency can reduce aggression tendencies. Based on our review, we predict that HA will moderate those effects with less attention shift in novel/unexpected situations, failure to adjust behaviours when confronted with conflict stimuli, and failure to show reduced aggression after receiving mitigating information.

Therefore, future studies should combine a process-oriented framework, together with a multi-level measurement approach (Scherer, 2019). This proposal can be linked with the already observed deficits in emotional granularity and in emotional dialecticism (see Section 2.2. on Appraisal). These steps, integrating cognitive processes and behavioural tasks (Robinson et al., 2019) will afford subtle indices of the key components of HA emotion deficits at the appraisal level.

3.6.3. Emotion awareness

Our assessment of alexithymia through the cognition–emotion interface is also consistent with emotion awareness theories, in particular the "three-process model" (Smith et al., 2018), which proposes three separate but interrelated neuro-cognitive processes that contribute to emotional knowledge and awareness. In the first process, internal emotion concept formation and access to emotion concepts in memory, is disrupted in alexithymia. Indeed, HA have impaired ability to access, communicate, and assimilate cognitive meanings of emotions into personal concepts and representations (particularly via DIF). Thus, having weak emotion concepts contributes to poorer verbal representations of emotions, and hinders the ability to connect experiences, thoughts, and memories, which is needed for effective emotion responding and communication with others.

Second, the three-process model proposes that appropriate emotion responding and emotion knowledge and awareness require generation of and response to physiological reactions to emotion (e.g. arousal). As our review showed, HA have difficulty detecting the cues needed to set cognitive priority (via EOT), deficits of emotional appraisal (via DDF), and particularly with negative emotion, elevated experiential avoidance, feelings of threat, and impulsive aggression (via DIF). Thus, HA are impaired in using physiological responses to emotions in conjunction with knowledge and experience to be able to understand and communicate about emotional experiences.

Finally, the three-process model proposes the importance of cognitive control over emotive states, through attention, working memory, and approach-avoidance strategies. Supporting the model, a dominant theme throughout this review is altered cognitive control in alexithymia, including prolonged automatic attention to negative and arousing stimuli (via DDF and EOT), a preference to avoid conscious attention and engagement with internal events, particularly when emotive (via EOT), and even generalised deficits of cognitive control (DIF-EOT interaction; e.g. Correro et al., 2021, this issue; Vermeulen et al., 2018).

Taken together, this review supports each part of the three-process model, indicating the value of this framework to guide future research in HA. As such, joint cognitive–behavioural studies that intentionally evaluate the three-process model would allow systematic testing of these dissociations. Such studies would delineate under what conditions underlying HA processes are outcomes of initial emotion dysregulation, dysfunctional avoidance strategies, or impulse control failure leading secondarily to suppression and experiential avoidance toward regulating emotions.

4. Conclusions

In the present article, we examined, for the first time, a long-standing unresolved contradiction between claims that alexithymia is related to emotion deficits versus other claims of emotional "over-responding" resulting from defensive reactions against experiencing overly intense feelings. Several conclusions emerge from our examination. First, we highlighted evidence that over-responding, while typically maladaptive (e.g. increased recall of illness words), can sometimes be beneficial (e.g. better positive memory in positive context). Second, although the existing literature explains alexithymia as always related to emotional contexts, our review uniquely delineated that there are clear patterns of deficits and over-responding in neutral contexts as well. This is essential for both clarifying cognitive-emotional functioning in alexithymia, and for guiding interventions. Third, our analysis of studies using the total score versus those examining the specific alexithymia facets revealed a facet-process relationship that underscores the importance of facet analysis. For example, deficits were predominant in cognitive processes, which had particularly clear links to early processes such as attention and appraisal that may have down-stream effects on other processes and behaviours. In contrast, behaviours such as impulsive aggression were tied to dysfunctional over-responding. These findings in alexithymia importantly highlight the importance of emotion processing even in normative populations. The vast majority of the studies included in this review employed participants without a diagnosable disorder. Thus, even those with no particular disorder can exhibit meaningful dysfunctions of emotion processing that influence functioning across the continuum of cognitive and behavioural functioning.

With this review we used alexithymia to draw attention to fundamental issues that personality traits offer to emotion research. Having limited or weak verbal representations of emotions increases the burden on attentional and memory processes, hindering the ability to connect to external and sensory experiences and make effective responses to them. Similarly, deficits in verbally elaborating feelings and an externally orienting style hinders connecting feelings to thoughts, memories and goals. This, in turn, impacts upon understanding of one's own emotion states and ability to communicate them with others (e.g. Barrett et al., 2007). These are furthermore foundational to developing appropriate emotion schemas and lexicon (Frijda, 1986; Lieberman et al., 2011) and effective interpersonal relationships (Izard et al., 2011). Altered automated processing and over-responding, particularly when intense, salient, or negative experiences are encountered, also contribute to difficulty in emotion processing, perhaps fostering negative feedback loops that reinforce threat anticipation, contributing overall to reduced emotion processing. The present review thus highlights the importance of alexithymia as a fundamental personality dimension in understanding the interplay between cognition and emotion.

Note

1. This particular study used the BVAQ instead of the TAS-20. The BVAQ scale involves a facet assessing poor fantasy life, which is closely related to externally oriented thinking (EOT).

Acknowledgements

Olivier Luminet is Research Director at the Fund for Scientific Research (FNRS-FRS) and full Professor at the UCLouvain, Belgium. Kristy Nielson is full Professor at the Department of Psychology, Marquette University, Milwaukee, WI. Nathan Ridout is Senior Lecturer in Psychology at Aston University, Birmingham, UK. The authors would like to thank the Editors of Cognition & Emotion, Sander Koole and Klaus Rothermund for their extensive comments and feedbacks throughout the process.

Disclosure statement

No potential conflict of interest was reported by the author(s).

Funding

This work was supported by Fund for Scientific Research (FNRS-FRS).

ORCID

Olivier Luminet http://orcid.org/0000-0002-1519-2178
Kristy A. Nielson http://orcid.org/0000-0001-8977-3138
Nathan Ridout http://orcid.org/0000-0002-7111-2996

References

Aaron, R. V., Snodgress, M. A., Blain, S. D., & Park, S. (2018). Affect labeling and other aspects of emotional experiences in relation to alexithymia following standardized emotion inductions. *Psychiatry Research*, *262*, 115–123. https://doi.org/10.1016/j.psychres.2018.02.014

Bagby, R. M., Carnovale, M., & Taylor, G. J. (2019). Bifactor analysis of the 20-item Toronto Alexithymia Scale: Replication in a community sample. *Psychotherapy and Psychosomatics*, *88* (suppl 1), 5.

Bagby, R. M., Parker, J. D. A., & Taylor, G. J. (1994). The twenty-item Toronto alexithymia scale-I. Item selection and cross-validation of the factor structure. *Journal of Psychosomatic Research*, *38*(1), 23–32. https://doi.org/10.1016/0022-3999(94)90005-1

Bagby, R. M., Parker, J. D. A., & Taylor, G. J. (2020). Twenty-five years with the 20-item Toronto Alexithymia scale. *Journal of Psychosomatic Research*, *131*, 109940. https://doi.org/10.1016/j.jpsychores.2020.109940

Bagby, R. M., Taylor, G. J., Parker, J. D. A., & Dickens, S. E. (2006). The development of the Toronto structured interview for alexithymia: Item selection, factor structure, reliability and concurrent validity. *Psychotherapy and Psychosomatics*, *75* (1), 25–39. https://doi.org/10.1159/000089224

Bagozzi, R. P., Wong, N., & Yi, Y. (1999). The role of culture and gender in the relationship between positive and negative affect. *Cognition and Emotion*, *13*(6), 641–672. https://doi.org/10.1080/026999399379023

Barrett, L. F., Gross, J., Christensen, T. C., & Benvenuto, M. (2001). Knowing what you're feeling and knowing what to do about it: Mapping the relation between emotion differentiation and emotion regulation. *Cognition and Emotion*, *15*(6), 713–724. https://doi.org/10.1080/02699930143000239

Barrett, L., Lindquist, K. A., & Gendron, M. (2007). Language as context for the perception of emotion. *Trends in Cognitive Sciences*, *11*(8), 327–332. https://doi.org/10.1016/j.tics.2007.06.003

Baudic, S., Jayr, C., Albi-Feldzer, A., Fermanian, J., Masselin-Dubois, A., Bouhassira, D., & Attal, N. (2016). Effect of alexithymia and emotional repression on postsurgical pain in women with breast cancer: A prospective longitudinal 12-month study. *The Journal of Pain*, *17*(1), 90–100. https://doi.org/10.1016/j.jpain.2015.10.001

Beresnevaite, M. (2000). Exploring the benefits of group psychotherapy in reducing alexithymia in coronary heart disease patients: A preliminary study. *Psychotherapy and Psychosomatics*, *69*(3), 117–122. https://doi.org/10.1159/000012378

Bermond, B., Oosterveld, P., & Vorst, H. C. (2015). Measures of alexithymia. In G. J. Boyle, D. H. Saklofske, & G. Matthews (Eds.), *Measures of personality and social psychological constructs* (pp. 227–256). Elsevier.

Binder, J. R., & Desai, R. H. (2011). The neurobiology of semantic memory. *Trends in Cognitive Sciences*, *15*(11), 527–536. 10.1016/j.tics.2011.10.001

Brandt, L., Pintzinger, N. M., & Tran, U. S. (2015). Abnormalities in automatic processing of illness-related stimuli in self-rated alexithymia. *PloS one*, *10*(6), e0129905. 10.1371/journal.pne.0129905

Brosch, T., Scherer, K. R., Grandjean, D. M., & Sander, D. (2013). The impact of emotion on perception, attention, memory, and decision-making. *Swiss Medical Weekly*, *143*, 13786. https://doi.org/10.4414/smw.2013.13786

Bucci, W. (1997). *Psychoanalysis and cognitive science: A multiple code theory*. Guilford Press.

Camia, C., Desmedt, O., & Luminet, O. (2020). Exploring autobiographical memory specificity and narrative emotional processing in alexithymia. *Narrative Inquiry, 30*(1), 59–79. https://doi.org/10.1075/ni.18089.kob

Ciarrochi, J., Kashdan, T. B., Leeson, P., Heaven, P., & Jordan, C. (2011). On being aware and accepting: A one-year longitudinal study into adolescent well-being. *Journal of Adolescence, 34*(4), 695–703. https://doi.org/10.1016/j.adolescence.2010.09.003

Cisler, J. M., & Koster, E. H. (2010). Mechanisms of attentional biases towards threat in anxiety disorders: An integrative review. *Clinical Psychology Review, 30*(2), 203–216. https://doi.org/10.1016/j.cpr.2009.11.003

Clyne, C., Latner, J. D., Gleaves, D. H., & Blampied, N. M. (2010). Treatment of emotional dysregulation in full syndrome and subthreshold binge eating disorder. *Eating Disorders, 18*(5), 408–424. https://doi.org/10.1080/10640266.2010.511930

Coffey, E., Berenbaurn, H., & Kerns, J. G. (2003). The dimensions of emotional intelligence, alexithymia, and mood awareness: Associations with personality and performance on an emotional stroop task. *Cognition and Emotion, 17*(4), 671–679. https://doi.org/10.1080/02699930302304

Correro II, A. N., Paitel, E. R., Byers, S. J., & Nielson, K. A. (2021). The role of alexithymia in memory and executive functioning across the lifespan. *Cognition and Emotion*, 1–16. https://doi.org/10.1080/02699931.2019.1659232

Davydov, D. M., Luminet, O., & Zech, E. (2013). An externally oriented style of thinking as a moderator of responses to affective films in women. *International Journal of Psychophysiology, 87*(2), 152–164. https://doi.org/10.1016/j.ijpsycho.2012.12.003

de Timary, P., Luts, A., Hers, D., & Luminet, O. (2008). Absolute and relative stability of alexithymia in alcoholic inpatients undergoing alcohol withdrawal: Relationship to depression and anxiety. *Psychiatry Research, 157*(1-3), 105–113. https://doi.org/10.1016/j.psychres.2006.12.008

de Timary, P., Roy, E., Luminet, O., Fillée, C., & Mikolajczak, M. (2008). Relationship between alexithymia, alexithymia factors and salivary cortisol in men exposed to a social stress test. *Psychoneuroendocrinology, 33*(8), 1160–1164. https://doi.org/10.1016/j.psyneuen.2008.06.005

Diener, E., Larsen, R. J., Levine, S., & Emmons, R. A. (1985b). Intensity and frequency: Dimensions underlying positive and negative affect. *Journal of Personality and Social Psychology, 48*(5), 1253–1265. https://doi.org/10.1037/0022-3514.48.5.1253

Diener, E., Sandvik, E., & Larsen, R. J. (1985a). Age and sex effects for emotional intensity. *Developmental Psychology, 21*(3), 542–546. https://doi.org/10.1037/0012-1649.21.3.542

DiStefano, R. A., & Koven, N. S. (2012). Dysfunctional emotion processing may explain visual memory deficits in alexithymia. *Personality and Individual Differences, 52*(5), 611–615. https://doi.org/10.1016/j.paid.2011.12.007

Donges, U. S., & Suslow, T. (2015). Alexithymia and memory for facial emotions. *Universitas Psychologica, 14*(1), 103–110. https://doi.org/10.11144/Javeriana.upsy14-1.amfe

Dressaire, D., Stone, C. B., Nielson, K. A., Guerdoux, E., Martin, S., Brouillet, D., & Luminet, O. (2015). Alexithymia impairs the cognitive control of negative material while facilitating the recall of neutral material in both younger and older adults. *Cognition and Emotion, 29*(3), 442–459. https://doi.org/10.1080/02699931.2014.919898

Edwards, E. R., Shivaji, S., Micek, A., & Wupperman, P. (2020). Distinguishing alexithymia and emotion differentiation conceptualizations through linguistic analysis. *Personality and Individual Differences, 157*. https://doi.org/10.1016/j.paid.2019.109801

Edwards, E. R., & Wupperman, P. (2017). Emotion regulation mediates effects of alexithymia and emotion differentiation on impulsive aggressive behavior. *Deviant Behavior, 38*(10), 1160–1171. https://doi.org/10.1080/01639625.2016.1241066

Ellsworth, P. C., & Scherer, K. R. (2003). Appraisal processes in emotion. In R. J. Davidson, K. R. Scherer, & H. Goldsmith (Eds.), *Handbook of affective sciences* (pp. 572–595). Oxford University Press.

Erbas, Y., Ceulemans, E., Lee Pe, M., Koval, P., & Kuppens, P. (2014). Negative emotion differentiation: Its personality and well-being correlates and a comparison of different assessment methods. *Cognition and Emotion, 28*(7), 1196–1213. https://doi.org/10.1080/02699931.2013.875890

Eysenck, M. W., Derakshan, N., Santos, R., & Calvo, M. G. (2007). Anxiety and cognitive performance: Attentional control theory. *Emotion, 7*(2), 336–353. https://doi.org/10.1037/1528-3542.7.2.336

Fantini-Hauwel, C., Luminet, O., & Vermeulen, N. (2015). Live happily live in hiding (from our affect): alexithymia influences affect intensity and affect frequency ratings in men. *Psychiatry Research, 230*(2), 637–642. https://doi.org/10.1016/j.psychres.2015.10.019

Field, A. (2009). *Discovering statistics using SPSS*. Sage Publications.

Frijda, N. H. (1986). *The emotions*. Cambridge University Press.

Frijda, N. H., Kuipers, P., & ter Schure, E. (1989). Relations among emotion, appraisal, and emotional action readiness. *Journal of Personality and Social Psychology, 57*(2), 212–228. https://doi.org/10.1037/0022-3514.57.2.212

Fujiwara, E. (2018). Looking at the eyes interferes with facial emotion recognition in alexithymia. *Journal of Abnormal Psychology, 127*(6), 571–577. https://doi.org/10.1037/abn0000361

Galderisi, S., Mancuso, F., Mucci, A., Garramone, S., Zamboli, R., & Maj, M. (2008). Alexithymia and cognitive dysfunctions in patients with panic disorder. *Psychotherapy and Psychosomatics, 77*(3), 182–188. https://doi.org/10.1159/000119738

Goerlich, K. S. (2018). Electrophysiology of alexithymia. In O. Luminet, G. J. Taylor, & R. M. Bagby (Eds.), *Alexithymia: Advances in research, theory, and clinical practice* (pp. 250–266). Cambridge University Press. https://doi.org/10.1017/9781108241595

Goerlich, K. S., & Aleman, A. (2018). Neuroimaging studies of alexithymia. In O. Luminet, G. J. Taylor, & R. M. Bagby (Eds.), *Alexithymia: Advances in research, theory, and clinical practice* (pp. 207–249). Cambridge University Press. https://doi.org/10.1017/9781108241595

Gross, J. J. (2014). *Handbook of emotion regulation*. Guilford.

Gross, J. J., & John, O. P. (2003). Individual differences in two emotion regulation processes: Implications for affect, relationships, and well-being. *Journal of Personality and Social Psychology, 85*(2), 348–362. https://doi.org/10.1037/0022-3514.85.2.348

Grynberg, D., Berthoz, S., & Bird, G. (2018). Social and interpersonal implications. In O. Luminet, G. J. Taylor, & R. M. Bagby (Eds.), *Alexithymia: Advances in research, theory, and clinical practice* (pp. 174–189). Cambridge University Press.

Grynberg, D., Chang, B., Corneille, O., Maurage, P., Vermeulen, N., Berthoz, S., & Luminet, O. (2012). Alexithymia and the processing of emotional facial expressions (EFEs): systematic review, unanswered questions and further perspectives. *PLoS ONE*, *7*(8), e42429. https://doi.org/10.1371/journal.pone.0042429

Grynberg, D., Vermeulen, N., & Luminet, O. (2014). Amplification of attentional blink by distress-related facial expressions: Relationships with alexithymia and affectivity. *International Journal of Psychology*, *49*(5), 371–380. https://doi.org/10.1002/ijop.12006

Gvirts, H. Z., & Dery, L. (2021). Alexithymia and reaching group consensus. *Cognition and Emotion*, 1–14. https://doi.org/10.1080/02699931.2019.1675600

Hayes, A. F. (2013). *Introduction to mediation: A regression-based approach*. The Guilford Press.

Hayes, S. C., Wilson, K. G., Gifford, E. V., Follette, V. M., & Strosahl, K. (1996). Experiential avoidance and behavioral disorders: A functional dimensional approach to diagnosis and treatment. *Journal of Consulting and Clinical Psychology*, *64*(6), 1152–1168. https://doi.org/10.1037/0022-006X.64.6.1152

Hobson, H., Brewer, R., Catmur, C., & Bird, G. (2019). The role of language in alexithymia: Moving towards a multiroute model of alexithymia. *Emotion Review*, *11*(3), 247–261. https://doi.org/10.1177/175407391983

Hoemann, K., & Feldman Barrett, L. (2019). Concepts dissolve artificial boundaries in the study of emotion and cognition, uniting body, brain, and mind. *Cognition and Emotion*, *33*(1), 67–76. 10.1080/02699931.2018.1535

Hogeveen, J., Bird, G., Chau, A., Krueger, F., & Grafman, J. (2016). Acquired alexithymia following damage to the anterior insula. *Neuropsychologia*, *82*, 142–148. https://doi.org/10.1016/j.neuropsychologia.2016.01.021

Honkalampi, K., De Berardis, D., Vellante, F., & Viinamäki, H. (2018). Relations between alexithymia and depressive and anxiety disorders and personality. In O. Luminet, G. J. Taylor, & R. M. Bagby (Eds.), *Alexithymia: Advances in research, theory, and clinical practice* (pp. 142–157). Cambridge University Press.

Hoppe, K. D., & Bogen, J. E. (1977). Alexithymia in twelve commissurotomized patients. *Psychotherapy and Psychosomatics*, *28*(1-4), 148–155. https://doi.org/10.1159/000287057

Hsing, C. K., Hofelich Mohr, A., Stansfield, R. B., & Preston, S. D. (2013). Alexithymia slows performance but preserves spontaneous semantic decoding of negative expressions in the emostroop task. *International Journal of Psychological Research*, *6*, 56–67. https://doi.org/10.21500/20112084.719

Hund, A. R., & Espelage, D. L. (2006). Childhood emotional abuse and disordered eating among undergraduate females: Mediating influence of alexithymia and distress. *Child Abuse & Neglect*, *30*(4), 393–407. https://doi.org/10.1016/j.chiabu.2005.11.003

Izard, C. E., Woodburn, E. M., Finlon, K. J., Krauthamer-Ewing, E. S., Grossman, S. R., & Seidenfeld, A. (2011). Emotion knowledge, emotion utilization, and emotion regulation. *Emotion Review*, *3*(1), 44–52. https://doi.org/10.1177/1754073910380972

Jacob, S., & Hautekeete, M. (1998). Alexithymia and memory: A more rigorous criterion for acceptance in recognition tasks? *Encéphale-Revue de Psychiatrie Clinique, Biologique et Thérapeutique*, *24*(3), 199–204.

Jakobson, L. S., & Pearson, P. M. (2021). Alexithymic traits predict the speed of classifying non-literal statements using nonverbal cues. *Cognition and Emotion*, 1–7. https://doi.org/10.1080/02699931.2020.1715346

Jelinek, L., Stockbauer, C., Randjbar, S., Kellner Michael, Ehring Thomas, Moritz, S. (2010). Characteristics and organization of the worst moment of trauma memories in posttraumatic stress disorder. *Behaviour Research and Therapy*, *48*(7), 680–685. https://doi.org/10.1016/j.brat.2010.03.014

John, O. P., & Gross, J. J. (2004). Healthy and unhealthy emotion regulation: Personality processes, individual differences, and life span development. *Journal of Personality*, *72*(6), 1301–1334. https://doi.org/10.1111/j.1467-6494.2004.00298.x

Kashdan, T. B., & Rottenberg, J. (2010). Psychological flexibility as a fundamental aspect of health. *Clinical Psychology Review*, *30*(7), 865–878. https://doi.org/10.1016/j.cpr.2010.03.001

Kauhanen, J., Kaplan, G. A., Cohen, R. D., Julkunen, J., & Salonen, J. T. (1996). Alexithymia and risk of death in middle-aged men. *Journal of Psychosomatic Research*, *41*(6), 541–549. https://doi.org/10.1016/S0022-3999(96)00226-7

Kensinger, E. A. (2009). Remembering the details: Effects of emotion. *Emotion Review*, *1*(2), 99–113. https://doi.org/10.1177/1754073908100432

Kingston, J., Clarke, S., & Remington, B. (2010). Experiential avoidance and problem behavior: A mediational analysis. *Behavior Modification*, *34*(2), 145–163. https://doi.org/10.1177/0145445510362575

Knapp, P. (1983). Emotions and bodily changes: A reassessment. In L. Temoshok, C. Van Dyke, & L. S. Zegans (Eds.), *Emotions in health and illness. Theoretical and research foundations* (pp. 15–27). Grune & Stratton.

Kojima, M., Frasure-Smith, N., & Lespérance, F. (2001). Alexithymia following myocardial infarction: Psychometric properties and correlates of the Toronto Alexithymia scale. *Journal of Psychosomatic Research*, *51*(3), 487–495. https://doi.org/10.1016/S0022-3999(01)00253-7

Koven, N. S. (2014). Abnormal valence differentiation in alexithymia. *Personality and Individual Differences*, *68*, 102–106. https://doi.org/10.1016/j.paid.2014.04.007

Kreitler, S. (2002). The psychosemantic approach to alexithymia. *Personality and Individual Differences*, *33*(3), 393–407. https://doi.org/10.1016/S0191-8869(01)00163-5

Krystal, H. (1982–83). alexithymia and the effectiveness of psychoanalytic treatment. *International Journal of Psychoanalytic Psychotherapy*, *9*, 354–378.

Krystal, H. (1988). *Integration and self-healing: Affect, trauma, alexithymia*. Analytic Press.

LaBar, K. S., & Cabeza, R. (2006). Cognitive neuroscience of emotional memory. *Nature Reviews Neuroscience*, *7*(1), 54–64. https://doi.org/10.1038/nrn1825

Laloyaux, J., Fantini, C., Lemaire, M., Luminet, O., & Larøi, F. (2015). Evidence of contrasting patterns for suppression and reappraisal emotion regulation strategies in alexithymia. *The Journal of Nervous and Mental Disease*, *203*(9), 709–717. https://doi.org/10.1097/NMD.0000000000000353

Lane, R. D., Reiman, E. M., Axelrod, B., Yun, L. S., Holmes, A., & Schwartz, G. E. (1998). Neural correlates of levels of emotional awareness: Evidence of an interaction between emotion and attention in the anterior cingulate cortex. *Journal of Cognitive Neuroscience*, *10*(4), 525–535. https://doi.org/10.1162/089892998562924

Lane, R. D., & Schwartz, G. (1987). Levels of emotional awareness: A cognitive developmental theory and its application to psychopathology. *American Journal of Psychiatry, 144*(2), 133–143. https://doi.org/10.1176/ajp.144.2.133

Larsen, R. J. (1985). Theory and measurement of affect intensity as an individual difference characteristic. *Journal of Research in Personality, 21*(1), 1–39. https://doi.org/10.1016/0092-6566(87)90023-7

Larwood, J. L., Vanman, E. J., & Dingle, G. A. (2021). Negative valence specific deficits in judgements of musical affective quality in alexithymia. *Cognition and Emotion*, 1–10. https://doi.org/10.1080/02699931.2019.1707514

Levine, L. J., & Edelstein, R. S. (2009). Emotion and memory narrowing: A review and goal-relevance approach. *Cognition and Emotion, 23*(5), 833–875. https://doi.org/10.1080/02699930902738863

Leweke, F., Bausch, S., Leichsenring, F., Walter, B., & Stingl, M. (2009). Alexithymia as a predictor of outcome of psychodynamically oriented inpatient treatment. *Psychotherapy Research, 19*(3), 323–331. https://doi.org/10.1080/10503300902870554

Liossi, C., Schoth, D. E., Bradley, B. P., & Mogg, K. (2009). Time-course of attentional bias for pain-related cues in chronic daily headache sufferers. *European Journal of Pain, 13*(9), 963–969. https://doi.org/10.1016/j.ejpain.2008.11.007

Lieberman, M. D., Inagaki, T. K., Tabibnia, G., & Crockett, M. J. (2011). Subjective responses to emotional stimuli during labeling, reappraisal, and distraction. *Emotion*, 11(3), 468–480. doi:10.1037/a0023503

Luminet, O., Bagby, R. M., & Taylor, G. J. (2001). An evaluation of the absolute and relative stability of alexithymia in patients with major depression. *Psychotherapy and Psychosomatics, 70*(5), 254–260. https://doi.org/10.1159/000056263

Luminet, O., Bagby, R. M., Wagner, H. L., Taylor, G. J., & Parker, J. D. A. (1999). Relation between alexithymia and the Five Factor Model of personality: A facet level analysis. *Journal of Personality Assessment, 73*(3), 345–358. https://doi.org/10.1207/S15327752JPA7303_4

Luminet, O., Cordovil de Sousa Uva, M., Fantini, C., & de Timary, P. (2016). The association between depression and craving in alcohol dependency is moderated by gender and by alexithymia factors. *Psychiatry Research, 239*, 28–38. https://doi.org/10.1016/j.psychres.2016.02.062

Luminet, O., Grynberg, D., Ruzette, N., & Mikolajczak, M. (2011). Personality-dependent effects of oxytocin: Greater social benefits for high alexithymia scorers. *Biological Psychology, 87*(3), 401–406. https://doi.org/10.1016/j.biopsycho.2011.05.005

Luminet, O., Rimé, B., Bagby, R. M., & Taylor, G. J. (2004). A multimodal investigation of emotional responding in alexithymia. *Cognition and Emotion, 18*(6), 741–766. https://doi.org/10.1080/02699930341000275

Luminet, O., Rokbani, L., Ogez, D., & Jadoulle, V. (2007). An evaluation of the absolute and relative stability of alexithymia in women with breast cancer. *Journal of Psychosomatic Research, 62*(6), 641–648. https://doi.org/10.1016/j.jpsychores.2007.01.003

Luminet, O., Vermeulen, N., Demaret, C., Taylor, G. J., & Bagby, R. M. (2006). Alexithymia and levels of processing: Evidence for an overall deficit in remembering emotion words. *Journal of Research in Personality, 40*(5), 713–733. https://doi.org/10.1016/j.jrp.2005.09.001

Luminet, O., Zech, E., Rimé, B., & Wagner, H. L. (2000). Predicting cognitive and social consequences of emotional episodes: The contribution of emotional intensity, the Five Factor Model and alexithymia. *Journal of Research in Personality, 34*(4), 471–497. https://doi.org/10.1006/jrpe.2000.2286

Lundh, L. G., Johnsson, A., Sundqvist, K., & Olsson, H. (2002). Alexithymia, memory of emotion, emotional awareness, and perfectionism. *Emotion, 2*(4), 361–379. https://doi.org/10.1037/1528-3542.2.4.361

Lundh, L. G., & Simonsson-Sarnecki, M. (2002). Alexithymia and cognitive bias for emotional information. *Personality and Individual Differences, 32*(6), 1063–1075. https://doi.org/10.1016/S0191-8869(01)00110-6

MacLean, P. D. (1949). Psychosomatic disease and the « visceral brain » - recent developments bearing on the papez theory of emotion. *Psychosomatic Medicine, 11*(6), 338–353. https://doi.org/10.1097/00006842-194911000-00003

MacLeod, C. (2019). Anxiety-linked attentional bias: Backward glances and future glimpses. *Cognition and Emotion, 33*(1), 139–145. https://doi.org/10.1080/02699931.2018.1551190

Mann, L. S., Wise, T. N., Trinidad, A., & Kohanski, R. (1994). Alexithymia, affect recognition, and the 5-factor model of personality in normal subjects. *Psychological Reports, 74*(2), 563–567. https://doi.org/10.2466/pr0.1994.74.2.563

Marchesi, C., Ossola, P., Tonna, M., & De Panfilis, C. (2014). The TAS-20 more likely measures negative affects rather than alexithymia itself in patients with major depression, panic disorder, eating disorders and substance use disorders. *Comprehensive Psychiatry, 55*(4), 972–978. https://doi.org/10.1016/j.comppsych.2013.12.008

Mather, M., & Sutherland, M. R. (2011). Arousal-biased competition in perception and memory. *Perspectives on Psychological Science, 6*(2), 114–133. https://doi.org/10.1177/1745691611400234

McDougall, J. (1982–83). Alexithymia, psychosomatosis, and psychosis. *International Journal of Psychoanalytic Psychotherapy, 9*, 379–388.

Meganck, R., Vanheule, S., Inslegers, R., & Desmet, M. (2009). Alexithymia and interpersonal problems: A study of natural language use. *Personality and Individual Differences, 47*(8), 990–995. https://doi.org/10.1016/j.paid.2009.08.005

Meltzer, M. A., & Nielson, K. A. (2010). Memory for emotionally provocative words in alexithymia: A role for stimulus relevance. *Consciousness and Cognition, 19*(4), 1062–1068. https://doi.org/10.1016/j.concog.2010.05.008

Miller, G. A., & Chapman, J. P. (2001). Misunderstanding analysis of covariance. *Journal of Abnormal Psychology, 110*(1), 40–48. https://doi.org/10.1037/0021-843X.110.1.40

Montebarocci, O., & Surcinelli, P. (2018). Correlations between TSIA and TAS-20 and their relation to self-reported negative affect: A study using a multi-method approach in the assessment of alexithymia in a nonclinical sample from Italy. *Psychiatry Research, 270*, 187–193. https://doi.org/10.1016/j.psychres.2018.09.036

Morie, K. P., & Ridout, N. (2018). Alexithymia and maladaptive regulatory behaviors in substance use disorders and eating disorders. In O. Luminet, G. J. Taylor, & R. M. Bagby (Eds.), *Alexithymia: Advances in research, theory, and clinical practice* (pp. 158–174). Cambridge University Press.

Mueller, J., Alpers, G. W., & Reim, N. (2006). Dissociation of rated emotional valence and Stroop interference in observer-rated alexithymia. *Journal of Psychosomatic Research*, *61*(2), 261–269. https://doi.org/10.1016/j.jpsychores.2006.02.017

Muir, K., Madill, A., & Brown, C. (2017). Individual differences in emotional processing and autobiographical memory: Interoceptive awareness and alexithymia in the fading affect bias. *Cognition and Emotion*, *31*(7), 1392–1404. https://doi.org/10.1080/02699931.2016.1225005

Muller, J., Bühner, M., Ziegler, M., & Sahin, L. (2008). Are alexithymia, ambivalence over emotional expression, and social insecurity overlapping constructs? *Journal of Psychosomatic Research*, *64*(3), 319–325. https://doi.org/10.1016/j.jpsychores.2007.10.005

Nemiah, J. C. (1977). Alexithymia. Theoretical considerations. *Psychotherapy and Psychosomatics*, *28*(1-4), 199–206. https://doi.org/10.1159/000287064

Nemiah, J. C., & Sifneos, P. E. (1970). Psychosomatic illness: A problem in communication. *Psychotherapy and Psychosomatics*, *18*(1-6), 154–160. https://doi.org/10.1159/000286074

Nielson, K. A., & Meltzer, M. A. (2009). Modulation of long-term memory by arousal in alexithymia: The role of interpretation. *Consciousness and Cognition*, *18*(3), 786–793. https://doi.org/10.1016/j.concog.2009.06.001

Nowakowski, M. E., McFarlane, T., & Cassin, S. (2013). Alexithymia and eating disorders: A critical review of the literature. *Journal of Eating Disorders*, *1*(1), 21. https://doi.org/10.1186/2050-2974-1-21

Ogrodniczuk, J. S., Kealy, D., Hadjipavlou, G. A., & Cameron, K. (2018). In O. Luminet, G. J. Taylor & R. M. Bagby (Eds.), *Alexithymia: Advances in research, theory, and clinical practice* (pp. 190–206). Cambridge University Press.

Paez, D., Velasco, C., & Gonzalez, J. L. (1999). Expressive writing and the role of alexithymia as a dispositional deficit in self-disclosure and psychological health. *Journal of Personality and Social Psychology*, *77*(3), 630–641. https://doi.org/10.1037/0022-3514.77.3.630

Panayiotou, G., Leonidou, C., Constantinou, E., Hart, J., Rinehart, K. L., Sy, J. T., & Björgvinsson, T. (2015). Do alexithymic individuals avoid their feelings? Experiential avoidance mediates the association between alexithymia, psychosomatic, and depressive symptoms in a community and a clinical sample. *Comprehensive Psychiatry*, *56*, 206–216. https://doi.org/10.1016/j.comppsych.2014.09.006

Panayiotou, G., Panteli, M., & Vlemincx, E. (2018). Processing emotions in alexithymia. A systematic review of physiological markers. In O. Luminet, G. J. Taylor, & R. M. Bagby (Eds.), *Alexithymia: Advances in research, theory, and clinical practice* (pp. 291–320). Cambridge University Press.

Panayiotou, G., Panteli, M., & Vlemincx, E. (2021). Adaptive and maladaptive emotion processing and regulation, and the case for alexithymia. *Cognition and Emotion*, 1–19. https://doi.org/10.1080/02699931.2019.1671322

Pandey, R. (1995). Stroop interference effect of emotion-arousing words in alexithymia. *Journal of the Indian Academy of Applied Psychology*, *21*(1), 21–28.

Papciak, A. S., Feuerstein, M., & Spiegel, J. A. (1985). Stress reactivity in alexithymia: Decoupling of physiological and cognitive responses. *Journal of Human Stress*, *11*(3), 135–142. https://doi.org/10.1080/0097840X.1985.9936750

Parker, J. D. A., Bauermann, T. M., & Smith, C. T. (2000). Alexithymia and impoverished dream content: Evidence from rapid eye movement sleep awakenings. *Psychosomatic Medicine*, *62*(4), 486–491. https://doi.org/10.1097/00006842-200007000-00006

Parker, J., Taylor, G. J., & Bagby, R. M. (1993b). Alexithymia and the processing of emotional stimuli: An experimental study. *New Trends Experimental and Clinical Psychiatry*, *9*(1-2), 9–14.

Parker, J. D. A., Taylor, G. J., & Bagby, R. M. (1993a). Alexithymia and the recognition of facial expressions of emotion. *Psychotherapy and Psychosomatics*, *59*(3-4), 197–202. https://doi.org/10.1159/000288664

Parker, J. D. A., Taylor, G. J., & Bagby, R. M. (2003). The 20-item Toronto Alexithymia Scale: III. Reliability and factorial validity in a community population. *Journal of Psychosomatic Research*, *55*(3), 269–275. https://doi.org/10.1016/S0022-3999(02)00578-0

Pennebaker, J. W., & Smyth, J. M. (2016). *Opening up by writing it down: How expressive writing improves health and eases emotional pain*. Guilford Press.

Petersen, S. E., & Posner, M. I. (2012). The attention system of the human brain: 20 years after. *Annual Review of Neuroscience*, *35*(1), 73–89. https://doi.org/10.1146/annurev-neuro-062111-150525

Pollatos, O., & Gramann, K. (2011). Electrophysiological evidence of early processing deficits in alexithymia. *Biological Psychology*, *87*(1), 113–121. https://doi.org/10.1016/j.biopsycho.2011.02.016

Porcelli, P., Tulipani, C., Maiello, E., Cilenti, G., & Todarello, O. (2007). Alexithymia, coping,and illness behavior correlates of pain experience in cancer patients. *Psycho-oncology*, *16* (7), 644–650. https://doi.org/10.1002/pon.1115

Preacher, K. J., & Hayes, A. F. (2008). Assessing mediation in communication research. In A. F. Hayes, M. D. Slater, & L. B. Snyder (Eds.), *The Sage sourcebook of advanced data analysis methods for communication research* (pp. 13–54). Sage Publications.

Preece, D., Becerra, R., Allan, A., Robinson, K., & Dandy, J. (2017). Establishing the theoretical components of alexithymia via factor analysis: Introduction and validation of the attention-appraisal model of alexithymia. *Personality and Individual Differences*, *119*, 341–352. https://doi.org/10.1016/j.paid.2017.08.003

Preece, D., Becerra, R., Robinson, K., & Dandy, J. (2018). Assessing alexithymia: Psychometric properties and factorial invariance of the 20-item Toronto alexithymia scale in nonclinical and psychiatric samples. *Journal of Psychopathology and Behavioral Assessment*, *40*(2), 276–287. https://doi.org/10.1007/s10862-017-9634-6

Quirin, M., Robinson, M. D., Rauthmann, J. F., Kuhl, J., Read, S. J., Tops, M., & DeYoung, C. G. (2020). The dynamics of Personality approach (DPA): 20 tenets for uncovering the causal mechanisms of personality. *European Journal of Personality*, 34(6), 947–968. https://doi.org/10.1002/per.2295

Raichle, M. E. (2015). The brain's default mode network. *Annual Review of Neuroscience*, *38*(1), 433–447. https://doi.org/10.1146/annurev-neuro-071013-014030

Reise, S. P. (2012). The rediscovery of bifactor measurement models. *Multivariate Behavioral Research*, *47*(5), 667–696. https://doi.org/10.1080/00273171.2012.715555

Reker, M., Ohrmann, P., Rauch, A. V., Kugel, H., Bauer, J., Dannlowski, U., ... & Suslow, T. (2010). Individual differences in alexithymia and brain response to masked emotion faces. *Cortex*, 46(5), 658–667.

Ridout, N., Smith, J., & Hawkins, H. (2021). The influence of alexithymia on memory for emotional faces and realistic social interactions. *Cognition and Emotion*, 1–19. https://doi.org/10.1080/02699931.2020.1747991

Robinson, M. D., Klein, R. J., & Persich, M. R. (2019). Personality traits in action: A cognitive behavioral version of the social cognitive paradigm. *Personality and Individual Differences*, *147*, 214–222. https://doi.org/10.1016/j.paid.2019.04.041

Roedema, T. M., & Simons, R. F. (1999). Emotion-processing deficit in alexithymia. *Psychophysiology*, *36*(3), 379–387. https://doi.org/10.1017/S0048577299980290

Samur, D., Tops, M., Slapšinskaitė, R., & Koole, S. L. (2021). Getting lost in a story: How narrative engagement emerges from narrative perspective and individual differences in alexithymia. *Cognition and Emotion*, 1–13. https://doi.org/10.1080/02699931.2020.1732876

Scherer, K. R. (1999). Appraisal theory. In T. Dalgleish, & M. J. Power (Eds.), *Handbook of cognition and emotion* (pp. 637–663). Wiley.

Scherer, K. R. (2019). Studying appraisal-driven emotion processes: Taking stock and moving to the future. *Cognition and Emotion*, *33*(1), 31–40. https://doi.org/10.1080/02699931.2018.1510380

Scherer, K. R., & Moors, A. (2019). The emotion process: Event appraisal and component differentiation. *Annual Review of Psychology*, *70*(1), 719–745. https://doi.org/10.1146/annurev-psych-122216-011854

Schmidt, U., Jiwany, A., & Treasure, J. (1993). A controlled study of alexithymia in eating disorders. *Comprehensive Psychiatry*, *34*(1), 54–58. https://doi.org/10.1016/0010-440X(93)90036-4

Sekely, A., Bagby, R. M., & Porcelli, P. (2018a). Assessment of the alexithymia construct. In O. Luminet, G. J. Taylor, & R. M. Bagby (Eds.), *Alexithymia: Advances in research, theory, and clinical practice* (pp. 17–32). Cambridge University Press.

Sekely, A. S., Taylor, G. J., & Bagby, R. M. (2018b). Developing a short version of the Toronto structured interview for alexithymia using item response theory. *Psychiatry Research*, *266*, 218–227. https://doi.org/10.1016/j.psychres.2018.03.002

Senior, C., Hassel, S., Waheed, A., & Ridout, N. (2020). Naming emotions in motion: Alexithymic traits impact the perception of implied motion in facial displays of affect. *Emotion*, *20*(2), 311–316. https://doi.org/10.1037/emo0000546

Sharpe, E., Wallis, D. J., & Ridout, N. (2016). The influence of variations in eating disorder-related symptoms on processing of emotional faces in a non-clinical female sample: An eye-tracking study. *Psychiatry Research*, *240*, 321–327. https://doi.org/10.1016/j.psychres.2016.04.065

Sheppes, G., Suri, G., & Gross, J. J. (2015). Emotion regulation and psychopathology. *Annual Review of Clinical Psychology*, *11*(1), 379–405. https://doi.org/10.1146/annurev-clinpsy-032814-112739

Sifneos, P. E., Apfel-Savitz, R., & Frankel, F. H. (1977). The phenomenon of « alexithymia ». Observations in neurotic and psychosomatic patients. *Psychotherapy and Psychosomatics*, *28*(1-4), 47–57. https://doi.org/10.1159/000287043

Smith, S. M. (1994). Theoretical principles of context-dependent memory. In P. Morris, & Gruneberg M., *Theoretical aspects of memory* (Aspects of Memory, 2nd ed., Vol. 2, pp. 168–195). New York: Routledge.

Smith, R., Killgore, W. D., & Lane, R. D. (2018). The structure of emotional experience and its relation to trait emotional awareness: A theoretical review. *Emotion*, *18*(5), 670–692. https://doi.org/10.1037/emo0000376

Smyth, J. M., Anderson, C. F., Hockemeyer, J. R., & Stone, A. A. (2002). Does emotional nonexpressiveness or avoidance interfere with writing about stressful life events? An analysis in patients with chronic illness. *Psychology and Health*, *17*(5), 561–569. https://doi.org/10.1080/08870440290025777

Sugiura, Y. (2007). Responsibility to continue thinking and worrying: Evidence of incremental validity. *Behaviour Research and Therapy*, *45*(7), 1619–1628. https://doi.org/10.1016/j.brat.2006.08.001

Suslow, T. (1998). Alexithymia and automatic affective processing. *European Journal of Personality*, *12*(6), 433–443. https://doi.org/10.1002/(SICI)1099-0984(199811/12)12:6<433::AID-PER320>3.0.CO;2-O

Suslow, T., & Donges, U. S. (2017). Alexithymia components are differentially related to explicit negative affect but not associated with explicit positive affect or implicit affectivity. *Frontiers in Psychology*, *8*, 1758. https://doi.org/10.3389/fpsyg.2017.01758

Suslow, T., & Junghanns, K. (2002). Impairments of emotion situation priming in alexithymia. *Personality and Individual Differences*, *32*(3), 541–550. https://doi.org/10.1016/S0191-8869(01)00056-3

Suslow, T., Kersting, A., & Arolt, V. (2003). Alexithymia and incidental learning of emotional words. *Psychological Reports*, *93*(3_suppl), 1003–1012. https://doi.org/10.2466/pr0.2003.93.3f.1003

Takahashi, J., Hirano, T., & Gyoba, J. (2015). Effects of facial expressions on visual short-term memory in relation to alexithymia traits. *Personality and Individual Differences*, *83*, 128–135. https://doi.org/10.1016/j.paid.2015.04.010

Taylor, G. J. (2000). Recent developments in alexithymia theory and research. *The Canadian Journal of Psychiatry*, *45*(2), 134–142. https://doi.org/10.1177/070674370004500203

Taylor, G. J., & Bagby, R. M. (2013). Alexithymia and the five-factor model of personality. In T. A. Widiger, & CostaJr.P. T. (Eds.), *Personality Disorders and the Five Factor Model of Personality* (3rd ed., pp. 193–207). American Psychological Association.

Taylor, G. J., Bagby, R. M., & Parker, J. D. A. (1992). The Revised Toronto Alexithymia scale: Some reliability, validity, and normative data. *Psychotherapy and Psychosomatics*, *57*(1-2), 34–41. https://doi.org/10.1159/000288571

Taylor, G. J., Bagby, R. M., & Parker, J. D. A. (1997). *Disorders of affect regulation: Alexithymia in medical and psychiatric illness*. Cambridge University Press.

Taylor, G. J., Bagby, R. M., & Parker, J. D. A. (2016). What's in the name 'alexithymia'? A commentary on "affective agnosia: Expansion of the alexithymia construct and a new opportunity to integrate and extend freud's legacy.". *Neuroscience and Biobehavioral Reviews*, *68*, 1006–1020. https://doi.org/10.1016/j.neubiorev.2016.05.025

Taylor, G. J., Ryan, D., & Bagby, R. M. (1985). Toward the development of a new self-report alexithymia scale. *Psychotherapy and Psychosomatics*, *44*(4), 191–199. https://doi.org/10.1159/000287912

Taylor, G. J., Bagby, R. M., & Luminet, O. (2000). Assessment of alexithymia: Self-report and observer-rated measures. In J.

D. A. Parker and R. Bar-On (Eds.), *The handbook of emotional intelligence* (pp. 301–319). San Francisco, CA: Jossey Bass.

Terock, J., Janowitz, D., Spitzer, C., Miertsch, M., Freyberger, H. J., & Grabe, H. J. (2015). Alexithymia and self-directedness as predictors of psychopathology and psychotherapeutic treatment outcome. *Comprehensive Psychiatry*, *62*, 34–41. https://doi.org/10.1016/j.comppsych.2015.06.007

Terock, J., Van der Auwera, S., Janowitz, D., Klinger-König, J., Schmidt, C. O., Freyberger, H. J., & Grabe, H. J. (2019). The relation of alexithymia, chronic perceived stress and declarative memory performance: Results from the general population. *Psychiatry Research*, *271*, 405–411. https://doi.org/10.1016/j.psychres.2018.12.024

Teten, A. L., Miller, L. A., Bailey, S. D., Dunn, N. J., & Kent, T. A. (2008). Empathic deficits and alexithymia in trauma-related impulsive aggression. *Behavior Sciences and the Law*, *26*(6), 823–832. https://doi.org/10.1002/bsl.843

Tolmunen, T., Lehto, S. M., Heliste, M., Kurl Sudhir, Kauhanen Jussi (2010). Alexithymia is associated with increased cardiovascular mortality in middle aged Finnish men. *Psychosomatic Medicine*, *72*(2), 187–191. https://doi.org/10.1097/PSY.0b013e3181c65d00

Tull, M. T., Medaglia, E., & Roemer, L. (2005). An investigation of the construct validity of the 20-item Toronto Alexithymia Scale through the use of a verbalization task. *Journal of Psychosomatic Research*, *59*(2), 77–84. https://doi.org/10.1016/j.jpsychores.2005.02.016

Vanheule, S. (2008). Challenges for alexithymia research: A commentary on "the construct of alexithymia: Associations with defense mechanisms". *Journal of Clinical Psychology*, *64*(3), 332–337. https://doi.org/10.1002/jclp.20467

Vanheule, S., Meganck, R., & Desmet, M. (2011). Alexithymia, social detachment and cognitive processing. *Psychiatry Research*, *190*(1), 49–51. https://doi.org/10.1016/j.psychres.2010.06.032

Velotti, P., Garofalo, C., Petrocchi, C., Cavallo, F., Popolo, R., & Dimaggio, G. (2016). Alexithymia, emotion dysregulation, impulsivity and aggression: A multiple mediation model. *Psychiatry Research*, *237*, 296–303. https://doi.org/10.1016/j.psychres.2016.01.025

Venta, A., Hart, J., & Sharp, C. (2013). The relation between experiential avoidance, alexithymia and emotion regulation in inpatient adolescents. *Clinical Child Psychology and Psychiatry*, *18*(3), 398–410. https://doi.org/10.1177/1359104512455815

Vermeulen, N. (2021). Alexithymia disrupts verbal short-term memory. *Cognition and Emotion*, 1–10. https://doi.org/10.1080/02699931.2019.1701418

Vermeulen, N., Bayot, M., Mermillod, M., & Grynberg, D. (2019). Alexithymia disrupts the beneficial influence of arousal on attention: Evidence from the attentional blink. *Personality Disorders: Theory, Research, and Treatment*, *10*(6), 545–550. https://doi.org/10.1037/per0000351

Vermeulen, N., Domachowska, I., & Nielson, K. A. (2018). Memory and executive functions in alexithymia. In O. Luminet, G. J. Taylor, & R. M. Bagby (Eds.), *Alexithymia: Advances in research, theory, and clinical practice* (pp. 49–77). Cambridge University Press.

Vermeulen, N., & Luminet, O. (2009). Alexithymia factors and memory performances for neutral and emotional words. *Personality and Individual Differences*, *47*(4), 305–309. https://doi.org/10.1016/j.paid.2009.03.018

Vermeulen, N., Luminet, O., & Corneille, O. (2006). Alexithymia and the automatic processing of affective information: Evidence from the affective priming paradigm. *Cognition and Emotion*, *20*(1), 64–91. https://doi.org/10.1080/02699930500304654

Vermeulen, N., Toussaint, J., & Luminet, O. (2010). The influence of alexithymia and music on the incidental memory for emotion words. *European Journal of Personality*, *24*(6), 551–568. https://doi.org/10.1002/per.758

Wagner, H., & Lee, V. (2008). Alexithymia and individual differences in emotional expression. *Journal of Research in Personality*, *42*(1), 83–95. https://doi.org/10.1016/j.jrp.2007.04.001

Webb, T. L., Miles, E., & Sheeran, P. (2012). Dealing with feeling: A meta-analysis of the effectiveness of strategies derived from the process model of emotion regulation. *Psychological Bulletin*, *138*(4), 775–808. https://doi.org/10.1037/a0027600

Welding, C., & Samur, D. (2018). Language processing in alexithymia. In O. Luminet, G. J. Taylor, & R. M. Bagby (Eds.), *Alexithymia: Advances in research, theory, and clinical practice* (pp. 90–104). Cambridge University Press. https://doi.org/10.1017/9781108241595

Wiebe, A., Kersting, A., & Suslow, T. (2017). Deployment of attention to emotional pictures varies as a function of externally oriented thinking: An eye tracking investigation. *Journal of Behavior Therapy and Experimental Psychiatry*, *55*, 1–5. https://doi.org/10.1016/j.jbtep.2016.11.001

Williams, C., & Wood, R. L. (2010). Alexithymia and emotional empathy following traumatic brain injury. *Journal of Clinical and Experimental Neuropsychology*, *32*(3), 259–267. https://doi.org/10.1080/13803390902976940

Wotschack, C., & Klann-Delius, G. (2013). Alexithymia and the conceptualization of emotions: A study of language use and semantic knowledge. *Journal of Research in Personality*, *47*(5), 514–523. https://doi.org/10.1016/j.jrp.2013.01.011

Yiend, J. (2010). The effects of emotion on attention: A review of attentional processing of emotional information. *Cognition and Emotion*, *24*(1), 3–47. https://doi.org/10.1080/02699930903205698

Zech, E., Luminet, O., Rimé, B., & Wagner, H. L. (1999). Alexithymia and its measurement. Confirmatory factor analyses of the twenty-item Toronto Alexithymia Scale and the Bermond-Vorst alexithymia questionnaire. *European Journal of Personality*, *13*(6), 511–532. https://doi.org/10.1002/(SICI)1099-0984(199911/12)13:6<511::AID-PER347>3.0.CO;2-0

Adaptive and maladaptive emotion processing and regulation, and the case of alexithymia

Georgia Panayiotou, Maria Panteli and Elke Vlemincx

ABSTRACT

In this conceptual review, we discuss models of emotion and its regulation and identify a spectrum of processes that characterise adaptive adjustment to the affective environment. We describe a *dynamic-phasic model* of emotion processing and regulation, focusing on five stages: *anticipation, response, recovery, habituation and rest* as part of a cascade of responses to emotional challenges, as these become progressively expected, proximal, chronic or repeated. We argue for the need to investigate beyond simple reactivity to emotional stimuli, in order to understand mental and physical health conditions where emotional dysregulation plays a role. We propose that a hallmark of an effective and adaptive emotion regulation system is its flexibility, in the service of life goals and values. Consistent with McEwen's model (1998, *Stress, adaptation, and disease: Allostasis and allostatic load. Annals of the New York Academy of Sciences*, *840*(1), 33–44), inflexible emotion regulation can lead to increased allostatic load, from frequent stress, inadequate reactivity, failed shutdown and habituation, which may result in physical and mental illness. Alexithymia exemplifies inflexible emotion regulation, with dysfunctions potentially across all stages of emotion processing, both psychologically and physiologically. These maladaptive processes and their consequence on allostatic load potentially explain the association between alexithymia and physical and mental illness.

Alexithymia involves difficulties in identifying, differentiating and describing emotions, and externally oriented thinking and has been linked to physical and mental health problems. Research examining emotional dysregulation in alexithymia has focused on subjective and physiological *reactivity* during emotional challenges, as the many studies on this topic, reviewed by Panayiotou, Panteli, and Vlemincx (2018b), show. However, emotion processing and regulation entail a wider spectrum of psychological and physiological processes. In this paper, we examine how these processes may explain the link between alexithymia and poor mental and physical health.

We draw from theories of emotion (Lang, 1979; Watson & Tellegen, 1985), emotion processing (Baumann, Kaschel, & Kuhl, 2007; Davidson, Jackson, & Kalin, 2000; Fanselow, 1994; Skinner & Zimmer-Gembeck, 2007) and regulation (Aldao, Sheppes, & Gross, 2015; Kashdan & Rottenberg, 2010; Koole, 2009), to argue that to understand alexithymia (and other conditions involving emotion difficulties) the full range of emotional processes must be considered.[1] We discuss a dynamic-phasic perspective, addressing (dys)regulation during five essential phases: *anticipation* of emotion stimuli, *reactivity* to these, *recovery* after a stimulus is no longer present, *habituation* to repeated stimuli, and *rest* in the absence of emotional events.

Within this framework, we focus on flexibility as a premise for adaptive emotion regulation.[2] Flexible emotion regulation allows these five phases to unfold fluidly, in a manner consistent with goals, needs and values, synchronised with situational demands, promoting physical and psychological health. Behaviourally, this constitutes psychological flexibility, i.e. *the capacity to persist with and change behavior in a manner that incorporates conscious and open contact with thoughts and feelings, and that is consistent with one's values and goals* (Scott, McCracken, & Norton, 2015, p. 286). Physiologically, it means adjusting autonomic, endocrine and neuromuscular responses to match situational demands and accomplish these goals.

To the contrary, inflexible regulation disrupts adaptive processes through rigid use of strategies to modulate psychological and physiological responses irrespective of the situation, one's goals and values. For example, strategies that down-regulate negative affect, like avoidance (or poor emotional awareness, as in alexithymia), bring relief from stressors in the short-run (Davydov, 2017; Davydov, Stewart, Ritchie, & Chaudieu, 2010). However, when used inflexibly, in the long-run, they predict psychological and physical dysfunction (Stabbe, Rolffs, & Rogge, 2019; Tavakoli, Broyles, Reid, Sandoval, & Correa-Fernández, 2019), through progressive disengagement from meaningful and reinforcing activities, goals, needs and values (Scott & McCracken, 2015). Individuals high, compared to those low, in psychological flexibility have greater emotional clarity (Salovey, Mayer, Goldman, Turvey, & Palfai, 1995), autonomy, competency (Johnston & Finney, 2010) and vitality (Kubzansky & Thurston, 2007) and fewer health problems. We rely on the well-established model of allostatic load (McEwen, 1998) to discuss how inflexibility in managing affect at any of the five phases, indexed by various markers of stress accumulation, may explain the association between alexithymia (and other emotional disorders) and somatic and mental illness.

What are emotions?

Emotions are subjective, physiological, expressive, and functional phenomena reflecting motivational tendencies of approach toward appetitive and withdrawal from aversive stimuli (Bradley & Lang, 2000; Davidson et al., 2000). Lang's (1979) Bio-Informational Theory describes emotions as action dispositions, which instigate behaviours, in response to emotional events, even before one is aware of an emotion or consciously selects appropriate action. This early response involves activation of physiological processes that mobilise autonomic, somatomotor, endocrine and metabolic systems (Phillips, Drevets, Rauch, & Lane, 2003).

In studying emotions in psychopathology and conditions like alexithymia, most research has focused on reactivity to emotional stimuli. Going beyond reactivity, however, several theorists (e.g. Baumann et al., 2007; Davidson et al., 2000; Fanselow, 1994; Lang, Bradley, & Cuthbert, 1997; Skinner & Zimmer-Gembeck, 2007) describe how emotional responses vary along a "cascade" of stages, that unfold as the eliciting event becomes more imminent, threatening or proximal in time and space. According to Fanselow (1994), "pre-encounter" takes place when harm is distant or unlikely, eliciting anticipation, vigilance and risk assessment, whereas "post-encounter" occurs when actual or perceived threat is detected, evoking freezing and orienting, to prevent encounter with threat. When actually facing threat ("circa-strike"), active fight or flight are initiated. Specific patterns of the dynamic, fluctuating trajectories of emotions are suggested by Kuppens and Verduyn (e.g. 2017) to reflect emotion dysregulation and illness vulnerability, while Davidson (2015) and Trull, Lane, Koval, and Ebner-Priemer (2015) stress the need to study individual differences in affective dynamics in order to understand psychopathology and well-being.

Unfolding emotional processes

We propose a dynamic-phasic approach to studying emotion processing, focusing on *anticipation, response, recovery, habituation*, and *rest* (Figure 1). These stages are not delineated by sharp boundaries, but smoothly evolve into one another, not always in sequence (e.g. a predator may surge while the

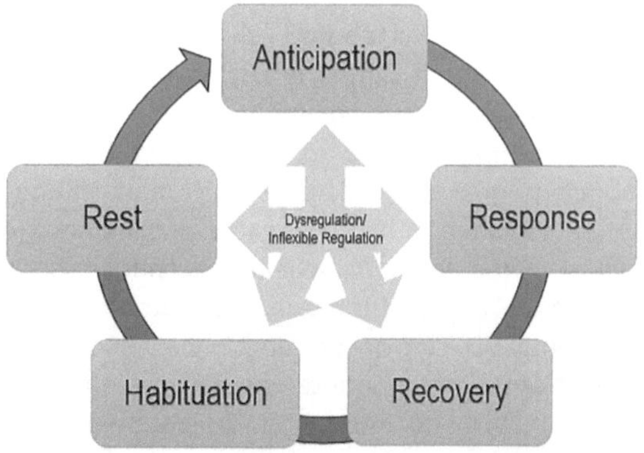

Figure 1. A dynamic-phasic model of emotion processing.

organism recovers from a previous attack, without the chance for rest or anticipation). Studying each stage, involving processes serving different survival functions, can inform conclusions regarding when and under what circumstances emotion dysregulation occurs.

Anticipation

Organisms anticipate challenges that can be foreseen, using contextual cues to predict upcoming motivationally relevant stimuli based on previous learning and memory (Cravo, Rohenkohl, Santos, & Nobre, 2017), in order to minimise bodily disruption and optimise perception and action generation (Mossbridge, Tressoldi, & Utts, 2012). However, one's ability for anticipation is influenced by characteristics of the cueing environment and individual differences. Worry, rumination and anxiety may lead to chronic arousal and hypervigilance (Verkuil, Brosschot, Putman, & Thayer, 2009), unnecessarily depleting resources, whereas attentional avoidance impairs anticipation of potentially relevant stimuli.

Response

Organisms react to perceived emotional stimuli, based on their identification and appraisal (Phillips et al., 2003). Individual differences, e.g. in anxiety, affect appraisals and may produce attention biases, higher engagement and difficulty in disengagement from threatening stimuli (Cisler & Koster, 2010). Also, stimulus and task characteristics influence perception, evaluation (Grynberg, Chang, et al., 2012) and response, including the presence of competing stimuli (i.e. affective priming; task perceptual load), the subjective meaning of a stimulus, its modality, intensity, salience, familiarity, concreteness and integrity. In this complex context, the individual must attend to significant stimuli, ignore insignificant ones and initiate appropriate coping.

Flexible and adaptive emotional functioning means producing goal-appropriate, timely and fittingly intense responses, rather than reacting invariably, irrespective of the emotional events' proximity and significance (Waugh, Thompson, & Gotlib, 2011). Consistently derailing or interrupting the smooth evolution of emotional responses because of unwillingness or inability to engage or disengage with an event, irrespective of its relevance for survival or other goals, can increase allostatic load. Flexibility should pertain to all aspects of emotional responses. Poor valence granulation (e.g. anxious individuals invariably perceiving facial expressions as disapproving) will result in disproportionate approach/withdrawal behaviours, such as unnecessary social withdrawal. Excessive or deficient arousal (e.g. consistently perceiving situations as threatening) can interfere with attention deployment, performance, and learning, depletion of resources, increased risk exposure or reduced reinforcement opportunities.

Essential for adequate reactivity is appropriate appraisal of one's ability to cope (Carver & Scheier, 1988). Emotional challenges that are appraised to exceed coping resources may elicit low physiological reactivity as in depression, melancholia, generalised anxiety or PTSD (Liu, Sarapas, & Shankman, 2016; McTeague & Lang, 2012). This freezing response is adaptive for short-term escape (Porges, 2001), but can accumulate stress in the long-run.

Finally, adaptive reactivity itself evolves dynamically, dependent on the activity of different physiological and neural systems, in response to contextual requirements. For example, during a novel stimulus, heart rate accelerates for the first 4–6s, followed by deceleration in 17–23s, involving sensory intake and release from parasympathetic control, and then by secondary, sympathetically mediated, acceleration at 31–76s (del Paso, Godoy, & Vila, 1993) reflecting mental processing and action preparation (Bradley & Lang, 2000). Parallel processes occur in the electrodermal, facial and other systems.

Responding inflexibly as if all stimuli at all times are equally significant, threatening, appetitive, or indifferent, irrespective of their proximity and relevance to immediate or long-term goals, characterises conditions like anxiety (extreme threat responses), depression (lack of pleasure even from previously desired activities), psychopathy (lack of fear, even in danger), and alexithymia (low emotional response irrespective of stimulus significance). Such inflexible responding may disrupt psychological and physiological processes (McEwen, 2007), triggering mental and physical illness progression, or disengagement from goals, needs, values and relationships.

Recovery

Reactivity is adaptive for survival, only while the emotional stimulus is or will be present. Once the stimulus ends, one should recover and return to resting state, in order to conserve energy and restore homeostasis (Zautra, 2009). Good recovery involves quickly regaining equilibrium physiologically and psychologically, by deactivating the sympathetic and activating the parasympathetic system (Appelhans & Luecken, 2006), and is essential to make resources available for exploration, need satisfaction, life goals and novel challenges. Inability to inhibit reactivity and disengage from stressors can cause exhaustion through tonic hyperarousal (McEwen, 1998). Slowed recovery and "difficulty in processing safety signals" (Pieper, Brosschot, van der Leeden, & Thayer, 2007) as often found in anxiety, can result in exhaustion and desensitisation from responding to later, real threat.

Habituation

Habituation describes the process of becoming less reactive toward repeated or familiar stimuli that no longer carry the same novelty and significance (Grissom & Bhatnagar, 2009; Rankin et al., 2009). Habituation rates depend on the intensity and familiarity of the stimulus; less intense and more familiar stimuli produce stronger habituation (Herman, 2013). Although habituation, strictly speaking, results from non-associative learning processes, it may become dependent on context through associative learning, being thus affected by memory and learning processes. Whereas fast habituation has been linked to health (Bower, Low, Moskowitz, Sepah, & Epel, 2008) habituating too slowly is connected to PTSD, (Shalev et al., 2000), anxiety (Frith, Stevens, Johnstone, & Crow, 1982) and depression in fibromyalgia (de Tommaso et al., 2011); habituating too fast has been linked to suicide propensity in depression (Jandl, Steyer, & Kaschka, 2010; Sarchiapone et al., 2017).

Resting state

When an imminent challenge is not present or anticipated, the adaptive response is to recuperate and conserve resources. Intense emotional and physiological activation during such times is inefficient, deters one from pursuing goals and experiencing life, while remaining mindful of and open to new opportunities and challenges, and characterises conditions like anxiety and depression (Abercrombie et al., 1998).

Flexible emotion regulation

Humans can adjust their emotional reactions along dimensions of valence, arousal, and approach/avoidance, before, during or after an emotional event (Koole, 2009). Persevering with a strategy to modulate affect, irrespective of the context and one's goals, can incur mental and physical costs. There is evidence that reappraisal strategies predict positive health outcomes and well-being, whereas avoidance, suppression and rumination are less adaptive, predicting depression, eating disorders, substance use and anxiety (Aldao, Nolen-Hoeksema, & Schweizer, 2010). However, even "adaptive" strategies can be inappropriate for certain situations (Sheppes, Scheibe, Suri, & Gross, 2011), while strategies considered "maladaptive" are sometimes conducive to health. We, and others, suggest that adaptive emotion regulation depends on synchrony with the context and one's needs, goals and values (Bonanno, Papa, Lalande, Westphal, & Coifman, 2004; Kashdan & Rottenberg, 2010), and thus no strategy is inherently good or bad.

Adaptive emotion regulation requires psychological, behavioural and physiological processes and strategies to change fluidly as the situation evolves and new demands arise (Aldao et al., 2015; Leonidou, Panayiotou, Bati, & Karekla, 2019). Physiologically, homeostatic feedback and feedforward processes must be flexibly enlisted (Friedman, 2007). Allostasis defines such dynamic regulatory processes that allow bodily systems to meet situational demands (McEwen, 1998). Although allostasis is essential to optimal bodily functioning, it comes with a cost, called allostatic load, defined as the cumulative wear and tear on the body as a result of adaptation (McEwen, 2007). Under normal circumstances and for most individuals, adaptive allostasis involves neuroendocrine (e.g. cortisol, (nor)epinephrine), cardiovascular (e.g. blood pressure, heart rate), metabolic (e.g. glucose, insulin) and immune (e.g. cytokines; Kano, Grabe, & Terock, 2018; McEwen, 1998) response fluctuations. However, when one's affective response does not fit the situation, the organism may incur allostatic load and illness vulnerability, via malfunctions in neuroendocrine (e.g. emotional and cognitive deficits), cardiovascular (e.g. atherosclerosis, myocardial infarction), metabolic (e.g. diabetes, obesity) and immune systems (immune suppression; Juster, McEwen, & Lupien, 2010). In the long run, allostatic load can exhaust mediating stress systems, reduce functionality of effector systems (cardiovascular, respiratory, gastrointestinal) and predispose to disease (McEwen, 1998, 2007).

In sum, emotion processing and regulation must be flexible, producing psychological and physiological responses that are timely and commensurate to the situation. Flexibility requires a wide repertoire of strategies and the ability to select and implement those contextually appropriate. The next section describes how alexithymia may involve low flexibility and dysregulation, potentially along all five stages of processing, leading to accumulation of allostatic load that may explain its link to negative physical and psychological outcomes. The section also notes areas where current evidence is inconclusive, necessitating additional research.

Emotional dysregulation in alexithymia

The focus of research on the response stage of processing has influenced theorising about alexithymia. Based on early observations of high autonomic reactivity but low emotional awareness in alexithymia, the "blindfeel" hypothesis was proposed (Lane, Ahern, Schwartz, & Kaszniak, 1997). Later evidence proved to be quite mixed, and in fact seems to weigh in the opposite direction, of high or normal subjective responses paired with low physiological arousal (Panayiotou et al., 2018b). Hence, emotion-processing deficits in alexithymia remain elusive making theorising difficult and hindering development of interventions. Adopting a dynamic-phasic approach, may broaden the scope of research, clarifying the forms of emotion dysregulation associated with this trait. As an example, this approach can be used to assess hypotheses that alexithymia involves a defensive way of dealing with emotions or experiential avoidance (Krystal, 2015; Panayiotou, Leonidou, Constantinou, & Michaelides, 2018a; Panayiotou et al., 2015). Such avoidance might take the form of low physiological and/or subjective reactivity during the response stage. Null findings when testing this hypothesis can be further explored through examination of all five phases. They might be due to reactivity being too high during baseline or anticipation, masking the expected effects. Findings of inappropriate reactivity during the response stage may in turn, generate further predictions about delayed recovery, poor habituation to repeated exposure, heightened anticipation of future exposures, and high tonic reactivity during rest. Even within the response stage, a dynamic perspective would prompt micro-analysis of responses to identify moment-to-moment dynamic response changes within very short time windows, to observe the engagement, maintenance and disengagement of processes such as orienting, vigilance, selective attention, sustained attention and arousal. It is possible, that, as predicted by vigilance-avoidance models of anxiety, early hypervigilance and hyperreactivity is followed by attentional withdrawal and blunted responses in alexithymia as well, but only a dynamic approach would unveil this.

Indeed, the extant literature suggests that alexithymia may entail emotion dysregulation across all or most of the five phases, resulting in allostatic load and illness (Honkalampi, De Berardis, Vellante, & Viinamäki, 2018; Porcelli & Taylor, 2018). Allostatic load may accumulate along four main markers of maladaptation: *frequent stress exposure, inadequate response, failed shutdown*, and *failure to habituate* (McEwen, 1998; McEwen & Gianaros, 2010). We next review evidence for these markers in alexithymia, discuss how these fit within our dynamic-phasic framework and highlight areas where additional research is clearly needed.

Anticipation

Hypervigilance to and over-perception of emotional stimuli or failure to adequately anticipate them using prior learning, can result in unnecessary stress exposure, inefficient coping and stress accumulation (Grupe & Nitschke, 2013), contributing to *frequent stress* (Loewenstein & Lerner, 2003). Inadequate anticipation may also disrupt social relationships, creating new interpersonal stressors. Some of the few studies examining anticipatory processes in alexithymia support hypervigilance to and enhanced the anticipation of emotional stimuli (Delle-Vigne, Kornreich, Verbanck, & Campanella, 2014), with increased physiological arousal (Fukunishi, Sei, Morita, & Rahe, 1999; Panayiotou & Constantinou, 2017). de Timary, Roy, Luminet, Fillée, and Mikolajczak (2008) found that difficulty in describing feelings was associated with increased cortisol levels during stress anticipation, but not during stress exposure. Two studies showed increased skin conductance to a first exposure to an emotional stimulus, but no alexithymia effects during later exposures, (Grynberg, Davydov, Vermeulen, & Luminet, 2012; Rabavilas, 1987), suggesting hyper-reactivity to novelty; this perhaps could reflect increased vigilance. Byrne and Ditto (2005) found increased blood pressure in alexithymia during stress anticipation.

Some contradictory results also exist: Pollatos et al. (2011) and Starita, Làdavas, and Di Pellegrino (2016) found decreased skin conductance in alexithymic participants before a public speaking stressor and aversive electrical stimulation respectively. Bokeriia, Golukhova, Polunina, Davydov, and Kruglova (2008) reported reduced baseline heart rate in alexithymic patients awaiting cardiac surgery.

Anticipation deficits may relate to difficulties in learning and memory (Luminet, Vermeulen, Demaret, Taylor, & Bagby, 2006; Vermeulen, Domachowska, & Nielson, 2018) leading to failed recognition of predictors of repeated emotional events (Rankin et al., 2009). However, further research is needed to document anticipation deficits and link them to these observed difficulties, as dysregulation during anticipation remains a rather under-studied domain. Future, well-designed studies should control the amount and type of information conveyed by cues predicting repeated emotional stimuli, while differentiating clearly between inappropriate reactivity during anticipation, baseline, and exposure phases.

Response

Emotional hyper- and hypo-reactivity, i.e. *inadequate response*, is an important source of allostatic load (McEwen, 1998), possibly due to poor evaluation of the stimulus as potentially threatening (valence) or its proximity/intensity (arousal), and deficits in learning and memory, as found in alexithymia (Luminet et al., 2006; Vermeulen, Toussaint, & Luminet, 2010). They may also relate to deficiencies in deploying attention appropriately during perception, to initiate reflexes and behaviour. Limited available electrophysiological and neuroimaging evidence indeed suggests poor early encoding, differentiation, recognition and granulation of emotional stimuli in alexithymia, (see systematic review, Grynberg et al., 2012): Pollatos and Gramann (2011) showed reduced P1 amplitudes to emotional pictures, suggesting early perceptual difficulties that may deter later processing and awareness. No emotional modulation of the N190, indicating poor encoding of fearful postures was also found (Borhani, Borgomaneri, Làdavas, & Bertini, 2016), as well as delayed N2b component, showing delayed attentional disengagement and shifting toward new information (Vermeulen, Luminet, De Sousa, & Campanella, 2008). Contradictory evidence of enhanced evoked potentials during early processing in alexithymia (Delle-Vigne et al., 2014; Schäfer, Schneider, Tress, & Franz, 2007) has been interpreted as a need to deploy greater cognitive resources for emotion perception. fMRI studies concur with poor attention allocation and encoding, showing lower activation of emotional brain areas in alexithymia during brief presentations of facial expressions (Grynberg, Chang, et al., 2012).

Ample research now supports hypo-reactivity in alexithymia across physiological systems. Although some findings show equivalent autonomic responses to controls, and some show hyper-reactivity, a substantial corpus of studies (reviewed in Panayiotou et al., 2018b) shows reduced cardiovascular and electrodermal responses to emotional challenges, indexing limited sympathetic activation, energy mobilisation and action preparation that potentially impairs coping and awareness, leading to inadequate emotional responding. Specifically, the sympatho-adreno-medullary (SAM) system responds to acute stress by releasing catecholamines, allowing energy mobilisation, through glucose and fat release, increased respiration, heart rate and blood flow (see Kano et al., 2018). Hypo-reactivity may indicate inadequate fight-flight responses, increasing risk to the organism. Stress also activates the hypothalamic pituitary adrenal (HPA)-axis and glucocorticoid production, which acutely inhibits pro-inflammatory cytokine production, preventing inflammation (Juster et al., 2010). A deficient immune response elevates risk for physical and psychiatric disease, as immune responses fight infections and maintain health (McEwen, 2007). However, findings on endocrine responses in alexithymia remain inconclusive, with some studies suggesting HPA axis hyper-reactivity during stress, and others supporting no relationship between alexithymia and neuroendocrine activity (Kano et al., 2018). Somewhat more consistently, findings suggest HPA hyporeactivity during baselines, which may result from prolonged stress and repetitive HPA axis overstimulation (Kano et al., 2018). Thus, the impact of observed hypo-reactivity in alexithymia on primary mediators of allostatic load needs to be further examined in order to delineate illness pathways.

Recovery

Difficulties in returning to baseline when an emotional stimulus ends may result in *failed shutdown* (McEwen, 1998). For fast and adequate recovery, flexible attention shifting and response inhibition are essential.

Considering attention allocation deficits in alexithymia, compromised inhibitory and switching capacities could contribute to slow or inadequate recovery from stressors (Gotlib & Joormann, 2010), tonic hyperarousal and *failed shutdown*, leading to greater allostatic load. Further, given that emotion modulation is facilitated by the ability to represent affect symbolically and connect it to past experiences, memory and learning deficits in alexithymia (Darrow & Follette, 2014; Luminet et al., 2006) may compromise the ability to update one's evaluations of and responses to emotional information (e.g. that a feared stimulus has moved to a safe distance).

In effect, evidence for recovery difficulties in alexithymia is inconclusive, with few studies specifically addressing this issue. Many studies report similarities in physiological responses between high and low alexithymic individuals following music (Grynberg et al., 2012), public speech (Eastabrook, Lanteigne, & Hollenstein, 2013; Pollatos et al., 2011), Stroop tasks (Connelly & Denney, 2007), and other emotional, cognitive and stress tasks (e.g. Martínez Sánchez & García, 2011; Martínez Sánchez, Ortiz Soria, & Ato García, 2001). Nevertheless, a few studies support no or slow recovery in alexithymia. Davydov, Luminet, and Zech (2013) found that participants high in externally oriented thinking had no return to baseline after a sad-avoidance film; Gündel et al. (2004) showed that alexithymic spasmodic torticollis patients had increased skin conductance during recovery from affective stimuli. However, these findings must be seen cautiously, as alexithymic participants showed poor change from baseline during emotional stimulation.

Altogether, some evidence of aberrant recovery in alexithymia exists, but most findings support normal physiological recovery (Panayiotou et al., 2018b). In the future, the methodological issues of differences in baselines preceding, and reactivity during emotional tasks need to be better accounted to draw firm conclusions regarding recovery dysregulation in alexithymia, a phase of processing for which data are currently inconclusive.

Habituation

Memory deficits in alexithymia (Luminet et al., 2006; Vermeulen et al., 2010), and difficulties in learning from experience (Darrow & Follette, 2014) may lead to continued reactivity in response to repeated emotional exposures, and contexts that have become associated with these, as if the stimulus continued to carry the same novelty and significance. Evidence for *failure to habituate* (McEwen & Gianaros, 2010) in alexithymia is limited, with some results suggesting reduced habituation compared to controls, while other studies showing stronger habituation (see Panayiotou et al., 2018b). Luminet, Rimé, Bagby, and Taylor (2004), showed that difficulty in describing feelings was positively correlated with heart rate both at exposure and re-exposure suggesting lack of habituation. Bogdanov et al. (2013) found delayed skin conductance habituation in alexithymia during a computer game.

In contrast, Starita et al. (2016) provide evidence for faster extinction of electrodermal responses when cues were no longer followed by aversive electrical stimulation in high compared to moderate or low alexithymic participants, indicating stronger habituation. Grynberg et al. (2012) and Rabavilas (1987) showed that alexithymic participants exhibited high autonomic reactivity during a first exposure to an affective stimulus, but findings became nonsignificant during subsequent exposures, suggesting the presence of fast habituation. Habituating too fast may represent a form of dysregulation as one may not fully process a significant stimulus or override necessary coping too quickly, placing oneself at risk (Sarchiapone et al., 2017). Thus, although dysregulation during habituation is another potential route to continued stress exposure in alexithymia, current evidence is mixed, and it is unclear if it converges towards habituation being too fast or too slow, necessitating further research.

Rest

Failed shutdown can also result from increased activity during resting or baseline states. Increased tonic arousal may result from hypervigilance to threat and inability to process safety signals (Panayiotou & Constantinou, 2017), along with reduced inhibitory capacities (Delle-Vigne et al., 2014), resulting in chronic activation of SAM and HPA systems. Although acute release of glucocorticoids inhibits the production of pro-inflammatory cytokines, chronic release of glucocorticoids by the HPA-axis enhances pro-inflammatory cytokines production, resulting in immune response suppression. Prolonged glucocorticoid release has been implicated in Cushing's disease, dementia, sleep deprivation, depression and anxiety, and seems to cause atrophy in the prefrontal cortex, which may instigate mental disorders (McEwen, 2007). Chronic SAM activation contributes to strokes, hypertension and heart disease (Fredrikson & Matthews, 1990) and susceptibility to infections (Cohen & Rodriguez, 1995) via chronic sympathetic arousal and low parasympathetic control. Currently, a few studies provide evidence for baseline hypofunction of the HPA axis in alexithymia (Kano et al., 2018); this however, may be a result of chronic hyper-activation which desensitises the endocrine system. Chronic arousal may also affect illness perceptions, causing bodily sensations, which may be misinterpreted as illness symptoms (Leonidou & Panayiotou, 2018), explaining in part the link between alexithymia and somatisation.

With regards to physiological arousal during rest in alexithymia, several studies suggest increased cardiovascular or electrodermal activity (Davydov et al., 2013; Eastabrook et al., 2013; Gündel et al., 2004; Martínez Sánchez & García, 2011; Panayiotou & Constantinou, 2017), although many studies find equivalent, and a few reduced tonic arousal compared to control participants (Panayiotou et al., 2018b). Depending on the instructions given to participants, baselines may represent either rest or anticipation, necessitating more studies with experimental designs more clearly differentiating between rest and other phases of processing.

Inflexible emotion regulation strategies

Research on self-reported emotion regulation strategies suggests inflexible regulation in alexithymia, leading to *frequent stress*. Alexithymia reliably correlates positively with strategies known to generally increase the severity and frequency of unwanted thoughts and feelings including non-acceptance, experiential avoidance and suppression, and negatively with active coping and reappraisal (Ghorbani, Khosravani, Bastan, & Ardakani, 2017; Panayiotou et al., 2018a). Further, alexithymic individuals may have a limited repertoire of emotion regulation skills (Darrow & Follette, 2014). Reduced corrective learning due to inflexible use of ineffective coping can compromise decision making, solidification of coping repertoires, resilience during future challenges and social effectiveness (Aldao et al., 2010; Craske, 2015; Kashdan & Rottenberg, 2010) incurring increased allostatic load and compromised physical and mental health. In line with this hypothesis, research suggests that reliance on avoidance, mediates the association between alexithymia and depression, psychosomatic symptoms and social anxiety (Panayiotou, 2018; Panayiotou et al., 2015).

Summary and conclusions

In this conceptual review, we first argue for a dynamic-phasic perspective to the study of emotion processing and regulation in order to understand the complex etiologies of conditions and disorders involving emotional difficulties. The case of alexithymia nicely demonstrates this point, as much research has focused primarily on the response stage of emotion processing, whereas limited evidence regarding anticipation, recovery, habituation and rest, hints to the possibility that dysregulation may occur during these phases as well. The proposed dynamic phasic approach contributes to a future research agenda, aiming to examine emotional processes throughout the cascade of responses to emotion challenges, setting *a priori* hypotheses and launching appropriate designs to address them, in order to understand emotion dysregulation in alexithymia, and other disorders. In future designs, phases must be clearly delineated, manipulated and compared within-subject, so that, (1) rest and anticipation are clearly distinguishable, (2) emotional reactivity is assessed as difference from rest and anticipation (using stimuli and challenges varying in valence and arousal), (3) recovery is evaluated as return from an active response to a stimulus, (4) habituation is examined to repeated stimulation. Comparing activity elicited by each of these phases between participants with different levels of alexithymia (while controlling for confounding traits such as anxiety and depression) will enhance understanding of which aspects of emotional stimuli (valence, arousal, social/non-social) and which processes underlying emotion regulation (e.g. attention, learning, memory) are deficient in alexithymia. A future agenda can also utilise additional markers of anticipation (e.g. eye fixations), habituation (e.g. skin conductance responses to acoustic startle; Walker et al., 2019) or startle reflex habituation; (Panayiotou & Constantinou, 2017) or recovery (e.g. face-locked P3 component; Morriss, Taylor, Roesch, & van Reekum, 2013). Because psychological and physiological mechanisms within each stage are dynamic, analysis of moment to moment responses is also necessary, including ecological momentary assessment of emotion regulation, subjective experience, cognitions, behaviours and physiological responses in real-life settings (Shiffman, Stone, & Hufford, 2008).

The second argument made in this paper concerns the need for a flexible emotion regulation system that helps one adjust to the changing demands of the environment, while serving one's values, goals and needs. In a future research agenda for alexithymia, questions relevant to flexibility involve the appropriateness of valence evaluations and levels of arousal for the time and stage of processing, considering the significance and proximity of the stimulus, and the ability to modulate responses accordingly. Inflexibility at the psychological and physiological level and in the use of dispositional coping should also be examined in relation to its effect on immune, neuro-endocrine, cardiovascular and muscular systems, to identify specific disease progression mechanisms. For example, alexithymic hypo-reactivity during the response stage may result in system insensitivity; when chronically unresponsive to emotional stimuli, the HPA and SAM systems don't 'practice' and desensitise, which further impairs phasic responding to emotional stimuli. This pattern of 'desensitization' is commonly seen, in the form of blunted physiological reactivity to stressors, in depression, PTSD and trauma (e.g. McTeague & Lang, 2012). On the other hand, excessive stress exposure, due to mechanisms described above, could lead to disease through acute surges in autonomic parameters, such as heart rate or blood pressure leading to atherosclerosis and/or myocardial infarction (McEwen, 1998). Chronic activation of glucocorticoids reduces immune responding to acute challenges (Irwin & Miller, 2007), documented in alexithymia (see review Uher, 2010), which can also in part explain the high prevalence of alexithymia in mental (Honkalampi et al., 2018; Morie & Ridout, 2018) and physical illness (see reviews Porcelli & Taylor, 2018; Uher, 2010) and medically unexplained symptoms (De Gucht, Fischler, & Heiser, 2004). In the long term, inappropriate levels of activation during various stages of processing may become the new body norm, via alteration of allostatic set points, further increasing inflexibility, physiological dysregulation and illness risk (Herman, 2013).

Progress in the treatment and prevention of alexithymia and associated disorders can be more forthcoming when central pathogenic mechanisms are identified and targeted. Psychological and physiological inflexibility may present such a target. Training in diverse emotion regulation skills may address difficulties at different stages of processing (e.g. exposure for improved habituation, mindfulness and relaxation training for difficulties at rest, thought restructuring skills for recovery), permitting alexithymic individuals to more fully process emotional challenges through improved awareness, tolerance, acceptance and flexibility, in ways consistent with the situation and one's life goals, needs and values.

Notes

1. We use the term emotion regulation to broadly encompass efforts to change emotions, and refer to emotional processing as the unfolding of responses from the time before an emotional event occurs until it is no longer present.
2. In addition to inflexibility, there are potentially other characteristics of suboptimal emotion regulation, e.g. decoupled responses among response systems (as found in alexithymia; see Panayiotou et al., 2018b) but these, and their relation to the model presented here are beyond the scope of this discussion.

Disclosure statement

No potential conflict of interest was reported by the authors.

References

Abercrombie, H. C., Schaefer, S. M., Larson, C. L., Oakes, T. R., Lindgren, K. A., Holden, J. E., ... Benca, R. M. (1998). Metabolic rate in the right amygdala predicts negative affect in depressed patients. *Neuroreport*, *9*(14), 3301–3307.

Aldao, A., Nolen-Hoeksema, S., & Schweizer, S. (2010). Emotion-regulation strategies across psychopathology: A meta-analytic review. *Clinical Psychology Review*, *30*(2), 217–237.

Aldao, A., Sheppes, G., & Gross, J. J. (2015). Emotion regulation flexibility. *Cognitive Therapy and Research*, *39*(3), 263–278.

Appelhans, B. M., & Luecken, L. J. (2006). Heart rate variability as an index of regulated emotional responding. *Review of General Psychology*, *10*(3), 229–240.

Baumann, N., Kaschel, R., & Kuhl, J. (2007). Affect sensitivity and affect regulation in dealing with positive and negative affect. *Journal of Research in Personality*, *41*(1), 239–248.

Bogdanov, V. B., Bogdanova, O. V., Gorlov, D. S., Gorgo, Y. P., Dirckx, J. J., Makarchuk, M. Y., ... Critchley, H. (2013). Alexithymia and empathy predict changes in autonomic arousal during affective stimulation. *Cognitive and Behavioral Neurology*, *26*(3), 121–132.

Bokeriia, L. A., Golukhova, E. Z., Polunina, A. G., Davydov, D. M., & Kruglova, M. V. (2008). Alexithymia, depression and heart rate in candidates for cardiac surgery. *International Journal of Cardiology*, *126*(3), 448–449.

Bonanno, G. A., Papa, A., Lalande, K., Westphal, M., & Coifman, K. (2004). The importance of being flexible: The ability to both enhance and suppress emotional expression predicts long-term adjustment. *Psychological Science*, *15*(7), 482–487.

Borhani, K., Borgomaneri, S., Làdavas, E., & Bertini, C. (2016). The effect of alexithymia on early visual processing of emotional body postures. *Biological Psychology*, *115*, 1–8.

Bower, J. E., Low, C. A., Moskowitz, J. T., Sepah, S., & Epel, E. (2008). Benefit finding and physical health: Positive psychological changes and enhanced allostasis. *Social and Personality Psychology Compass, 2*(1), 223–244.

Bradley, M. M., & Lang, P. J. (2000). Emotion and motivation. *Handbook of Psychophysiology, 2*, 602–642.

Byrne, N., & Ditto, B. (2005). Alexithymia, cardiovascular reactivity, and symptom reporting during blood donation. *Psychosomatic Medicine, 67*(3), 471–475.

Carver, C. S., & Scheier, M. F. (1988). A control-process perspective on anxiety. *Anxiety Research, 1*(1), 17–22.

Cisler, J. M., & Koster, E. H. (2010). Mechanisms of attentional biases towards threat in anxiety disorders: An integrative review. *Clinical Psychology Review, 30*(2), 203–216.

Cohen, S., & Rodriguez, M. S. (1995). Pathways linking affective disturbances and physical disorders. *Health Psychology, 14* (5), 374–380.

Connelly, M., & Denney, D. R. (2007). Regulation of emotions during experimental stress in alexithymia. *Journal of Psychosomatic Research, 62*(6), 649–656.

Craske, M. (2015). Optimizing exposure therapy for anxiety disorders: An inhibitory learning and inhibitory regulation approach. *Verhaltenstherapie, 25*(2), 134–143.

Cravo, A. M., Rohenkohl, G., Santos, K. M., & Nobre, A. C. (2017). Temporal anticipation based on memory. *Journal of Cognitive Neuroscience, 29*(12), 2081–2089.

Darrow, S. M., & Follette, W. C. (2014). A behavior analytic interpretation of alexithymia. *Journal of Contextual Behavioral Science, 3*(2), 98–108.

Davidson, R. J. (2015). Comment: Affective chronometry has come of age. *Emotion Review, 7*(4), 368–370.

Davidson, R. J., Jackson, D. C., & Kalin, N. H. (2000). Emotion, plasticity, context, and regulation: Perspectives from affective neuroscience. *Psychological Bulletin, 126*(6), 890–909.

Davydov, D. M. (2017). Alexithymia as a health risk and resilience factor. *Journal of Psychosomatic Research, 101*, 66–67.

Davydov, D. M., Luminet, O., & Zech, E. (2013). An externally oriented style of thinking as a moderator of responses to affective films in women. *International Journal of Psychophysiology, 87*(2), 152–164.

Davydov, D. M., Stewart, R., Ritchie, K., & Chaudieu, I. (2010). Resilience and mental health. *Clinical Psychology Review, 30* (5), 479–495.

De Gucht, V., Fischler, B., & Heiser, W. (2004). Neuroticism, alexithymia, negative affect, and positive affect as determinants of medically unexplained symptoms. *Personality and Individual Differences, 36*(7), 1655–1667.

Delle-Vigne, D., Kornreich, C., Verbanck, P., & Campanella, S. (2014). Subclinical alexithymia modulates early audio-visual perceptive and attentional event-related potentials. *Frontiers in Human Neuroscience, 8*, 106.

del Paso, G. A. R., Godoy, J., & Vila, J. (1993). Respiratory sinus arrhythmia as an index of parasympathetic cardiac control during the cardiac defense response. *Biological Psychology, 35*(1), 17–35.

de Timary, P., Roy, E., Luminet, O., Fillée, C., & Mikolajczak, M. (2008). Relationship between alexithymia, alexithymia factors and salivary cortisol in men exposed to a social stress test. *Psychoneuroendocrinology, 33*(8), 1160–1164.

de Tommaso, M., Federici, A., Santostasi, R., Calabrese, R., Vecchio, E., Lapadula, G., ... Livrea, P. (2011). Laser-evoked potentials habituation in fibromyalgia. *The Journal of Pain, 12*, 116–124.

Eastabrook, J. M., Lanteigne, D. M., & Hollenstein, T. (2013). Decoupling between physiological, self-reported, and expressed emotional responses in alexithymia. *Personality and Individual Differences, 55*(8), 978–982.

Fanselow, M. S. (1994). Neural organization of the defensive behavior system responsible for fear. *Psychonomic Bulletin & Review, 1*(4), 429–438.

Fredrikson, M., & Matthews, K. A. (1990). Cardiovascular responses to behvioral stress and hypertension: A meta-analytic review. *Annals of Behavioral Medicine, 12*(1), 30–39.

Friedman, B. H. (2007). An autonomic flexibility–neurovisceral integration model of anxiety and cardiac vagal tone. *Biological Psychology, 74*(2), 185–199.

Frith, C. D., Stevens, M., Johnstone, E. C., & Crow, T. J. (1982). Skin conductance habituation during acute episodes of schizophrenia: Qualitative differences from anxious and depressed patients. *Psychological Medicine, 12*(3), 575–583.

Fukunishi, I., Sei, H., Morita, Y., & Rahe, R. H. (1999). Sympathetic activity in alexithymics with mother's low care. *Journal of Psychosomatic Research, 46*(6), 579–589.

Ghorbani, F., Khosravani, V., Bastan, F. S., & Ardakani, R. J. (2017). The alexithymia, emotion regulation, emotion regulation difficulties, positive and negative affects, and suicidal risk in alcohol-dependent outpatients. *Psychiatry Research, 252*, 223–230.

Gotlib, I. H., & Joormann, J. (2010). Cognition and depression: Current status and future directions. *Annual Review of Clinical Psychology, 6*, 285–312.

Grissom, N., & Bhatnagar, S. (2009). Habituation to repeated stress: Get used to it. *Neurobiology of Learning and Memory, 92*(2), 215–224.

Grupe, D. W., & Nitschke, J. B. (2013). Uncertainty and anticipation in anxiety: An integrated neurobiological and psychological perspective. *Nature Reviews Neuroscience, 14*(7), 488–501.

Grynberg, D., Chang, B., Corneille, O., Maurage, P., Vermeulen, N., Berthoz, S., & Luminet, O. (2012). Alexithymia and the processing of emotional facial expressions (EFEs): Systematic review, unanswered questions and further perspectives. *PloS One, 7* (8), e42429.

Grynberg, D., Davydov, D. M., Vermeulen, N., & Luminet, O. (2012). Alexithymia is associated with an augmenter profile, but not only: Evidence for anticipation to arousing music. *Scandinavian Journal of Psychology, 53*(5), 375–381.

Gündel, H., Greiner, A., Ceballos-Baumann, A. O., Ladwig, K. H., Von Rad, M., Förstl, H., & Jahn, T. (2004). Alexithymia is no risk factor for exacerbation in spasmodic torticollis patients. *Journal of Psychosomatic Research, 56*(6), 699–705.

Herman, J. (2013). Neural control of chronic stress adaptation. *Frontiers in Behavioral Neuroscience, 7*, 61.

Honkalampi, K., De Berardis, D., Vellante, F., & Viinamäki, H. (2018). Relations depressive between and anxiety alexithymia disorders and alexithymia. In O. Luminet, R. M. Bagby, & G. J. Taylor (Eds.), *Alexithymia: Advances in research, theory, and clinical practice* (pp. 142–157). Cambridge: Cambridge University Press.

Irwin, M. R., & Miller, A. H. (2007). Depressive disorders and immunity: 20 years of progress and discovery. *Brain, Behavior, and Immunity, 21*(4), 374–383.

Jandl, M., Steyer, J., & Kaschka, W. P. (2010). Suicide risk markers in major depressive disorder: A study of electrodermal activity and event-related potentials. *Journal of Affective Disorders, 123*(1–3), 138–149.

Johnston, M. M., & Finney, S. J. (2010). Measuring basic needs satisfaction: Evaluating previous research and conducting new psychometric evaluations of the basic needs satisfaction in general scale. *Contemporary Educational Psychology, 35*(4), 280–296.

Juster, R.-P., McEwen, B. S., & Lupien, S. J. (2010). Allostatic load biomarkers of chronic stress and impact on health and cognition. *Neuroscience & Biobehavioral Reviews, 35*(1), 2–16.

Kano, M., Grabe, H. J., & Terock, J. (2018). Genetic immune factors system and functioning endocrine associated and alexithymia. In O. Luminet, R. M. Bagby, & G. J. Taylor (Eds.), *Alexithymia: Advances in research, theory, and clinical practice* (pp. 267–289). Cambridge: Cambridge University Press.

Kashdan, T. B., & Rottenberg, J. (2010). Psychological flexibility as a fundamental aspect of health. *Clinical Psychology Review, 30* (7), 865–878.

Koole, S. L. (2009). The psychology of emotion regulation: An integrative review. *Cognition and Emotion, 23*(1), 4–41.

Krystal, H. (2015). *Integration and self healing: Affect, trauma, alexithymia.* New York: Routledge.

Kubzansky, L. D., & Thurston, R. C. (2007). Emotional vitality and incident coronary heart disease. *Archives of General Psychiatry, 64*(12), 1393–1401.

Kuppens, P., & Verduyn, P. (2017). Emotion dynamics. *Current Opinion in Psychology, 17*, 22–26.

Lane, R. D., Ahern, G. L., Schwartz, G. E., & Kaszniak, A. W. (1997). Is alexithymia the emotional equivalent of blindsight? *Biological Psychiatry, 42*(9), 834–844.

Lang, P. J. (1979). A bio-informational theory of emotional imagery. *Psychophysiology, 16*(6), 495–512.

Lang, P. J., Bradley, M. M., & Cuthbert, B. N. (1997). Motivated attention: Affect, activation, and action. In P. J. Lang, R. F. Simons, & M. T. Balaban (Eds.), *Attention and orienting: Sensory and motivational processes* (pp. 97–135). Mahwah, NJ: Lawrence Erlbaum Associates Publishers.

Leonidou, C., & Panayiotou, G. (2018). How do illness-anxious individuals process health-threatening information? A systematic review of evidence for the cognitive-behavioral model. *Journal of Psychosomatic Research, 111*, 100–115.

Leonidou, C., Panayiotou, G., Bati, A., & Karekla, M. (2019). Coping with psychosomatic symptoms: The buffering role of psychological flexibility and impact on quality of life. *Journal of Health Psychology, 24*, 175–187.

Liu, H., Sarapas, C., & Shankman, S. A. (2016). Anticipatory reward deficits in melancholia. *Journal of Abnormal Psychology, 125* (5), 631–640.

Loewenstein, G., & Lerner, J. S. . (2003). The role of affect in decision making. In R. J. Davidson, K. R. Scherer, & H. H. Goldsmith (Eds.), *Handbook of affective sciences* (pp. 619–642). New York: Oxford University Press.

Luminet, O., Rimé, B., Bagby, R. M., & Taylor, G. (2004). A multimodal investigation of emotional responding in alexithymia. *Cognition and Emotion, 18*(6), 741–766.

Luminet, O., Vermeulen, N., Demaret, C., Taylor, G. J., & Bagby, R. M. (2006). Alexithymia and levels of processing: Evidence for an overall deficit in remembering emotion words. *Journal of Research in Personality, 40*(5), 713–733.

Martínez Sánchez, F. M., & García, M. A. (2011). Sympathetic reactivity to experimentally induced stress in alexithymia. *Anales de Psicología/Annals of Psychology, 27*(3), 757–762.

Martínez Sánchez, F., Ortiz Soria, B., & Ato García, M. (2001). Subjective and autonomic stress responses in alexithymia. *Psicothema, 13*(1), 57–62.

McEwen, B. S. (1998). Stress, adaptation, and disease: Allostasis and allostatic load. *Annals of the New York Academy of Sciences, 840*(1), 33–44.

McEwen, B. S. (2007). Physiology and neurobiology of stress and adaptation: Central role of the brain. *Physiological Reviews, 87* (3), 873–904.

McEwen, B. S., & Gianaros, P. J. (2010). Central role of the brain in stress and adaptation: Links to socioeconomic status, health, and disease. *Annals of the New York Academy of Sciences, 1186*(1), 190–222.

McTeague, L. M., & Lang, P. J. (2012). The anxiety spectrum and the reflex physiology of defense: From circumscribed fear to broad distress. *Depression and Anxiety, 29*(4), 264–281.

Morie, K. P., & Ridout, N. (2018). Alexithymia and maladaptive regulatory behaviors in substance use disorders and eating disorders. In O. Luminet, R. M. Bagby, & G. J. Taylor (Eds.), *Alexithymia: Advances in research, theory, and clinical practice* (pp. 158–173). Cambridge: Cambridge University Press.

Morriss, J., Taylor, A. N., Roesch, E. B., & van Reekum, C. M. (2013). Still feeling it: The time course of emotional recovery from an attentional perspective. *Frontiers in Human Neuroscience, 7*, 201.

Mossbridge, J., Tressoldi, P. E., & Utts, J. (2012). Predictive physiological anticipation preceding seemingly unpredictable stimuli: A meta-analysis. *Frontiers in Psychology, 3*, 390.

Panayiotou, G. (2018). Alexithymia as a core trait in psychosomatic and other psychological disorders. In C. Charis & G. Panayiotou (Eds.), *Somatoform and other psychosomatic disorders* (pp. 89–106). Cham: Springer.

Panayiotou, G., & Constantinou, E. (2017). Emotion dysregulation in alexithymia: Startle reactivity to fearful affective imagery and its relation to heart rate variability. *Psychophysiology, 54*, 1323–1334.

Panayiotou, G., Leonidou, C., Constantinou, E., Hart, J., Rinehart, K. L., Sy, J. T., & Björgvinsson, T. (2015). Do alexithymic individuals avoid their feelings? Experiential avoidance mediates the association between alexithymia, psychosomatic, and depressive symptoms in a community and a clinical sample. *Comprehensive Psychiatry, 56*, 206–216.

Panayiotou, G., Leonidou, C., Constantinou, E., & Michaelides, M. P. (2018a). Self-Awareness in alexithymia and associations with social anxiety. *Current Psychology*, 1–10. Retrieved from https://link.springer.com/article/10.1007

Panayiotou, G., Panteli, M., & Vlemincx, E. (2018b). Processing emotions in alexithymia: A systematic review of physiological markers. In O. Luminet, R. M. Bagby, & G. J. Taylor (Eds.), *Alexithymia: Advances in research, theory, and clinical practice* (pp. 291–320). Cambridge: Cambridge University Press.

Phillips, M. L., Drevets, W. C., Rauch, S. L., & Lane, R. (2003). Neurobiology of emotion perception I: The neural basis of normal emotion perception. *Biological Psychiatry, 54*(5), 504–514.

Pieper, S., Brosschot, J. F., van der Leeden, R., & Thayer, J. F. (2007). Cardiac effects of momentary assessed worry episodes and stressful events. *Psychosomatic Medicine, 69*(9), 901–909.

Pollatos, O., & Gramann, K. (2011). Electrophysiological evidence of early processing deficits in alexithymia. *Biological Psychology, 87*(1), 113–121.

Pollatos, O., Werner, N. S., Duschek, S., Schandry, R., Matthias, E., Traut-Mattausch, E., & Herbert, B. M. (2011). Differential effects of alexithymia subscales on autonomic reactivity and anxiety during social stress. *Journal of Psychosomatic Research*, *70*(6), 525–533.

Porcelli, P., & Taylor, G. J. (2018). Alexithymia and physical illness: A psychosomatic approach. In O. Luminet, R. M. Bagby, & G. J. Taylor (Eds.), *Alexithymia: Advances in research, theory, and clinical practice* (pp. 105–126). Cambridge: Cambridge University Press.

Porges, S. W. (2001). The polyvagal theory: Phylogenetic substrates of a social nervous system. *International Journal of Psychophysiology*, *42*(2), 123–146.

Rabavilas, A. D. (1987). Electrodermal activity in low and high alexithymia neurotic patients. *Psychotherapy and Psychosomatics*, *47*(2), 101–104.

Rankin, C. H., Abrams, T., Barry, R. J., Bhatnagar, S., Clayton, D. F., Colombo, J., … Marsland, S. (2009). Habituation revisited: An updated and revised description of the behavioral characteristics of habituation. *Neurobiology of Learning and Memory*, *92* (2), 135–138.

Salovey, P., Mayer, J. D., Goldman, S. L., Turvey, C., & Palfai, T. P. (1995). Emotional attention, clarity, and repair: Exploring emotional intelligence using the trait meta-mood scale. In J. W. Pennebaker (Ed.), *Emotion, disclosure, & health* (pp. 125–154). Washington, DC: American Psychological Association.

Sarchiapone, M., Iosue, M., Carli, V., Amore, M., Baca-Garcia, E., Batra, A., … Gusmao, R. (2017). EUDOR-A multi-centre research program: A naturalistic, European multi-centre clinical study of EDOR test in adult patients with primary depression. *BMC Psychiatry*, *17*(1), 108.

Schäfer, R., Schneider, C., Tress, W., & Franz, M. (2007). Cortical augmenting in alexithymic subjects after unpleasant acoustic stimulation. *Journal of Psychosomatic Research*, *63*(4), 357–364.

Scott, W., & McCracken, L. M. (2015). Psychological flexibility, acceptance and commitment therapy, and chronic pain. *Current Opinion in Psychology*, *2*, 91–96.

Scott, W., McCracken, L. M., & Norton, S. (2015). A confirmatory factor analysis of facets of psychological flexibility in a sample of people seeking treatment for chronic pain. *Annals of Behavioral Medicine*, *50*(2), 285–296.

Shalev, A. Y., Peri, T., Brandes, D., Freedman, S., Orr, S. P., & Pitman, R. K. (2000). Auditory startle response in trauma survivors with posttraumatic stress disorder: A prospective study. *American Journal of Psychiatry*, *157*(2), 255–261.

Sheppes, G., Scheibe, S., Suri, G., & Gross, J. J. (2011). Emotion-regulation choice. *Psychological Science*, *22*(11), 1391–1396.

Shiffman, S., Stone, A. A., & Hufford, M. R. (2008). Ecological momentary assessment. *Annual Review of Clinical Psychology*, *4*, 1–32.

Skinner, E. A., & Zimmer-Gembeck, M. J. (2007). The development of coping. *Annual Review of Psychology*, *58*, 119–144.

Stabbe, O. K., Rolffs, J. L., & Rogge, R. D. (2019). Flexibly and/or inflexibly embracing life: Identifying fundamental approaches to life with latent profile analyses on the dimensions of the hexaflex model. *Journal of Contextual Behavioral Science*, *12*, 106–118.

Starita, F., Làdavas, E., & Di Pellegrino, G. (2016). Reduced anticipation of negative emotional events in alexithymia. *Scientific Reports*, *6*, 27664.

Tavakoli, N., Broyles, A., Reid, E. K., Sandoval, J. R., & Correa-Fernández, V. (2019). Psychological inflexibility as it relates to stress, worry, generalized anxiety, and somatization in an ethnically diverse sample of college students. *Journal of Contextual Behavioral Science*, *11*, 1–5.

Trull, T. J., Lane, S. P., Koval, P., & Ebner-Priemer, U. W. (2015). Affective dynamics in psychopathology. *Emotion Review*, *7* (4), 355–361.

Uher, T. (2010). Alexithymia and immune dysregulation: A critical review. *Activitas Nervosa Superior*, *52*(1), 40–44.

Verkuil, B., Brosschot, J. F., Putman, P., & Thayer, J. F. (2009). Interacting effects of worry and anxiety on attentional disengagement from threat. *Behaviour Research and Therapy*, *47*(2), 146–152.

Vermeulen, N., Domachowska, I., & Nielson, K. A. (2018). Memory and executive functions. In O. Luminet, R. M. Bagby, & G. J. Taylor (Eds.), *Alexithymia: Advances in research, theory, and clinical practice* (pp. 78–89). Cambridge: Cambridge University Press.

Vermeulen, N., Luminet, O., De Sousa, M. C., & Campanella, S. (2008). Categorical perception of anger is disrupted in alexithymia: Evidence from a visual ERP study. *Cognition and Emotion*, *22*(6), 1052–1067.

Vermeulen, N., Toussaint, J., & Luminet, O. (2010). The influence of alexithymia and music on the incidental memory for emotion words. *European Journal of Personality*, *24*(6), 551–568.

Walker, F. R., Thomson, A., Pfingst, K., Vlemincx, E., Aidman, E., & Nalivaiko, E. (2019). Habituation of the electrodermal response – a biological correlate of resilience? *PloS One*, *14*(1), e0210078.

Watson, D., & Tellegen, A. (1985). Toward a consensual structure of mood. *Psychological Bulletin*, *98*(2), 219–235.

Waugh, C. E., Thompson, R. J., & Gotlib, I. H. (2011). Flexible emotional responsiveness in trait resilience. *Emotion*, *11*(5), 1059–1067.

Zautra, A. J. (2009). Resilience: One part recovery, two parts sustainability. *Journal of Personality*, *77*(6), 1935–1943.

Negative valence specific deficits in judgements of musical affective quality in alexithymia

Joel L. Larwood, Eric J. Vanman and Genevieve A. Dingle

ABSTRACT

Alexithymia is characterised by a lack of words for emotional experiences and it has been implicated in deficits in emotion processing. Research in this area has typically focused on judgements of discrete emotions rather than of affect, which is a precursor to emotion construction. In the current study, higher alexithymia was predicted to be related to more neutral judgements of valence and arousal of music representing a range of emotions. Participants ($N = 162$) listened to ten 15-second musical pieces that represented five target emotions (happy, sad, tender, angry, and fearful) and rated the valence and arousal of each. Participants also listed emotion words they knew to be expressed in music. Analyses revealed that alexithymia was not related to the number of emotion words generated but was related to valence-specific affect judgements of music. Participants higher in alexithymia rated sad, angry, and fearful pieces as more neutral in valence and arousal. Alexithymia was not related to ratings of valence or arousal for happy and tender pieces. These findings suggest that perceptual deficits in alexithymia may be specific to negative emotions. Our results are consistent with the idea that alexithymia is related to the direction of attention away from negative stimuli.

Negative valence-specific deficits in judgements of musical affective quality in alexithymia

Alexithymia is a sub-clinical personality trait primarily characterised by a lack of words for emotional experiences. It consists of three facets: difficulty identifying feelings, difficulty describing feelings, and an externally oriented thinking style (Bagby, Parker, & Taylor, 1994). Difficulty identifying and describing feelings reflects cognitive deficits in the processing of emotions and emotional information (Goerlich-Dobre, Votinov, Habel, Pripfl, & Lamm, 2015). Alexithymia is also related to a reduced perceived, but not objective, ability to monitor bodily sensations (Zamariola, Vlemincx, Corneille, & Luminet, 2018). Higher levels of alexithymia are related to reduced capacity for forming mental representations of emotions and reduced ability to accurately label emotions (Grynberg et al., 2012a; Ihme et al., 2014). These difficulties observed in alexithymia are particularly relevant within constructionist theories of emotion.

Barrett (2006, 2017) proposed that emotions are constructed in relation to bodily sensations, situational context, and knowledge of what constitutes a specific emotion, such as sadness or anger. Emotional ability is supported by the use of emotion words, which organise conceptual information and reduce uncertainty about an experience (Barrett, Lindquist, & Gendron, 2007). Vital but not sufficient for the emotion construction process is the awareness of core affect (Barrett, 2017; Russell, 2003). Core affect consists of two dimensions: valence (how pleasant or unpleasant a feeling or object is) and arousal (how energising or activating a feeling or object is). Russell (2003) proposed that all objects and events have an affective quality, and therefore can be considered along the dimensions of valence and arousal. However, not all objects or events will allow for a change in experienced core affect or emotion experience (see also

Frijda, 2016). For instance, a landscape may be judged as having an affective quality but this judgement of affective quality will not necessarily lead to an affective or emotional experience. For an emotion to be either experienced or perceived, the affective quality must be categorised into an emotion through an act of conceptualisation. This conceptualisation process involves considering previous instances of an emotion and evaluating them against the current situation (Barrett, 2006). Emotion judgements, therefore, have two key elements: affective judgements, and integration of these judgements with existing linguistically supported concepts.

Barrett (2006) proposed that people with alexithymia have difficulty with conceptualising core affect into an emotion category. Emotion concepts are informed by past experiences. Accordingly, the conceptual deficits seen in alexithymia may stem from an earlier deficit in affect judgement and a lack of integration of affective information with emotion concepts. A meta-analysis on neural activation during emotional stimuli presentation (van der Velde et al., 2013) found that higher alexithymia scores were related to increased activation in the anterior cingulate gyrus for easy or observational tasks but decreased activation for demanding tasks (i.e. emotion ratings). Furthermore, decreased activation in the amygdala and dorsomedial prefrontal cortex (dmPFC) was found during negative stimuli presentation, in addition to decreased activation of anterior insula during positive stimuli presentation. Reduced grey-matter volume has been found in the left middle temporal gyrus but this does not correspond to reduced activation during stimulus presentation (Grabe et al., 2014; van der Velde et al., 2013).

According to constructionist theory, neural areas are involved in the cognitive production of emotion through the integration of interoceptive (internal) and exteroceptive (external) sensations (Lindquist, Wager, Kober, Bliss-Moreau, & Barrett, 2012). Internal and external sensory processing are facilitated by the anterior cingulate cortex (realisation of core affect), amygdala (attending to salient external cues), and anterior insula (interoceptive awareness) (Lindquist et al., 2012). Finally, the dmPFC supports emotion concept knowledge. It is not just the linguistic or conceptual networks of the brain that are compromised in alexithymia but also areas that correspond to attending to and realising core affect.

In a systematic review, Grynberg et al. (2012a) highlighted reduced accuracy in the labelling of facial emotions in people with alexithymia. Measures of depression and anxiety explained some of the variance in these results. However, the reduced accuracy in labelling facial emotions may also stem from poor emotion concept representation. This is consistent with findings in the dmPFC and left temporal lobe. Emotion processing deficits in alexithymia have additionally been associated with reduced sensitivity to perceptual cues. For example, Vermeulen, Luminet, Cordovil De Sousa, and Campanella (2008) and Aftanas, Varlamov, Reva, and Pavlov (2003) concluded that higher alexithymia scores corresponded with reduced attention to emotional stimuli. However, Franz, Schaefer, Schneider, Sitte, and Bachor (2004) found no ERP indicators of reduced emotion perception in people with alexithymia but did find people with higher alexithymia were less likely to linguistically refer to emotions. Considering this body of literature, there are grounds to support the idea that alexithymia is characterised by reduced emotional attention and spontaneous categorisation of emotional stimuli. Parker, Prkachin, and Prkachin (2005) suggested that task time constraints further reduce the performance of people higher in alexithymia during emotional tasks. However, deficits in the processing of visual stimuli over extended time periods have been found on the affective dimension of valence in alexithymia (Luminet, Rimé, Bagby, & Taylor, 2004; Vanman, Dawson, & Brennan, 1998).

For an emotion to be judged, the stimulus must be considered emotionally relevant. Scherer (2005) posited that music is judged as emotional without serving a behavioural purpose. Consistent with this, Juslin and Laukka (2004) found emotions to be readily judged in musical excerpts. Alexithymia has been associated with reduced sensitivity to discrepancy between musical stimuli and primed emotion words (Goerlich, Witteman, Aleman, & Martens, 2011). However, this alexithymia effect may have been over-estimated due to the short presentation period (Parker et al., 2005). Musical stimuli presented for longer periods of time have been judged and verbalised less accurately by people with higher levels of alexithymia – even when negative mood and autism traits have been controlled for (Allen, Davis, & Hill, 2013; Bayot et al., 2014; Heaton et al., 2012; Punkanen, Eerola, & Erkkilä, 2011; Taruffi, Allen, Downing, & Heaton, 2017).

Researchers have yet to examine the judgement of affect in musical emotions in relation to alexithymia. Allen et al. (2013) suggested judgements of musical emotion are first influenced by perceived affective quality. However, the authors only studied categorical emotion judgements. Cespedes-Guevara and Eerola (2018) also argued that musical emotions are constructed around affective qualities, past experiences, and associations with the music. Vermeulen, Toussaint, and Luminet (2010) found that music influenced cognitive processing for people with higher levels of alexithymia such that negative music reduced the encoding of semantic information. It is, therefore, possible that negative emotions are still readily experienced and integrated during behavioural tasks. However, these results do not demonstrate whether the deficits seen in emotional judgements in alexithymia stem from difficulties at an affective level or at a higher level of emotion conceptualisation.

Music is an ideal stimulus type to investigate the contribution of alexithymia on emotion judgements because it is readily processed as emotionally relevant. Neurological findings suggest that alexithymia is negatively related to activity in brain regions employed in both the encoding of affective information and integration of affective information with conceptual knowledge. The purpose of the present study was to investigate whether the deficits observed in higher levels of alexithymia lie in judgements of affective quality (valence/arousal). Participants were asked to recall emotion words associated with music. Musical stimuli representing five emotion categories of different valence and arousal combinations (happy, tender, sad, angry, fearful) were then presented. We hypothesised that people higher in alexithymia would (a) have reduced recall of emotion words for music, and (b) would judge arousal and valence of all musical stimuli as more neutral than participants lower in alexithymia.[4] No specific hypotheses were made about individual facets of alexithymia; however, relationships between alexithymia facets and other variables were explored. These *post-hoc* analyses were conducted following reviewer suggestions because differential processes have been found for the facets of alexithymia and negative mood (see Grynberg et al., 2012a).

Method

Participants

One-hundred and sixty-two participants were sampled using the online recruitment platform *Prolific* (http://prolific.co). Participants were aged 18–25 years ($M = 21.52$, $SD = 1.94$) and 91 were females. To be eligible for the study, participants had to be aged 18–25 and residents of the United Kingdom, with no additional exclusion criteria applied. Participants were paid £1.25 for their participation in the online survey (15 minutes at £5 an hour) and the study was advertised as "exploring music and emotions".

Stimuli and measures

Musical Emotion Concepts. In a text box participants freely responded to the following prompt: "In this box please write as many emotions as you can think of that are expressed in music". Linguistic Inquiry Word Count software (Pennebaker, Boyd, Jordan, & Blackburn, 2015) was used to count the number of words listed and the proportion of positive and negative emotion words. The proportion of positive and negative words was then converted to a count of positive and negative emotion words that were summed to give the total number of emotion words.

Musical stimuli. Ten pieces of music representing five emotions (happiness, tenderness,[1] anger, fear, and sadness) were taken from the film soundtrack list provided by Eerola and Vuoskoski (2011).[2] All pieces were 15 seconds in duration and instrumental only.

Affective judgements. Participants were given the instruction to rate the emotion of the music on two semantic differential scales. The first scale measured valence and was measured from −3 (negative) to 3 (positive) and the second measured arousal from −3 (low energy) to 3 (high energy). The valence and arousal judged for each target emotion was the average valence and arousal score for the two musical pieces representing the given target emotion.

Alexithymia. Alexithymia was measured using the 20-item Toronto Alexithymia Scale (TAS-20; Bagby et al., 1994). The TAS-20 is widely used to measure alexithymia and demonstrated good internal consistency in the current sample, Cronbach's alpha = .84. The difficulty describing feelings and difficulty identifying feelings subscales demonstrated good internal consistency, Cronbach's alphas > .80, while the externally oriented subscale demonstrated weak internal consistency, Cronbach's alpha = .37.

Depression. Depression was measured using the depression subscale of the Depression Anxiety and Stress Scale (DASS; Lovibond & Lovibond, 1995). The DASS is widely used by health professionals to assess for depression and was originally collected in the data set for another project. The depression subscale of the DASS showed excellent internal consistency, Cronbach's alpha = .94. The stress and anxiety subscales were not analysed for this study.

Procedure

The study was completed online using the Qualtrics survey platform. After providing consent, participants were asked to complete the measure of musical emotion concepts, 60 seconds was allowed for this before the page automatically advanced. They were then instructed to listen to each musical piece and make a rating of their judgement of the affect in the musical piece using the sliders showing the semantic differential scale. Participants then listened to and rated all ten musical pieces in a randomised order before completing alexithymia and demographic measures. Additional mood and personality measures were collected for a separate study.[3]

Ethical approval

Ethical approval for the study was given by the Faculty of Health and Behavioural Sciences at The University of Queensland.

Results

Considering first the hypothesised relationship between emotion word generation and alexithymia, zero-order correlations were examined between total alexithymia scores and total number of emotion words. No correlation was found between these two measures. Although not hypothesised, we explored the correlations between subscales of alexithymia and positive and negative word frequency. The correlation matrix can be seen in Table 1, along with descriptive statistics. Only one significant relationship between an alexithymia facet and lexicon count was found, whereby difficulty describing feelings negatively related to positive music emotion lexicon. However, this relationship was no longer significant when controlling for depression, $p = .531$.

Two mixed general linear models with participant set as a grouping variable were conducted. Alexithymia, musical piece target emotion and their interaction were entered as predictors in the model and descriptive statistics for ratings of each target emotion can be seen in Table 2. Ratings of valence were assessed in the first model. Model results are presented in Table 3, with simple slope estimates provided along with a graphical representation in Figure 1. Alexithymia scores were inconsistently related to ratings of valence across stimuli. For negatively valenced music, alexithymia was related to more neutral judgements of valence. However, no relationship was found between alexithymia and positively valenced music on judgements of valence. Likewise, alexithymia did not predict arousal ratings for all target emotions. The model results are also reported in Table 3 and shown in Figure 2 along with simple slope estimates. Alexithymia related to higher arousal judgements for sad music and lower arousal judgements for angry and fearful music with no relation found for happy or tender music. The inclusion of depression as a control variable did not

Table 1. Means, standard deviations, and correlations with confidence intervals for relationships between alexithymia and words listed.

Variable	*M*	*SD*	Range	1	2	3	4	5	6	7
1. Alexithymia	54.31	11.91	26–81							
2. Externally Oriented Thinking	20.19	3.93	10–31	.58** [.47, .68]						
3. Difficulty Describing Feelings	15.56	4.70	5–24	.84** [.79, .88]	.26** [.11, .40]					
4. Difficulty Identifying Feelings	18.57	6.32	7–34	.89** [.86, .92]	.28** [.13, .42]	.68** [.59, .76]				
5. Depression	5.81	5.12	0–18	.55** [.43, .65]	.17* [.02, .32]	.54** [.42, .64]	.52** [.40, .62]			
6. Positive emotion words listed	2.99	1.47	0–9	−.13 [−.28, .03]	.05 [−.11, .20]	−.19* [−.33, −.03]	−.13 [−.28, .02]	−.17* [−.32, −.02]		
7. Negative emotion words listed	3.68	2.12	0–11	.02 [−.14, .17]	.03 [−.13, .18]	.05 [−.11, .20]	−.02 [−.17, .14]	.05 [−.11, .20]	.20* [.05, .34]	
8. Total Emotion words listed	6.67	2.81	0–15	−.05 [−.20, .10]	.05 [−.11, .20]	−.06 [−.21, .10]	−.08 [−.23, .07]	−.05 [−.20, .10]	.67** [.58, .75]	.86** [.81, .89]

Notes: Confidence Intervals for each correlation are presented in square brackets. Sixty−one participants were below the cut off of 51 for non-alexithymic. *$p < .05$, **$p < .01$.

Table 2. Descriptive statistics of perception of valence and arousal for each music emotion category.

	Valence	Arousal
Sad	−0.96 (*1.16*)	−1.23 (*1.13*)
Happy	2.21 (*0.91*)	2.14 (*0.88*)
Fearful	−1.47 (*1.09*)	0.69 (*1.28*)
Tender	0.75 (*1.10*)	−0.50 (*1.04*)
Angry	−1.00 (*1.13*)	1.16 (*1.36*)

Note: Data presented as Mean (*standard deviation*) with scores ranging from −3 (negative valence/low arousal) to + 3 (positive valence/high arousal)

improve model fit for valence or arousal ratings (Table 4) and follow up analyses were subsequently not conducted on the models including depression.

Discussion

Alexithymia has been related to reduced accuracy in the perception and judgement of emotional stimuli on a categorical level. However, less is known about how alexithymia influences the judgements of a song's affective quality. The current study investigated how total alexithymia scores related to affective quality judgements of musical stimuli for different emotions. Past studies on musical stimuli have shown deficits in the processing of emotional stimuli over short (<1sec) and long (>10 secs) time periods. However, these studies have not evaluated the influence of alexithymia on judgements of core affect – a vital process for the construction of emotion.

The results did not support the first hypothesis that higher alexithymia would be related to fewer emotion words recalled as conveyed by music. However, exploratory analyses revealed a negative relationship between the difficulty describing feelings subscale and the number of positive emotions listed as being present in music. To the best of our knowledge, this is the first study to investigate emotion word generation in the context of music. Past literature has focused on frequency of words used to describe previous events and found alexithymia to predict a reduced range of emotion words (Wagner & Lee, 2008; Wotschack & Klann-Delius, 2013). Consistent with this, Luminet et al. (2004) found the facet of difficulty describing feelings to predict reduced use of emotion words for films. This suggests that people who struggle to explicitly label feelings may also struggle to encode or recall categorical emotional information regarding music. In our study, the relationship was nullified when depression was controlled for, consistent with research showing a positive memory bias associated with depression (Gotlib, Joormann, & Foland-Ross, 2014).

Contrary to our results, Luminet, Vermeulen, Demaret, Taylor, and Bagby (2006) found alexithymia to be related to difficulties in recalling previously presented emotion words. Accordingly, task factors may influence the recall of emotion words. Considering our measurement approach, we are only able to make claims about the recall of words known to be associated with musical emotions. This measurement does not capture the complexity of the emotion concept held, or how easily the emotion concept is accessed and integrated with core affect.

The primary purpose of this study was to evaluate whether alexithymic deficits are present in the

Table 3. GLMM output for ratings of valence and arousal with tender music condition set as referent level.

	Valence			Arousal		
Predictors	Estimates	CI	*p*	Estimates	CI	*p*
(Intercept)	0.86	0.09–1.62	**0.029**	−0.71	−1.52–0.10	0.087
Alexithymia	−0.00	−0.02–0.01	0.776	0.00	−0.01–0.02	0.600
Sad	−3.26	−4.30 – −2.22	**<0.001**	−2.14	−3.25 – −1.03	**<0.001**
Happy	1.87	0.83–2.91	**<0.001**	3.02	1.92–4.13	**<0.001**
Fearful	−3.38	−4.42 – −2.34	**<0.001**	2.32	1.22–3.43	**<0.001**
Angry	−2.80	−3.84 – −1.76	**<0.001**	3.49	2.39–4.60	**<0.001**
Alexithymia*Happy	−0.01	−0.03–0.01	0.441	−0.01	−0.03–0.01	0.479
Alexithymia*Sad	0.03	0.01–0.05	**0.003**	0.03	0.01–0.05	**0.010**
Alexithymia*Fearful	0.02	0.00–0.04	**0.025**	−0.02	−0.04 – −0.00	**0.039**
Alexithymia*Angry	0.02	0.00–0.04	**0.044**	−0.03	−0.05 – −0.01	**0.001**
Random Effects						
σ^2	1.04			1.18		
τ_{00}	0.10_{id}			0.09_{id}		
ICC	0.08_{id}			0.07_{id}		
Observations	810			810		
Marginal R^2/Conditional R^2	0.631/0.662			0.539/0.572		

Note: Tender was set as the referent condition as it is the emotion category closest to neutral arousal and valence.

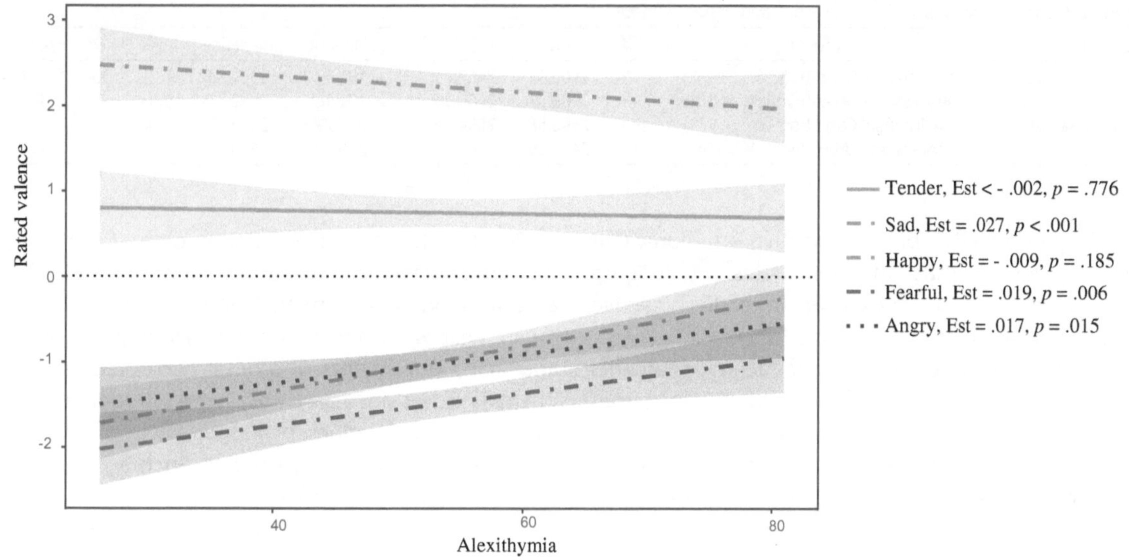

Figure 1. Simple slopes of alexithymia at each level of target emotion for judgements of valence. Note: 95% confidence interval is indicated by coloured bands.

judgement of affective quality (valence/arousal). Results did not support our second hypothesis that higher alexithymia scores would predict more neutral judgements of valence and arousal alike. Higher alexithymia only predicted more neutral judgements of valence and arousal when the target emotion of the song was negatively valenced (i.e. sad, angry, and fearful music). As a result, affect processing or judgement of negative emotions may be impaired for people with higher alexithymia, even when a greater period of time is allowed for processing. This is consistent with research on nonverbal emotions in alexithymia. Bayot et al. (2014) found that total alexithymia scores were related to reduced

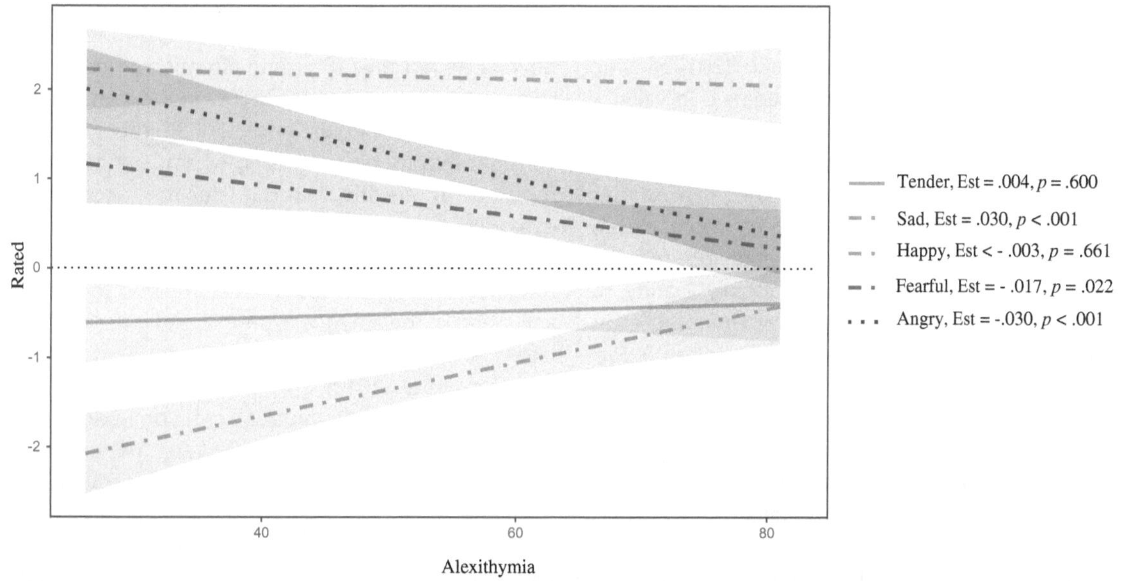

Figure 2. Simple slopes of alexithymia at each level of target emotion for judgements of arousal. Note: 95% confidence interval is indicated by coloured bands.

Table 4. Model comparison with and without depression in model.

Dependent variable	Model	*Df*	AIC	BIC	logLiklihood	deviance	χ^2	*Df*	$p(>\chi^2)$
Valence Rating	Alexithymia*Condition	12	2406.34	2462.71	−1191.17	2382.34		NA	NA
	Depression + Alexithymia*Condition	13	2408.31	2469.38	−1191.16	2382.31	0.03	1	0.87
Arousal Rating	Alexithymia*Condition	12	2498.58	2554.94	−1237.29	2474.58	NA	NA	NA
	Depression + Alexithymia*Condition	13	2499.56	2560.62	−1236.78	2473.56	1.02	1	0.31

accuracy in negative but not positive emotions. Our results suggest that the difficulties in judging musical emotions are present at the earlier affective judgement phase of construction.

Alexithymia may be related to reduced judgements of valence and arousal but only when the target emotion of the stimulus is negative. Our results contradict past findings of a global deficit in valence perception (Luminet et al., 2004; Vanman et al., 1998). Discrepancy in statistical power may explain these results. In previous studies, alexithymia was dichotomised and therefore less sensitive to a higher-order interaction with stimulus valence. Our study also specifically tested different target emotions that previous studies by Luminet et al. (2004) and Vanman et al. (1998) did not. There may still be a true effect of alexithymia on positively valenced affect judgements that our study was not sensitive to finding. This interpretation would still be consistent with the moderation found in the current study. This is the case as the moderation indicates the effect of alexithymia on valence and arousal ratings was stronger for negatively valenced stimuli than positively valenced stimuli.

Our results are also inconsistent with Grynberg, Davydov, Vermeulen, and Luminet (2012b) who found songs high in arousal and negative in valence lead to increased negative mood in people with higher alexithymia scores. However, this result deals with emotional consequences of negative stimuli rather than judgements and may be more closely related to the poor emotion regulation observed in alexithymia (Preece, Becerra, Robinson, Dandy, & Allan, 2018). A systematic review by Grynberg et al. (2012a) suggested a global deficit in emotion judgements in alexithymia but did not compare differences in effect sizes. A meta-regression study would be well suited to establishing whether the deficit in alexithymia is indeed valence specific or if the deficit is global but larger for negatively valenced emotions. Alternatively, there may be no moderating effect of valence, which would indicate our significant interaction was a false positive.

Perhaps the most interesting finding of our study was that, when the target emotion was negative, arousal judgements moved towards neutral. This meant that when target arousal was high (i.e. anger and fear), judgements of arousal decreased as alexithymia scores increased but when target arousal was low (i.e. sadness), judgements of arousal increased with alexithymia scores. Such a finding, to the best of our knowledge, is novel in the literature. It suggests that alexithymia relates to a multi-dimensional blunting of affective judgements or a shift towards stimuli being seen as less intense in their affective quality in terms of valence and arousal when they are negatively valenced. In the context of previous findings that have looked at categorical rather than dimensional judgements it may be that the emotion judgement deficits in alexithymia are seen early in the construction process (i.e. before emotional labelling). Our results are also consistent with those of Roedema and Simons (1999) who showed alexithymia to influence arousal judgements when all stimuli were negative.

Our findings can be interpreted in the context of patterns of neural activation in alexithymia. Previous ERP studies have suggested that people higher in alexithymia do not give the same attention or processing to emotional stimuli as those low in the trait (Aftanas et al., 2003; Vermeulen et al., 2008). These findings consider automatic processing which is known to be reduced in alexithymia but do not account for extended processing as was the case in our study. Turning to the facial processing and alexithymia literature, negatively valenced faces are related to reduced activation of the amygdala, dmPFC and anterior cingulate when the task involved making judgements (van der Velde et al., 2013). This reduced activation is also likely present during musical emotion judgements, given the regions of interest are not modality specific. Therefore, potential reduced activation of the dmPFC, anterior cingulate, and amygdala may explain the blunted judgments of the negatively valenced stimuli in our study (Lindquist et al., 2012; Posner et al., 2009).

Alexithymia is related to reduced attention to emotive stimuli and it may be that this is particularly the case for negative emotions (Suslow, Junghanns, Donges, & Arolt, 2001). Musical emotion perception can lead to an emotional response (Juslin & Laukka, 2004). Therefore, the direction of attention away from negative stimuli may explain our results. People with higher levels of alexithymia have a reduced ability to effectively regulate emotions and are less able to manage any negative emotion that may follow negative emotion processing (Preece et al., 2018). Our findings that alexithymia dampens the affective judgements of negative stimuli can be understood in terms of participants avoiding negative emotional experiences. Such a regulation-based motivation would not be required for positive emotional stimuli as positive emotions are more readily tolerated. Despite the reduced processing of negatively valenced stimuli in alexithymia, negative affect is higher in people with alexithymia (da Silva, Vasco, & Watson, 2017). Furthermore, emotional avoidance has been linked to alexithymia and may contribute to psychopathologies as well as the reduced ability to regulate emotions (Panayiotou et al., 2015; Venta, Hart, & Sharp, 2013).

Future applied research on mitigating the effects of alexithymia could focus on directing attention toward negative cues in music. Past research has considered music listening as a way to practice labelling emotions where experiences with a piece of music are explicitly integrated with an emotion concept (Dingle, Sharman, & Larwood, 2019). Future studies should look to manipulate attentional focus during negative stimuli presentation to establish whether judgements of affective stimuli can be expanded in people with higher alexithymia scores. Research looking to increase affective processing of negative stimuli would then provide grounds for deliberate efforts to expand emotion knowledge in alexithymia. This may aid negative emotion differentiation, which is reduced in alexithymia while positive emotion differentiation is not affected (Aaron, Snodgress, Blain, & Park, 2018).

Although this study does provide insight into how alexithymia may influence the emotion construction process, it is not without limitations. The initial measure relating to emotion words for music only provided an indication of the knowledge of the word. A consequence of this is that affective judgements cannot be specifically related to emotion differentiation ability. It is likely that the depth of emotion concept knowledge would have an additive effect in predicting emotional differentiation. Therefore, future studies should investigate not just the size of the emotional lexicon but also the specificity of knowledge about each listed emotion (e.g. remorse as an emotion experienced after acting in a way you later regret) as well as differential judgements of emotions (e.g. remorse as distinct from sadness; Barrett, Gross, Conner Christensen, & Benvenuto, 2001). Future studies could also explicitly relate judgements of core affect to categorical emotion perception and differentiation.

Finally, we did not control for previous associations with the musical stimuli or liking of the stimuli, which is known to influence perceptions of valence (Eerola & Vuoskoski, 2013). The initial validation of the stimulus set used in the current study does, however, indicate that familiarity with the pieces is low and that this was unlikely to influence ratings (Eerola & Vuoskoski, 2011). The validation study did not measure liking and therefore the influence of liking remains unaccounted for in this study. Future studies using musical stimuli should measure participant's levels of liking and add it as a control variable in analyses involving affective judgments.

Despite these limitations, the current study provides evidence for higher alexithymia scores contributing to more neutral affective judgments of negatively valenced musical stimuli. This is in line with the functional neuroanatomy of emotion construction and subsequent broader constructionist theory. The results suggest that the difficulties in applying words to emotions in alexithymia may have their origins in affective difficulties. Therefore, difficulties observed in alexithymia may be considered as affective as well as conceptual. These affective difficulties may be a product of the diversion of attention away from negative affective cues.

Notes

1. Tender was described in relation to music by Zentner, Grandjean, and Scherer (2008) as being a positively valenced emotion described by softness, longing, nostalgia and dreamy.
2. The songs had the following numbers in Vuoskoski and Eerola (2011). sad: 31, 109; angry: 1, 69, fearful, 11, 14; happy: 23, 105; tender: 41, 42.
3. The OSF project showing the original data set division can be seen at https://osf.io/gvy4b/
4. The pre-registration of this study can be viewed at https://osf.io/3myru/wiki/home/ a link to stimulus and analysis script can be found at https://osf.io/tf29j/.

Acknowledgements

The authors would like to acknowledge Anna Hickling for their helpful comments on the manuscript.

Disclosure statement

No potential conflict of interest was reported by the authors.

Funding

Joel Larwood is supported by a Commonwealth of Australia research training program scholarship (RTP).

ORCID

Joel L. Larwood http://orcid.org/0000-0002-4522-6447
Eric J. Vanman http://orcid.org/0000-0001-7014-6951
Genevieve A. Dingle http://orcid.org/0000-0002-4915-169X

References

Aaron, R. V., Snodgress, M. A., Blain, S. D., & Park, S. (2018). Affect labelling and other aspects of emotional experiences inrelation to alexithymia following standardized emotion inductions. *Psychiatry Research*, *262*, 114–123. https://doi.org/10.1016/J.PSYCHRES.2018.02.014

Aftanas, L. I., Varlamov, A. A., Reva, N. V., & Pavlov, S. V. (2003). Disruption of early event-related theta synchronization of human EEG in alexithymics viewing affective pictures. *Neuroscience Letters*, *340*(1), 57–60. doi:10.1016/S0304-3940(03)00070-3

Allen, R., Davis, R., & Hill, E. (2013). The effects of autism and alexithymia on physiological and verbal responsiveness to music. *Journal of Autism and Developmental Disorders*, *43*(2), 432–444. doi:10.1007/s10803-012-1587-8

Bagby, R. M., Parker, J. D. A., & Taylor, G. J. (1994). The twenty-item Toronto Alexithymia Scale-I. Item selection and cross-validation of the factor structure. *Journal of Psychosomatic Research*, *38*(1), 23–32. doi:10.1016/0022-3999(94)90005-1

Barrett, L. F. (2006). Solving the emotion paradox: Categorization and the experience of emotion. *Personality and Social Psychology Review*, *10*, 20–46. doi:10.1207/s15327957pspr1001_2

Barrett, L. F. (2017). *How emotions are made: The secret life of the brain*. New York, NY: Houghton Mifflin Harcourt.

Barrett, L. F., Gross, J., Conner Christensen, T., & Benvenuto, M. (2001). Knowing what you're feeling and knowing what to do about it: Mapping the relation between emotion differentiation and emotion regulation. *Cognition & Emotion*, *15*(6), 713–724. doi:10.1080/02699930143000239

Barrett, L. F., Lindquist, K. A., & Gendron, M. (2007). Language as context for the perception of emotion. *Trends in Cognitive Sciences*, *11*(8), 327–332. doi:10.1016/j.tics.2007.06.003

Bayot, M., Pleyers, G., Kotsou, I., Lefèvre, N., Sauter, D. A., & Vermeulen, N. (2014). Joint effect of alexithymia and mood on the categorization of nonverbal emotional vocalizations. *Psychiatry Research*, *216*(2), 242–247. doi:10.1016/j.psychres.2013.12.007

Cespedes-Guevara, J., & Eerola, T. (2018). Music communicates affects, not basic emotions – A constructionist account of attribution of emotional meanings to music. *Frontiers in Psychology*, *9*, 215. doi:10.3389/fpsyg.2018.00215

da Silva, A. N., Vasco, A. B., & Watson, J. C. (2017). Alexithymia and emotional processing: A mediation model. *Journal of Clinical Psychology*, doi:10.1002/jclp.22422

Dingle, G. A., Sharman, L. S., & Larwood, J. L. (2019). Young people's use of music for emotional immersion. In K. Skewes-McFerran, P. Derrington, & S. Saarikallio (Eds.), *Handbook of music and adolescence* (pp. 25–37). Oxford: Oxford University Press.

Eerola, T., & Vuoskoski, J. K. (2011). A comparison of the discrete and dimensional models of emotion in music. *Psychology of Music*, *39*(1), 18–49. doi:10.1177/0305735610362821

Eerola, T., & Vuoskoski, J. K. (2013). A review of music and emotion studies: Approaches, emotion models, and stimuli. *Music Perception: An Interdisciplinary Journal*, *30*(3), 307–340. doi:10.1525/mp.2012.30.3.307

Franz, M., Schaefer, R., Schneider, C., Sitte, W., & Bachor, J. (2004). Visual event-related potentials in subjects with alexithymia: Modified processing of emotional aversive information? *American Journal of Psychiatry*, *161*(4), 728–735. doi:10.1176/appi.ajp.161.4.728

Frijda, N. H. (2016). The evolutionary emergence of what we call "emotions". *Cognition and Emotion*, *30*(4), 609–620. doi:10.1080/02699931.2016.1145106

Goerlich-Dobre, K. S., Votinov, M., Habel, U., Pripfl, J., & Lamm, C. (2015). Neuroanatomical profiles of alexithymia dimensions and subtypes. *Human Brain Mapping*, *36*(10), 3805–3818. doi:10.1002/hbm.22879

Goerlich, K. S., Witteman, J., Aleman, A., & Martens, S. (2011). Hearing feelings: Affective categorization of music and speech in alexithymia, an ERP study. *PloS One*, *6*(5), e19501. doi:10.1371/journal.pone.0019501

Gotlib, I. H., Joorman, J., & Forland-Ross, L. C. (2014). Understanding familial risk for depression: A 25-year perspective. *Perspectives on Psychological Science*, *9*(1), 94–108. https://doi.org/10.1177/1745691613513469

Grabe, H. J., Wittfeld, K., Hegenscheid, K., Hosten, N., Lotze, M., Janowitz, D., … Freyberger, H. J. (2014). Alexithymia and brain gray matter volumes in a general population sample. *Human Brain Mapping*, *35*(12), 5932–5945. doi:10.1002/hbm.22595

Grynberg, D., Chang, B., Corneille, O., Maurage, P., Vermeulen, N., Berthoz, S., & Luminet, O. (2012a). Alexithymia and the processing of emotional facial expressions (EFEs): Systematic review, unanswered questions and further perspectives. *PLOS ONE*, *7*(8), e42429. doi:10.1371/journal.pone.0042429

Grynberg, D., Davydov, D. M., Vermeulen, N., & Luminet, O. (2012b). Alexithymia is associated with an augmenter profile, but not only: Evidence for anticipation to arousing music. *Scandinavian Journal of Psychology*, *53*(5), 375–381. doi:10.1111/j.1467-9450.2012.00962.x

Heaton, P., Reichenbacher, L., Sauter, D., Allen, R., Scott, S., & Hill, E. (2012). Measuring the effects of alexithymia on perception of emotional vocalizations in autistic spectrum disorder and typical development. *Psychological Medicine*, *42*(11), 2453–2459. doi:10.1017/S0033291712000621

Ihme, K., Sacher, J., Lichev, V., Rosenberg, N., Kugel, H., Rufer, M., ... Suslow, T. (2014). Alexithymic features and the labeling of brief emotional facial expressions – An fMRI study. *Neuropsychologia, 64,* 289–299. doi:10.1016/j.neuropsychologia.2014.09.044

Juslin, P. N., & Laukka, P. (2004). Expression, perception, and induction of musical emotions: A review and a questionnaire study of everyday listening. *Journal of New Music Research, 33* (3), 217–238. doi:10.1080/0929821042000317813

Lindquist, K. A., Wager, T. D., Kober, H., Bliss-Moreau, E., & Barrett, L. F. (2012). The brain basis of emotion: A meta-analytic review. *Behavioral and Brain Sciences, 35*(3), 121–143. doi:10.1017/S0140525X11000446

Lovibond, S. H., & Lovibond, P. H. (1995). *Manual for the depression anxiety stress scales* (2nd ed). Sydney: Psychology Foundation.

Luminet, O., Rimé, B., Bagby, R. M., & Taylor, G. (2004). A multimodal investigation of emotional responding in alexithymia. *Cognition & Emotion, 18*(6), 741–766. doi:10.1080/02699930341000275

Luminet, O., Vermeulen, N., Demaret, C., Taylor, G. J., & Bagby, R. M. (2006). Alexithymia and levels of processing: Evidence for an overall deficit in remembering emotion words. *Journal of Research in Personality, 40*(5), 713–733. doi:10.1016/j.jrp.2005.09.001

Panayiotou, G., Leonidou, C., Constantinou, E., Hart, J., Rinehart, K. L., Sy, J. T., & Björgvinsson, T. (2015). Do alexithymic individuals avoid their feelings? Experiential avoidance mediates the association between alexithymia, psychosomatic, and depressive symptoms in a community and a clinical sample. *Comprehensive Psychiatry, 56,* 206–216. doi:10.1016/j.comppsych.2014.09.006

Parker, P. D., Prkachin, K. M., & Prkachin, G. C. (2005). Processing of facial expressions of negative emotion in alexithymia: The influence of temporal constraint. *Journal of Personality, 73*(4), 1087–1107. doi:10.1111/j.1467-6494.2005.00339.x

Pennebaker, J. W., Boyd, R. L., Jordan, K., & Blackburn, K. (2015). *The development and psychometric properties of LIWC2015.* Austin, TX: University of Texas at Austin.

Preece, D., Becerra, R., Robinson, K., Dandy, J., & Allen, A. (2018). The psychometric assessment of alexithymia: Development and validation of the Perth Alexithymia Questionnaire. *Personality and Individual Differences, 132,* 32–44. https://doi.org/10/1016/j.paid.2018.05.011

Posner, J., Russell, J. A., Gerber, A., Gorman, D., Colibazzi, T., Yu, S., ... Peterson, B. S. (2009). The neurophysiological bases of emotion: An fMRI study of the affective circumplex using emotion-denoting words. *Human Brain Mapping, 30,* 883–895. doi:10.1002/hbm.20553

Punkanen, M., Eerola, T., & Erkkilä, J. (2011). Biased emotional recognition in depression: Perception of emotions in music by depressed patients. *Journal of Affective Disorders, 130*(1–2), 118–126. doi:10.1016/j.jad.2010.10.034

Roedema, T. M., & Simons, R. F. (1999). Emotion-processing deficit in alexithymia. *Psychophysiology, 36*(3), doi:10.1017/S0048577299980290

Russell, J. A. (2003). Core affect and the psychological construction of emotion. *Psychological Review, 110,* 145–172. doi:10.1037/0033-295X.110.1.145

Scherer, K. R. (2005). What are emotions? And how can they be measured? *Social Science Information, 44*(4), 695–729. doi:10.1177/0539018405058216

Suslow, T., Junghanns, K., Donges, U.-S., & Arolt, V. (2001). Alexithymia and automatic processing of verbal and facial affect stimuli. *Cahiers de Psychologie Cognitive/Current Psychology of Cognition, 20*(5), 297–324.

Taruffi, L., Allen, R., Downing, J., & Heaton, P. (2017). Individual differences in music-perceived emotions. *Music Perception: An Interdisciplinary Journal, 34*(3), Retrieved from http://mp.ucpress.edu/content/34/3/253.

van der Velde, J., Servaas, M. N., Goerlich, K. S., Bruggeman, R., Horton, P., Costafreda, S. G., & Aleman, A. (2013). Neural correlates of alexithymia: A meta-analysis of emotion processing studies. *Neuroscience and Biobehavioral Reviews, 37*(8), 1774–1785. doi:10.1016/j.neubiorev.2013.07.008

Vanman, E. J., Dawson, M. E., & Brennan, P. A. (1998). Affective reactions in the blink of an eye: Individual differences in subjective experience and physiological responses to emotional stimuli. *Personality and Social Psychology Bulletin, 24*(9), 994–1005. doi:10.1177/0146167298249007

Venta, A., Hart, J., & Sharp, C. (2013). The relation between experiential avoidance, alexithymia and emotion regulation in inpatient adolescents. *Clinical Child Psychology and Psychiatry, 18* (3), 398–410. doi:10.1177/1359104512455815

Vermeulen, N., Luminet, O., Cordovil De Sousa, M., & Campanella, S. (2008). Categorical perception of anger is disrupted in alexithymia: Evidence from a visual ERP study. *Cognition and Emotion, 22,* 1052–1067. doi:10.1080/02699930701597635

Vermeulen, N., Toussaint, J., & Luminet, O. (2010). The influence of alexithymia and music on the incidental memory for emotion words. *European Journal of Personality, 24*(6), 551–568. doi:10.1002/per.758

Wagner, H., & Lee, V. (2008). Alexithymia and individual differences in emotional expression. *Journal of Research in Personality, 42*(1), 83–95. doi:10.1016/j.jrp.2007.04.001

Wotschack, C., & Klann-Delius, G. (2013). Alexithymia and the conceptualization of emotions: A study of language use and semantic knowledge. *Journal of Research in Personality, 47,* 514–523. doi:10.1016/j.jrp.2013.01.011

Zamariola, G., Vlemincx, E., Corneille, O., & Luminet, O. (2018). Relationship between interoceptive accuracy, interoceptive sensibility, and alexithymia. *Personality and Individual Differences, 125,* 14–20. doi:10.1016/j.paid.2017.12.024

Zentner, M., Grandjean, D., & Scherer, K. R. (2008). Emotions evoked by the sound of music: Characterization, classification, and measurement. *Emotion, 8,* 494–521. doi:10.1037/1528-3542.8.4.494

Alexithymia and reaching group consensus

Hila Zahava Gvirts and Lihi Dery

ABSTRACT

One characteristic of human nature is the ability to align our behavior with others. Previous research has linked poor communication skills to alexithymia. This may suggest the possibility that individuals with high alexithymia do not adhere to the principles of social alignment. One form of cognitive alignment is consensus with a group. So far, little research attention has been given to the possible link between alexithymia and this form of cognitive social alignment. In this study, we address this gap by investigating the association between consensus-reaching abilities and alexithymia. A sample comprising of 122 participants completed the Toronto Alexithymia Scale and then played a specially designed game called "Consensus under a deadline". In each game, a participant played with either seven bots designed to act rationally and always seek a consensus, or with seven other participants. The participants were unaware who they were playing with. The results of the study confirm the link between alexithymia and impaired cognitive social alignment, showing that the alexithymia cognitive component (EOT) is associated with a deficit in reaching a consensus with humans (that sometimes act irrationally). However, this association was not evident when group members were bots (that always act rationally).

Alexithymia is a multifaceted construct comprising three components: (a) difficulty distinguishing between feelings and bodily sensations accompanying states of emotional arousal, (b) difficulty describing feelings, and (c) externally oriented thinking (Taylor & Bagby, 2000). While difficulties identifying and describing feelings are considered to tap the affective facet of alexithymia, the externally oriented thinking style is considered to reflect more of the "cognitive" dimension of alexithymia (Zackheim, 2007). This cognitive component is associated with a thinking style that directs thoughts and attention to external reality rather than internal focus and attention to emotional information (Franz et al., 2008).

The majority of the literature on alexithymia has focused on the intrapersonal domain, providing evidence supporting the association between alexithymia and a relationship with somatic complaints (Sifneos, 1973) and mental illness (Honkalampi, Saarinen, Hintikka, Virtanen, & Viinamäki, 1999; Leweke, Leichsenring, Kruse, & Hermes, 2012; Ospina et al., 2019; Taylor, Parker, Bagby, & Bourke, 1996). Although in recent years more studies examined the interpersonal outcomes associated with high alexithymia scores (Grynberg, Berthoz, & Bird, 2018; Joybari, 2014; Nicolò et al., 2011), the mechanisms underlying social difficulties in alexithymia have so far remained poorly understood (Grynberg et al., 2018).

One characteristic of human nature is social alignment. Social alignment has been conceptualised as the tendency to align with other members of the group in terms of thoughts and behaviour. In its basic form, it refers to motor alignment observed in various everyday social interactions such as when we unintentionally synchronise our walking pace with our partners (social motor synchrony, e.g. Sylos-Labini, d'Avella, Lacquaniti, & Ivanenko, 2018). Recently, Shamay-Tsoory, Saporta, Marton-Alper, and

Gvirts (2019) suggested two other "higher" forms of social alignment including emotional alignment (emotional contagion, e.g. Prochazkova & Kret, 2017) and cognitive alignment (e.g. conformity and consensus Coultas & van Leeuwen, 2015). Importantly, they proposed that these three levels of social alignment (motion, emotion, and cognition) represent a core mechanism of connectedness and rely on shared neural networks; therefore, triggering one behaviour activates all other behaviours and encourages likability, closeness and connectedness.

Notably, social alignment has been associated with a range of positive social outcomes (Kühn et al., 2010; McKelvey & Kerr, 1988; Rabinowitch & Knafo-Noam, 2015; Tarr, Launay, & Dunbar, 2016). It is, therefore, crucial to examine the possibility that individuals with high alexithymia traits may suffer from deficiencies in their capacity to achieve and enjoy social alignment. The literature on this topic has focused primarily on the link between alexithymia and emotional alignment (i.e. emotional contagion) with less research attention given to the two other forms of social alignment (motions and cognition). For example, high scorers on the "externally oriented thinking" scale were found to be related to reduced physiological reactivity in two film conditions (arousal-boosting and arousal-damping), while the content of the films evoked a similar subjective experience of sad feeling. In view of these findings, it was suggested that externally oriented thinking factor moderated emotional reactivity by decoupling the physiological domain of the emotional response from its subjective-experience domain which stayed unaffected (Davydov, Luminet, & Zech, 2013). More recently, a functional magnetic resonance imaging (fMRI) study showed that a higher score in the externally oriented thinking factor is associated with lower activation to masked happy faces but higher activation to masked fearful faces (Demers et al., 2019). In contrast, other facets of alexithymia did not show relationships with neural reactivity to masked emotional faces. The difficulties in accurate tuning of one's state with others were compared between a group of individuals with alexithymia and healthy controls. The results indicated that individuals with alexithymia rated painful stimuli as less painful than individuals without alexithymia and accordingly they displayed low vicarious responses to observed pain in the anterior cingulate associated with pain processing (Moriguchi et al., 2006). Taken together, this line of evidence supports the notion that individuals with alexithymia suffer from deficiencies in accurate tuning of their emotional state with the emotional state of others. In this context it is also important to note that individuals with high alexithymia were found to react with less corrugator imitation, especially toward angry faces (Sonnby-Borgström, 2009). Since imitation is considered close to the constructs of motor synchronisation (Shamay-Tsoory et al., 2019) these findings may be interpreted as supporting the notion that individual with alexithymia suffer from deficiencies in motor alignment. However, given that imitation leads to a shared affect that facilitates emotion recognition (Wallbott, 1991), it was argued that less corrugator imitation may interfere with the ability of individuals with alexithymia to share affect (Sonnby-Borgström, 2009). Thus, the fact that individuals with high alexithymia were found to react with less corrugator imitation may be interoperated as supporting the possibility that these individuals suffer from deficiencies in emotional alignment.

Regarding the link between motor alignment and alexithymia, no research has so far directly examined this topic. It is worth mentioning that a recent study employed the mirror game paradigm to examine whether participants with ASD are capable of creating highly synchronised motion (i.e. co-confident motion, see: Noy, Levit-Binun, & Golland, 2015) and whether this capability is related to their alexithymia traits. Their findings reveal a greater deficit of motor alignment in ASD subjects with higher alexithymia scores than among other ASD subjects with lower alexithymia scores (Brezis et al., 2017). These authors suggest that since impaired ability to recognise the emotions of others was argued to be associated with reduced empathy (Bird & Cook, 2013), it may also be associated with greater difficulties in physically synchronising with others.

As stated above, less research attention has been devoted to the possible link between cognitive alignment and alexithymia. One form of cognitive alignment is consensus with a group. Consensus is defined as a state of mutual agreement among members of a group where all opinions have been heard and addressed to the satisfaction of the group (Saint & Lawson, 1994). Considering a related construct, conformity with the group also refers to an act of fitting in with the group and does not require all members to think the same as others. Clear examples of consensus decisions are group decision-making by committees, juries, panels, etc. Notably, group consensus may also be observed in everyday situations including a group of friends discussing their next vacation destination; members of a university department choosing a day for a weekly seminar; a scientific committee deciding where to hold next year's conference; and a group of friends discussing where to go out. A deadline is a constraint faced by a group trying to form a consensus. For example, if a consensus is not reached by the deadline, the vacation will be postponed to an unknown date. In this case, reaching an agreement within a group before the deadline will most probably be beneficial to all members. Reaching a consensus necessitates a period of negotiation and communication to reach agreement on goals and objectives. Throughout this period, group members constantly monitor their preferences and the preferences of others to detect misalignment. Misalignment occurs when the preferable choice of an individual is different from the preferable choice of the majority of the group. In accordance with the social alignment model, this is an unpleasant state that often evokes distress and thus people are motivated to take steps to reduce it. As achieving alignment activates the reward system, the most preferable action would be to align with the majority of the group in order to reduce distress. Interestingly, while some members adhere to these principles by changing their own preference to the one chosen by the majority of the group members, others may try to change other members' preferences and to influence their choices (Mahardhika, Valls, Kanno, & Furuta, 2017). The fact that poor communication skills have been linked to alexithymia (Sevindi & Kumcagiz, 2018) may suggest the possibility that individuals with high alexithymia present inappropriate behaviour – one that does not adhere to the principles of social alignment.

Here, we sought to further contribute to the understanding of the interpersonal dimension of alexithymia by investigating the associations between alexithymia and a cognitive form of social alignment – consensus-reaching. To this end, we employed the "Consensus Under Deadline" (CUD) game (Yosef, Naamani-Dery, Obraztsova, Rabinovich, & Bannikova, 2017), an online voting game in which a group of people (termed "players") are required to reach a consensus under deadline. This task collects decisions of individuals within the group during the process of forming group consensus and, as such, may provide a valuable setting in which to study the link between alexithymia and consensus reaching. During the game, a sequential on-line voting process takes place, whereby players can change some of their preferences as the deadline approaches.

The game does not involve direct social interactions between the players and all the interaction is performed via an interactive on-line website. As inadvertent social cues such as mimics may influence social alignment (Faria, Dyer, Tosh, & Krause, 2010), the specific design of the task allowed us to investigate the association between alexithymia and reaching a consensus while excluding the effect of other social cues. In each game, participants are randomly assigned to a different group of eight players. The group members may be other genuine human players, but they may also be bots that were programmed to behave rationally – that is, in a manner that always promotes consensus-reaching. Individuals were not able to identify their fellow group members and were not even informed that bot players existed. Notably, games in which the player (unknowingly) played against bots were perceived by the player as conditions of high rational gameplay. We therefore assumed that during these games, the interaction between players was experienced as more harmonious (i.e. players were rational and built consensus more efficiently) in comparison with games where all players were humans.

Our study aimed to (1) assess the association between each player's components of alexithymia and his/her irrational behaviour in the consensus game, and (2) examine whether the association between alexithymia and irrational behaviour may be due to the irrationality of the other players. To this end, we compared a player's performance when playing with bots (a synchronised group acting rationally) vs. human (less synchronised group not always acting rationally).

In view of the social alignment model and previous findings that link alexithymia and the affective level of social alignment (Moriguchi et al., 2006), we hypothesised that alexithymia will be positively associated with deficiencies and difficulty in reaching a consensus with regard to the level of rationality of other players (i.e. playing with bots vs. playing with humans). Since there is limited research on this topic, we did not have a specific hypothesis about the effect of the level of rationality of other players on the association between alexithymia deficiencies and difficulty in reaching a consensus.

1. Method

1.1. Participants

One-hundred and twenty-two male and female students aged 21–35 years old were recruited for the study. All were students at a local university, and the incentive to participate was that they could earn up to five bonus points in a university course in which they were enrolled. They first completed the TAS-20 and then participated in the CUD game.

The power analysis for the planned experiments was based on our hope to find a correlation between the game type (bots or humans), the irrational behaviour, and the TAS scores. For two coefficients, Cohen's $f2 = 0.17$(effect size), $\alpha = 0.05$ and a power of 0.95, we needed to collect a sample of 91 participants. As reported, we ended up with 122 participants, out of whom 116 were valid, as 6 subjects did not fill in the TAS-20 questionnaire properly and were therefore excluded. The total cohort completing the study consisted of 76 females and 40 males. The mean age of participants was 24.102 (SD = 2.073, range 19–32).

1.2 Alexithymia assessment

We used the 20-item Toronto Alexithymia Scale (TAS-20), which is the most commonly used self-report measurement of alexithymia and has high reliability and validity (Parker, Taylor, & Bagby, 2003). The TAS-20 is a self-report scale that consists of 20 items. Items are rated using a 5-point Likert scale whereby 1 = strongly disagree and 5 = strongly agree. In addition to the total score, there are also scores for each one of the three dimensions of alexithymia: Difficulty Identifying Feelings (DIF), e.g. "I am often confused about what emotion I am feeling;" Difficulty Describing Feelings (DDF), e.g. "It is difficult for me to find the right words for my feelings;" and Externally Oriented Thinking (EOT), e.g. "I prefer talking to people about their daily activities rather than their feelings." Evidence of reliability and factorial validity of the TAS-20 has been established (Bagby, Parker, & Taylor, 1994; Bagby, Taylor, & Parker, 1994; Davydov et al., 2013; Parker et al., 2003). Cronbach's alpha's for the three TAS-20 subscales was 0.69. The subscales' Cronbach alpha's were above .70, except for EOT ($\alpha = .54$).

It has long been argued that the Cronbach alpha is a poor index of uni-dimensionality (Revelle, 1979; Zinbarg, Revelle, Yovel, & Li, 2005). This has even been argued by Cronbach himself (Cronbach, 1951, 1988). We, thus followed the recommendation of Revelle and Zinbarg (2009) and computed MacDonald's coefficient (2013). The reliability of the EOT subscale is not ideal, however, note that Hair, Black, Babin, Anderson, and Tatham (2010) suggest that while a value of 0.70 is generally agreed upon as an acceptable value, values as low as 0.60 may be acceptable for exploratory research.

Following this, we have calculated both Cronbach alpha and the Omega hierarchical for each of the TAS subscales. The Cronbach alpha is 0.81, 0.77 and 0.54 for DDF, DIF and EOT, respectively. The Omega hierarchical is 0.84, 0.85 and 0.65 for DDF, DIF and EOT, respectively.

Note that there are several previous studies in which the EOT was the only subscale that was found to be related to the dependent variable (Grynberg, Luminet, Corneille, Grèzes, & Berthoz, 2010; Vanheule, Meganck, & Desmet, 2011).

1.3 The CUD game

In order to identify actions that promote consensus-building, we used the CUD game, a time-limited iterative voting game (Bannikova, Naamani-Dery, Obraztsova, Rabinovich, & Rosenschein, 2016; Stamper, 1985). During the game, players are required to reach a consensus, i.e. unanimously choose a candidate out of five available alternatives, before some predefined deadline is reached.

Each game included eight players that are randomly assigned to the game. The players did not know the identities of the other players. Players were assigned to two types of groups:

(1) Eight human participants
(2) One human participant and seven bots. The bots were designed to play in a rational manner, according to an algorithm designed by Bannikova et al. (2016).

Each game includes five cards, each with a different animal image. The card values are displayed below the images (either 100, 80, 60, 40, or 20 points). While the same five cards are presented to all players, the rank order of the values of each card differs for each player. The players cannot see the card values of the other players, but they can see the current number of votes for each card (for example in Figure 1, four players chose the penguin image and two players chose the boar image).

To form a consensus, all players must unanimously select the same card before the deadline is reached. If no consensus is reached by the deadline, each player receives zero points. If a consensus is reached, players receive points according to the value of the chosen image. Therefore, each player receives a different amount of points.

This game simulates a realistic situation in which each member sees his or her personal advantage (in this case, choosing the card that has the highest points) but at the same time has the motivation to align with the other group members, as lack of agreement will lead to personal loss (zero points). For example, Figure 1 illustrates the cards of three of the players. In the present round, four players voted for the penguin. Each player has a different value for the penguin: 100 points for player #1, 80 points for player #2 and 60 points for player #3. If the card with the penguin image is chosen unanimously, then players 1, 2 and 3 will receive 100,80 and 60 points, respectively.

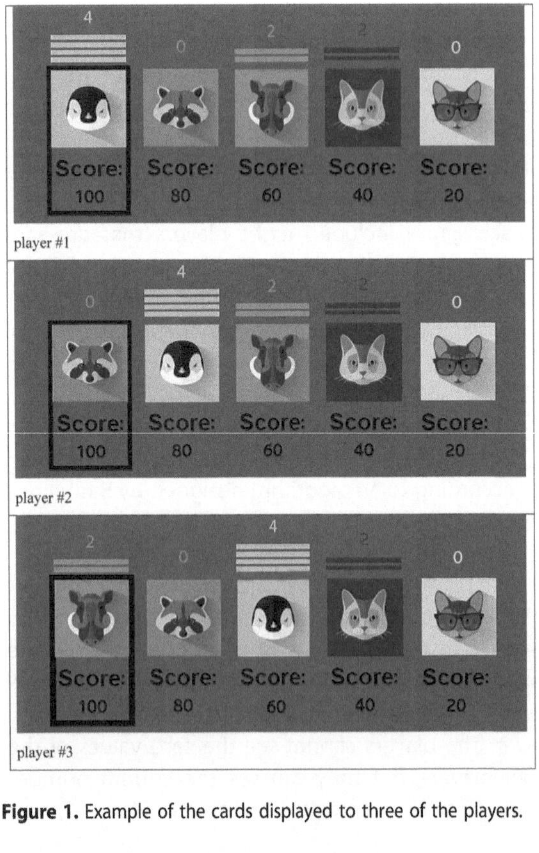

Figure 1. Example of the cards displayed to three of the players.

For each game, the deadline was set to 10 rounds, and each round was 15 seconds long. The game begins with the automatic selection of the highest preference of each voter. The current result is displayed. For example, if Figure 1 is displayed at the beginning of the game, it means that the penguin is the highest preference of four of the voters. For each round:

(1) Players who wish to change their selected card apply for a voting slot by selecting the card they would like to vote for.
(2) One player is chosen randomly from all of those who applied.
(3) The chosen player selects another card.
(4) The player screens are updated with the new number of votes per card.

The process continues in rounds until either a consensus is reached, or the deadline is reached (i.e. the end of 10 rounds), whichever comes first.

Figure 2 presents a screenshot of a player's screen upon game termination. In this case, a consensus was reached – all voters agreed on the penguin. Note that in order to boost motivation to reach a consensus, players were constantly reminded that a failure to reach a consensus results in zero game points and thus zero bonus in the course. This was done via a permanent message on the screen (the blue message in Figure 2).

1.3.1. Inappropriate and opposing alignment

According to the social alignment model, detection of misalignment means that if the most preferable choice for the player (i.e. the card that has a higher value for the player) is different from the most preferable choice by the majority of the group, he/ she will change their own choice and conform to the group. Rational behaviour is, therefore, defined as the tendency to conform to the group by voting for the card that was chosen by the majority of the group. In contrast to this rational behaviour, irrational behaviours are actions that do not promote consensus-building. Here, we define two types of irrational voting:

(1) Inappropriate alignment (IA) – the player is trying to change other members' preferences and to influence their choices. In this case, the player votes for a card that has a higher value for him/ her than the value of the card preferred by most

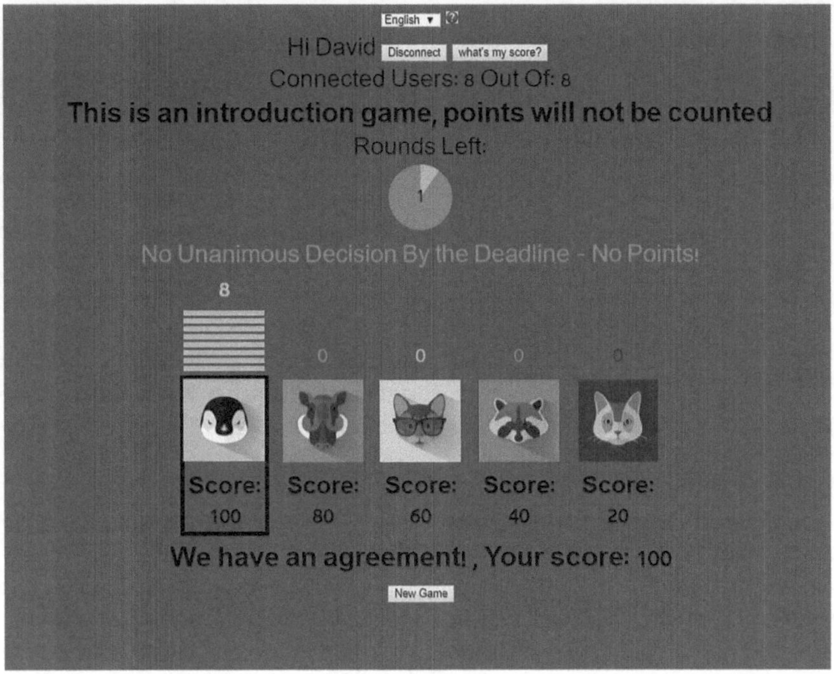

Figure 2. A consensus is reached.

players. Consider player #3 in Figure 1. The card preferred by most players is the penguin. This card has a value of 60 for player #3. An IA action would be to vote for the racoon which has a higher value (80) for him/her.

(2) Opposing alignment (OA) – the player votes for a card that has a lower value for him/her than the value of the card preferred by most players. Again, consider player #3 in Figure 1. An OA action would be to vote for one of the cards that has a lower value than the penguin (values 40 or 20).

An IA action reflects an attempt to earn more points by signaling to other group members to change their vote and to vote for a card that has a higher preference in terms of its value (points). However, given the time constraint, an attempt to change the choices of others will most probably harm the chances of reaching a consensus as the number of rounds is limited. This is especially true if one takes into account the fact that the other players do not know the motivation for performing the IA action, as they are not aware of the fact that the card that was chosen by the specific player holds a higher value for him. The OA action, on the other hand, does not seem to promote any motivation to maximise the number of points and it may simply reflect opposing alignment behaviour or anti-conformity.

The player signals were calculated after each round in each game. For each player, we summed the number of IA and OA actions he/she performed during all games.

1.4. Procedure

Subjects were required to complete the TAS-20 prior to their participation in the CUD game and were then invited to attend the CUD game at our university computer labs. Each lab was supervised by a research assistant who explained the game to the participants and was available to solve any difficulties that might arise, though no major problem was reported. Participants did not know with whom they were playing (i.e. who was with them in the same group). And, crucially, they were not aware that some of the games they were playing were being played with groups of bots. In fact, the participants were not even informed that the bot players existed.

As stated above, participant incentive was to earn points. At the beginning of the game, they were informed that they may participate in numerous games in order to be eligible for a bonus in a course in which they were enrolled. They were told that the maximum points they can earn are 1000 points and that every 200 points are equivalent to one bonus point in the course. Importantly, they were told that the maximum number of games they can play is 15. Thus, each player could play up to 15 games, but they could also play fewer games in case they reached the maximum number of points (i.e. 1000).

1.5. Statistical analysis

The number of IA and OA actions for each player in each game was recorded. The irrational actions (of type IA and OA) were considered separately for each player in each game, since a player might perform, for example, one IA action in one game, two OA actions in another game, and no irrational actions in a third game. As the irrational actions were not normally distributed, we turned the two types of irrational scores into binary variables (0 = rational choice, 1 = irrational choice). Consequently, any player that made an irrational choice in a game (one or more than one) was considered as an irrational player in that specific game. The average percentage of irrational choices of types IA or OA in games was 2.36% and 6.3%, respectively. Furthermore, 17.24% of the players performed irrational choices of type IA at some point, 27.59% performed irrational choices of type OA, and 29.31% of the players performed some type of irrational action (either IA or OA).

We divided our analyses into two parts:

(1) Individual level – examining the association between components of alexithymia and irrational behaviour in the consensus game and whether this association appears in both types of games: games that were played with humans and games that were played with bots (a harmonised group acting rationally).
(2) Group level – as stated earlier, during the process of reaching a consensus, each member influences the other members. This suggests that the composition of the group regarding their level of alexithymia traits may affect their ability to reach a consensus. We, therefore, conducted an exploratory analysis aimed at examining whether groups with a higher level of alexithymia traits had higher scores of irrational behaviours and whether the level of variability in alexithymia scores within groups can affect consensus reaching. To this end, groups were divided into subgroups according to the amount of high alexithymia (i.e. number of individuals with a TAS-20 total score ≥ 61) in the group. The average alexithymia scores and irrational behaviour scores (i.e. group average IA and group average OA) were calculated for each group.

For the individual analysis, we carried out a binary mixed model analysis with the irrational score as the dependent variable (0 = rational choice, 1 = irrational choice). The fixed effects were the game type (0 = games against humans, 1 = games against bots) and the three alexithymia factors (DIF, DDF and EOT). The participants were the random effect. This analysis was performed twice, each time with a different type of irrational behaviour as the dependent variable (i.e. IA or OA). In addition, we examined whether individuals improve over time, e.g. whether less IA and/or OA signals appear as individuals proceed to play more games. Here, we carried out a logistic regression general linear model analysis with the game number and the three alexithymia factors as independent variables. The analysis was performed twice, each time with a different type of irrational behaviour as the dependent variable (i.e. IA or OA).

For group analysis, as some of our continuous measures were clearly non-normally distributed (Kolmogorov–Smirnov test: $P < 0.10$), we chose the Bivariate Spearman correlations to assess the association between the average scores of the three different factors of alexithymia and average scores of the two types of irrational actions. Additionally, we assessed the association scores of irrational behaviours and convergence time (i.e. the period until consensus was reached). Since a higher level of heterogeneity across members in a group may have an effect on the different measures of group alignment, these analyses were conducted separately for each of the three sub-groups (defined according to the number of individuals with high alexithymia scores in the group). A multivariate analysis of variance (MANOVA) with group (number of levels was determined by the number sub-groups) as a between-subjects factor was performed to determine if a significant difference exists between the average irrational behaviour scores (i.e. group average IA and group average OA) of the sub-groups.

All analyses were performed using the statistical software SPSS (version 25), with *p*-values smaller than 0.05 considered as significant.

2. Results

Table 1 presents the mean (sd), minimum and maximum scores for each of the three alexithymia factors across groups (144 groups of 8 human players per group) and per individual (116 players). Since in each game, the human players were randomly assigned to a different group of eight players, the statistics are very similar.

Within a large community sample ($n = 1933$), Parker et al. (2003) found mean TAS-20 values of 45.57 ± 11.35 (total score). In our results, the mean TAS-20 total score was 45.87 ± 10.41. Therefore, our results are comparable with these findings and suggest that the TAS-20 total score in our sample is similar to the TAS-20 total score in the community samples.

2.1. Individual level

2.1.1. The CUD – inappropriate and opposing alignment signals

Out of 116 subjects, 12 subjects (10.3%) showed a TAS-20 total score ≥ 61 indicating high alexithymia. The binary mixed model with OA as the dependent variable revealed that only the EOT subscale predicted irrational voting ($F(1,224) = 4.885$, $p = 0.028$). The odds of performing irrational voting when interacting with humans were higher for participants who had high EOT scores (OR = 1.144, 95% CI [1.002–1.305]). This is reported in Table 2. In contrast, there was no significant impact on participants' EOT scores on the odds of performing irrational behaviour when interacting with bots (OR = 1.086, 95% CI [0.976–1.210]). Note that the binary mixed model with IA as the dependent variable revealed no significant effects (not presented).

2.1.2. Inappropriate and opposing alignment signals improvement

The logistic regression general linear model did not reveal any significant improvement of players over time. That is, it seems that the number of OA or IA signals does not decrease (or increase) as individuals play more games. These results are reported in supplementary material (Table 3 (OA as the dependent variable) and Table 4 (IA as the dependent variable)).

2.2 Group level – exploratory analysis

Out of a total of 144 games, 44.4% of the games had at least one player with a TAS-20 total score ≥61 indicating high alexithymia. There were 47 games in which one of the players had a high alexithymia score, 14 games in which two players and three games in which three players had a high alexithymia score. Note that since only three groups had three players with high alexithymia scores, these groups were excluded from the analysis at group level. Consequently, the analysis at group level was conducted on three types of sub-groups: (1) groups with one player who had high alexithymia (2) groups with two players who had high alexithymia scores and (3) groups with no members with high alexithymia scores.

The Spearman correlations for the association between the average scores of the three different factors of alexithymia and average scores of the two types of irrational actions were not significant. Likewise, the association between scores of irrational behaviours and convergence time was not significant (not presented).

Table 1. Descriptive statistics for TAS-20 factor scores for individual level (the 116 players) and for group level (mean scores for each of the 144 games of human groups).

	Mean (sd)		Minimum scores		Maximum scores	
	Individual level	Group level	Individual level	Group level	Individual level	Group level
DIF	14.09 (4.58)	14.09 (1.68)	7	8.78	29	21
DDF	12.42 (4.56)	12.41 (1.63)	5	6.59	25	19.08
EOT	19.36 (4.4)	19.3 (1.48)	9	13.41	31	25.97
Total	45.87 (10.41)	45.81 (10.11)	27	32.41	74	61.47

Notes: EOT, Externally oriented thinking; DDF, Difficulty describing feelings; DIF, Identifying feelings.

Table 2. Binary mixed model with OA as the dependent variable – fixed coefficients.

Model term	Coefficient	Std. Error	t	Sig.	95% Confidence interval		Exp (coefficient)	95% Confidence interval for exp (coefficient)	
					Lower	Upper		Lower	Upper
Intercept	−3.293	1.3071	−2.519	0.012	−5.869	−0.717	0.037	0.003	0.488
gameType = 1	1.129	1.1895	0.949	0.344	−1.215	3.473	3.093	0.297	32.243
gameType = 0	0[a]								
TAS EOT*[gameType = 1]	0.083	0.0545	1.522	0.129	−0.024	0.190	1.086	0.976	1.210
TAS EOT*[gameType = 0]*	0.134	0.0670	2.001	0.047	0.002	0.266	1.144	1.002	1.305
TAS EOT	0[a]								
TAS DDF*[gameType = 1]	0.031	0.0600	0.524	0.601	−0.087	0.150	1.032	0.917	1.161
TAS DDF*[gameType = 0]	−0.079	0.0702	−1.131	0.259	−0.218	0.059	0.924	0.804	1.061
TAS DDF	0[a]								
TAS DIF*[gameType = 1]	−0.094	0.0578	−1.632	0.104	−0.208	0.020	0.910	0.812	1.020
TAS DIF*[gameType = 0]	−0.016	0.0748	−0.217	0.828	−0.164	0.131	0.984	0.849	1.140
TAS DIF	0[a]								

Notes: IA, Inappropriate alignment; OA, Opposing alignment; EOT, Externally oriented thinking; DDF, Difficulty describing feelings; DIF, Identifying feelings, games against humans (game type = 0), games against bots (game type = 1).
[a]This coefficient is set to zero because it is redundant.
*$p < .05$.

Recall that in order to examine whether a higher level of heterogeneity across members in a group may have an effect on the different measures of group alignment, these correlations were also conducted separately for each of the sub-groups (defined according to the number of individuals with high alexithymia scores in the group). Our findings revealed significant positive correlation between convergence time and OA type of irrational behaviour, in groups with two players who had high alexithymia scores, suggesting that a group acting more irrationally needed more time to reach a consensus ($r = 0.534$, $p < 0.05$). Interestingly, this correlation was found to be non-significant for the two other sub-groups, that is when a group had less than two players with a high alexithymia score. Correlations between the average score of IA type of irrational behaviour and the three different factors of alexithymia or convergence time were non-significant, for all types of sub-groups. The MANOVA revealed non-significant difference between the average irrational behaviour scores (i.e. group average IA ($F(2,138) = 1.128$, $p = .326$) and group average OA ($F(2,138) = 1.139$, $p = .323$) of the three sub-groups.

3. Discussion

The present study was inspired by the social alignment model, which states that the three levels of social alignment (the motor, emotional and cognitive levels) are interrelated processes and rely on shared neural networks. The proposed model assumes that social alignment is beneficial to humans and promotes pro-social behaviour. Given that alexithymia is associated with difficulties in interpersonal relations (Grynberg et al., 2018; Joybari, 2014; Vanheule, Desmet, Meganck, & Bogaerts, 2007), we sought to examine whether these individuals suffer from deficiencies in their capacity to achieve social alignment. Previous findings showed that individuals with high alexithymia scores demonstrate impaired emotional contagion (Moriguchi et al., 2006), and that deficits in motor alignment in the autism spectrum disorder may be largely driven by alexithymia (Brezis et al., 2017). These findings suggest the possibility that alexithymia is associated with aberrant performance across all levels of social alignment (motion, emotion and cognition), although this possibility has not been thoroughly investigated. The aim of the current study was to examine the association between alexithymia and the ability to reach a consensus with the group (a form of cognitive social alignment). By comparing performance when playing with bots (a harmonised group acting rationally) vs. human (a less harmonised group not always acting rationally), we were able to examine whether the level of rationality of other players had any effect on the association between alexithymia and aberrant forms of cognitive alignment (i.e. behaviour that does not promote consensus-building).

The results of the present study confirm the hypothesised link between the alexithymia cognitive component (EOT) and impaired cognitive social alignment, showing that alexithymia is associated with a deficit in reaching a consensus with humans (i.e. irrational players). However, this association was not evident when group members were bots (i.e. rational players). Thus, individuals scoring high on the cognitive component of alexithymia, may have been affected by the actions of other group members. That is, their behaviour during the consensus building process may have been affected by the level of rational behaviour of other group members. Recall that bots were designed to always align their behaviours with the majority of the group, thus playing with a group of bots was experienced as playing with a highly harmonised group. Accordingly, one possible interpretation of our findings is that during games with bots, individuals scoring high on the cognitive component of alexithymia felt that a risk to harmonious social relations may occur if they acted irrationally. In an attempt to maintain group harmony, they inhibited actions that do not promote consensus building, as these actions might lead to potential confrontations or conflicts. By contrast, during games with humans, when group harmony was lower, individuals scoring high on the cognitive component of alexithymia might have realised that there are lower risks to the harmonious relationships and, therefore, did not inhibit actions that do not promote group consensus.

As noted earlier, according to the social alignment model, achieving alignment activates the reward system. Thus, the most preferable action would be to align with the majority of the group in order to reduce distress. The fact that during games with humans, these individuals did not adhere to these principles by changing their own preference to the one chosen by the majority of the group members, may further suggest that these individuals demonstrate a low reliance on the rewarding sensation associated with social alignment. Taken together, our findings suggest that when group harmony is very high (during games against bots) individuals scoring high on the cognitive component of alexithymia were concerned with maintaining group harmony. Thus, in this case, their tendency to align with the group was driven by the need to avoid potential confrontations or conflicts and not by the rewarding sensation associated with social alignment. By contrast, during games against humans in which the need to avoid conflict was lower, they present aberrant social alignment which may be due to low reliance on the rewarding sensation associated with social alignment.

The idea that individuals scoring high on the cognitive component of alexithymia are concerned with maintaining group harmony is supported by previous findings demonstrating that interdependent self-construals are positively associated with alexithymia, on the one hand, and with the need to maintain group harmony, on the other (Konrath, Grynberg, Corneille, Hammig, & Luminet, 2011). A more complete understanding of the links between alexithymia, interdependent self-construals and reaching a consensus might emerge from future research on the intricate relationships between these factors.

According to the social alignment model, the propensity towards alignment with others in terms of behaviours and cognitions is rooted in the rewarding sensation associated with social alignment (Shamay-Tsoory et al., 2019). Our findings raise the possibility that individuals scoring high on the cognitive component of alexithymia demonstrate a low reliance on the rewarding sensation associated with social alignment. As noted above, we speculate that the reason why in certain circumstances they tend to cognitively align with others may be rooted in their concern with maintaining group harmony.

Interestingly, the EOT subscale was the only subscale that was found to be positively associated with irrational behaviour. Specifically, the EOT was found to be associated with actions that reflect anti-conformity (OA). It is important to mention that in games with two players who had high alexithymia scores, a significant positive correlation was found between the OA type of irrational behaviour and the convergence time, suggesting that a group acting more irrationally requires more time and effort to build a consensus. Clearly, the fact that this association was significant only in groups with two players who had high alexithymia scores, but not for groups who had less than two players with a high alexithymia score, suggests that the composition of the group is a factor that can contribute to the effect of irrational behaviour on task performance (i.e. convergent time). Accordingly, having more group members with a high alexithymia score is expected to lead to a stronger association between irrational behaviour and task performance. Since game rounds are limited in number, long convergent time may eventually harm the chances of actually building a consensus. However, this interpretation requires caution, since this finding is the result of explanatory analysis (i.e. group analysis) and thus further research is needed in order to address the question of whether groups with more members with high alexithymia scores take more time to build a consensus, or indeed to reach one at all.

The EOT has been associated with several social cognition skills. A negative association was found between the EOT and the ability to assume the perspective of others in terms of their mental state (Grynberg et al., 2010). More recently, the EOT was found to uniquely predict variance in affective theory of mind (Demers & Koven, 2015). Finally, this subscale was found to be related to a pattern of social detachment, impaired cognitive processing (Vanheule et al., 2011) and interoceptive awareness (Herbert, Herbert, & Pollatos, 2011). Our findings add to this line of research by suggesting that the EOT is also associated with an impaired ability to reach mutual agreements with group of humans. It remains to be determined whether this association is moderated by variables such as detachment and impaired perspective-taking. Further research is required to articulate these links.

An exploratory analysis was conducted in order to examine whether the association between alexithymia and irrational behaviour may be due to the composition of the group regarding their level of alexithymia traits and whether higher level of heterogeneity in alexithymia scores within groups could lead to higher level of irrational behaviour. To this end, the games were divided according to group composition. This analysis did not show a significant association between alexithymia factors and irrational behaviour. Furthermore, the MANOVA revealed non-significant difference between the average irrational behaviour scores (i.e. group average IA and group average OA) of the sub-groups (defined according to the amount of high alexithymia players). However, it is possible that the sample size has led to reduced statistical power for this analysis. Indeed, group-level analysis was considered exploratory, as the sample size in this study was calculated to detect association for individual measures (e.g. alexithymia traits) and not group measures. Also, in the current study, we examined groups with no more than two alexithymia players. This has limited our ability to thoroughly examine whether higher level of heterogeneity in alexithymia scores within groups could decrease social alignment. Thus, further research is needed in order to thoroughly address the question of whether the composition of the group regarding their level of alexithymia may affect the ability to reach consensus. These studies should include a larger sample to allow manipulating the composition of the group in order to examine the relations between the heterogeneity in alexithymia scores within groups and social alignment.

Several limitations of the current study should be mentioned and, consequently, addressed in future studies. First, there may be other explanations to our findings. For example, it is possible that those with high levels of alexithymia behave more irrationally when the game is more difficult (because other players are behaving more irrationally). Alternatively, it is possible that those with high levels of alexithymia are more impulsive and try to gain a maximum of points in unclear situations. The interpretation of our findings also requires caution, in that other intervening factors may have influenced the results as we did not test for mood during the study and for other traits closely related to alexithymia. Furthermore, the EOT subscale score has unacceptably low levels of reliability, and many of the EOT items do not load on their intended factor in factor analysis (Kooiman, Spinhoven, & Trijsburg, 2002). Indeed, in line with previous studies (Cleland, Magura, Foote, Rosenblum, & Kosanke, 2005; Grynberg et al., 2010), the EOT scale yielded a low Cronbach's alpha. A possible limitation regarding the interpretation of the current results is the low internal consistency of the EOT factor. Future research of this type that is specifically interested in EOT could be improved by using a larger battery of self-report measures with EOT subscales that have higher reliability, such as the awareness subscale of the Difficulties in Emotion Regulation Scale (Gratz & Roemer, 2004) or the analysing subscale of the Bermond-Vorst Alexithymia Questionnaire (Vorst & Bermond, 2001).

Secondly, one source of potential bias in alexithymia studies is the complicated clinical picture created by the presence of psychiatric comorbidities or other emotional disturbances, such as depression and anxiety (Edel et al., 2010; Liss, Mailloux, & Erchull, 2008; Marchesi, Brusamonti, & Maggini, 2000). This bias was less likely to exist in the present study as we focused on a group of students and none of them reported suffering from mental illness. However, given that participants were not screened by a clinical psychologist, we cannot rule out the possibility that such conditions among the subjects impacted the results.

Thirdly, the participant's level of motivation was not measured in the current study, an especially relevant point as participants were earning five bonus points in a university course in which they were enrolled. Thus, the possibility that individuals with high alexithymia were acting less rationally because they were less motivated to make compromises cannot be rolled out. Future studies should, therefore, utilise measures of performance validity or compliance. Fourthly, deficits for higher alexithymia scores usually occur when the task is more difficult. Thus, it could be interesting for future studies to manipulate the complexity of the consensus reaching task in order to examine whether greater task difficulty enhances the link between alexithymia and reaching a consensus. Fifthly, it is important to note that our design is purely correlational, and we cannot determine the nature of the causal relationship between these variables. Nevertheless, it seems more logically plausible that differences in alexithymia influence the tendency to cognitive align with others and not vice versa.

Finally, while the main advantage of the CUD game is its ability to identify different type of voting that are not the most preferable choices in terms of their ability to promote consensus, the usage of the task has limited the external validity of our findings. One limit of the CUD game is that consensus is reached by a voting procedure without discussions between the participants, which is quite remote from what happens in human interactions. It would be interesting to examine the effect of visible group members on the link between alexithymia and reaching consensus, as this effect was not estimated by our experiment. Another game limit is the fact that individuals with higher levels of alexithymia were found to display deficits when the task difficulty was increased, such as when they were acting under time pressure (Ihme et al., 2014), suggesting the possibility that since time pressure in the CUD task is high it may influence our findings. In other words, it is possible that the irrational behaviour that was manifested during attempts at consensus-reaching was found because the CUD game contains a time constraint. While this may be relevant to some cases in which the time pressure is high such as in the example of reaching the end of a discussion time, future research is needed to assess the association between alexithymia and reaching a consensus when time constraint does not exist and under various deadlines. Moreover, while reaching a consensus in the CUD task was beneficial to all players (they could earn points bonus only if consensus was reached) in real life there are certain cases in which aligning with the group does not seem beneficial, and individuals may have good reasons to refuse the consensus. Future research should use a variety of ecologically valid social tasks to examine the social context in which group consensus may not be beneficial and how these different contexts may affect the link between alexithymia and reaching a consensus.

In conclusion, the significance of the current study lies in its suggestion that the cognitive component of alexithymia is associated with difficulties in reaching a consensus when harmony conditions are low (as occurs when playing unknowingly with a group of humans), but not when harmony conditions are high (as occurs when playing unknowingly with a group of bots). Further studies regarding alexithymia and consensus-reaching are needed. Nevertheless, we believe that the current study marks a step towards gaining a better understanding of the link between alexithymia and aberrant forms of social alignment. Given that social alignment plays a prominent role in interpersonal relations as it leads to closeness and likability (Shamay-Tsoory et al., 2019), studying the link between alexithymia and social alignment may contribute to greater and deeper understanding of the interpersonal outcomes associated with high alexithymia scores. Finally, the findings have implications for studying the association between reaching a consensus and several other psychological dimensions that have been found to be associated with alexithymia, e.g. ASD (Poquérusse, Pastore, Dellantonio, & Esposito, 2018).

Acknowledgments

The authors wish to thank David Ben-Yosef for his technical support in running the CUD game. Ornit Apelboim and Bar Ben Atiya for their help with this research project.

Disclosure statement

No potential conflict of interest was reported by the authors.

ORCID

Hila Zahava Gvirts http://orcid.org/0000-0002-3625-5959
Lihi Dery http://orcid.org/0000-0002-8710-3349

References

Bagby, R. M., Parker, J. D., & Taylor, G. J. (1994). The twenty-item Toronto Alexithymia Scale – I. Item selection and cross-validation of the factor structure. *Journal of Psychosomatic Research*, *38*(1), 23–32. doi:10.1016/0022-3999(94)90005-1

Bagby, R. M., Taylor, G. J., & Parker, J. D. (1994). The twenty-item Toronto Alexithymia Scale – II. Convergent, discriminant, and concurrent validity. *Journal of Psychosomatic Research*, *38*(1), 33–40. doi:10.1016/0022-3999(94)90006-X

Bannikova, M., Naamani-Dery, L., Obraztsova, S., Rabinovich, Z., & Rosenschein, J. S. (2016). Between fairness and a mistrial: Consensus under a deadline. *The 10th workshop on advances in preference handling (M-PREF)*. New-York, USA.

Bird, G., & Cook, R. (2013). Mixed emotions: The contribution of alexithymia to the emotional symptoms of autism. *Translational Psychiatry*, *3*(7), e285. doi:10.1038/tp.2013.61

Brezis, R.-S., Noy, L., Alony, T., Gotlieb, R., Cohen, R., Golland, Y., & Levit-Binnun, N. (2017). Patterns of joint improvisation in adults with autism spectrum disorder. *Frontiers in Psychology*, *8*, 1790. doi:10.3389/fpsyg.2017.01790

Cleland, C., Magura, S., Foote, J., Rosenblum, A., & Kosanke, N. (2005). Psychometric properties of the Toronto Alexithymia Scale (TAS-20) for substance users. *Journal of Psychosomatic Research*, *58*(3), 299–306. doi:10.1016/J.JPSYCHORES.2004.11.002

Coultas, J. C., & van Leeuwen, E. J. (2015). Conformity: Definitions, types, and evolutionary grounding. In V. Zeigler-Hill, L. L. Welling, & T. K. Shackelford (Eds.), *Evolutionary perspectives on social psychology* (pp. 189–202). Cham: Springer. doi:10.1007/978-3-319-12697-5_15

Cronbach, L. J. (1951). Coefficient alpha and the internal structure of tests. *Psychometrika*, *16*(3), 297–334. doi:10.1007/BF02310555

Cronbach, L. J. (1988). Internal consistency of tests: Analyses old and new. *Psychometrika*, *53*(1), 63–70. doi:10.1007/BF02294194

Davydov, D. M., Luminet, O., & Zech, E. (2013). An externally oriented style of thinking as a moderator of responses to affective films in women. *International Journal of Psychophysiology*, *87*(2), 152–164. doi:10.1016/j.ijpsycho.2012.12.003

Demers, L. A., & Koven, N. S. (2015). The relation of alexithymic traits to affective theory of mind. *American Journal of Psychology*, *128*(1), 31–42. doi:10.5406/amerjpsyc.128.1.0031

Demers, L. A., Schreiner, M. W., Hunt, R. H., Mueller, B. A., Klimes-Dougan, B., Thomas, K. M., & Cullen, K. R. (2019). Alexithymia is associated with neural reactivity to masked emotional faces in adolescents who self-harm. *Journal of Affective Disorders*, *249*, 253–261.

Edel, M. A., Rudel, A., Hubert, C., Scheele, D., Brüne, M., Juckel, G., & Assion, H. J. (2010). Alexithymia, emotion processing and social anxiety in adults with ADHD. *European Journal of Medical Research*, *15*(9), 403. doi:10.1186/2047-783x-15-9-403

Faria, J. J., Dyer, J. R., Tosh, C. R., & Krause, J. (2010). Leadership and social information use in human crowds. *Animal Behaviour*, *79*(4), 895–901. doi:10.1016/J.ANBEHAV.2009.12.039

Franz, M., Popp, K., Schaefer, R., Sitte, W., Schneider, C., Hardt, J., … Braehler, E. (2008). Alexithymia in the German general population. *Social Psychiatry and Psychiatric Epidemiology*, *43*(1), 54–62.

Gratz, K. L., & Roemer, L. (2004). Multidimensional assessment of emotion regulation and dysregulation: Development, factor structure, and initial validation of the difficulties in emotion regulation scale. *Journal of Psychopathology and Behavioral Assessment*, *26*, 41–54. Kluwer Academic Publishers-Plenum Publishers. doi:10.1023/B:JOBA.0000007455.08539.94

Grynberg, D., Berthoz, S., & Bird, G. (2018). Social and interpersonal implications of alexithymia. In O. Luminet, R. M. Bagby, & G. J. Taylor (Eds.), *Alexithymia: Advances in research, theory, and clinical practice* (pp. 174–189). Cambridge: Cambridge University Press. doi:10.1017/9781108241595.013

Grynberg, D., Luminet, O., Corneille, O., Grèzes, J., & Berthoz, S. (2010). Alexithymia in the interpersonal domain: A general deficit of empathy? *Personality and Individual Differences*, *49*(8), 845–850. doi:10.1016/j.paid.2010.07.013

Hair, J. F., Black, W. C., Babin, B. J., Anderson, R. E., & Tatham, R. (2010). *Multivariate data analysis* (7th ed.). Upper Saddle River, NJ: Pearson Prentice Hall.

Herbert, B. M., Herbert, C., & Pollatos, O. (2011). On the relationship between interoceptive awareness and alexithymia: Is interoceptive awareness related to emotional awareness? *Journal of Personality*, *79*(5), 1149–1175. doi:10.1111/j.1467-6494.2011.00717.x

Honkalampi, K., Saarinen, P., Hintikka, J., Virtanen, V., & Viinamäki, H. (1999). Factors associated with alexithymia in patients suffering from depression. *Psychotherapy and Psychosomatics*, *68*(5), 270–275. doi:10.1159/000012343

Ihme, K., Sacher, J., Lichev, V., Rosenberg, N., Kugel, H., Rufer, M., … Suslow, T. (2014). Alexithymia and the labeling of facial emotions: Response slowing and increased motor and somatosensory processing. *BMC Neuroscience*, *15*(1), 40. doi:10.1186/1471-2202-15-40

Joybari, M. T. (2014). Depression and interpersonal problems in adolescents: Their relationship with alexithymia and coping styles. *Iranian Journal of Psychiatry and Behavioral Sciences*, *8*(4), 38.

Konrath, S., Grynberg, D., Corneille, O., Hammig, S., & Luminet, O. (2011). On the social cost of interdependence: Alexithymia is enhanced among socially interdependent people. *Personality and Individual Differences*, *50*(2), 135–141. doi:10.1016/J.PAID.2010.09.008

Kooiman, C. G., Spinhoven, P., & Trijsburg, R. W. (2002). The assessment of alexithymia: A critical review of the literature and a psychometric study of the Toronto Alexithymia Scale-20. *Journal of Psychosomatic Research*, *53*(6), 1083–1090. doi:10.1016/S0022-3999(02)00348-3

Kühn, S., Müller, B. C. N., van der Leij, A., Dijksterhuis, A., Brass, M., & van Baaren, R. B. (2010). Neural correlates of emotional synchrony. *Social Cognitive and Affective Neuroscience*, *6*(3), 368–374. doi:10.1093/scan/nsq044

Leweke, F., Leichsenring, F., Kruse, J., & Hermes, S. (2012). Is alexithymia associated with specific mental disorders. *Psychopathology*, *45*(1), 22–28.

Liss, M., Mailloux, J., & Erchull, M. J. (2008). The relationships between sensory processing sensitivity, alexithymia, autism, depression, and anxiety. *Personality and Individual Differences*, *45*(3), 255–259. doi:10.1016/J.PAID.2008.04.009

Mahardhika, D., Valls, A. A., Kanno, T., & Furuta, K. (2017). Rational and non-rational influence in a time-constrained group decision making. In *Resilience: A new paradigm of nuclear safety* (pp. 279–287). Cham: Springer.

Marchesi, C., Brusamonti, E., & Maggini, C. (2000). Are alexithymia, depression, and anxiety distinct constructs in affective disorders? *Journal of Psychosomatic Research*, *49*(1), 43–49. doi:10.1016/S0022-3999(00)00084-2

McDonald, R. P. (2013). *Test theory: A unified treatment*. Sussex: Psychology Press.

McKelvey, W., & Kerr, N. H. (1988). Differences in conformity among friends and strangers. *Psychological Reports*, *62*(3), 759–762. doi:10.2466/pr0.1988.62.3.759

Moriguchi, Y., Ohnishi, T., Lane, R. D., Maeda, M., Mori, T., Nemoto, K., ... Komaki, G. (2006). Impaired self-awareness and theory of mind: An fMRI study of mentalizing in alexithymia. *NeuroImage*, *32*(3), 1472–1482. doi:10.1016/J.NEUROIMAGE.2006.04.186

Nicolò, G., Semerari, A., Lysaker, P. H., Dimaggio, G., Conti, L., D'Angerio, S., ... Carcione, A. (2011). Alexithymia in personality disorders: Correlations with symptoms and interpersonal functioning. *Psychiatry Research*, *190*(1), 37–42.

Noy, L., Levit-Binun, N., & Golland, Y. (2015). Being in the zone: Physiological markers of togetherness in joint improvisation. *Frontiers in Human Neuroscience*, *9*, 187. doi:10.3389/fnhum.2015.00187

Ospina, L. H., Shanahan, M., Perez-Rodriguez, M. M., Chan, C. C., Clari, R., & Burdick, K. E. (2019). Alexithymia predicts poorer social and everyday functioning in schizophrenia and bipolar disorder. *Psychiatry Research*, *273*, 218–226.

Parker, J. D., Taylor, G. J., & Bagby, R. M. (2003). The 20-item Toronto Alexithymia Scale: III. Reliability and factorial validity in a community population. *Journal of Psychosomatic Research*, *55*(3), 269–275. doi:10.1016/S0022-3999(02)00578-0

Poquérusse, J., Pastore, L., Dellantonio, S., & Esposito, G. (2018). Alexithymia and autism spectrum disorder: A complex relationship. *Frontiers in Psychology*, *9*(JUL), 1638. doi:10.3389/fpsyg.2018.01196

Prochazkova, E., & Kret, M. E. (2017). Connecting minds and sharing emotions through mimicry: A neurocognitive model of emotional contagion. *Neuroscience and Biobehavioral Reviews*, *80*, 99–114. doi:10.1016/j.neubiorev.2017.05.013

Rabinowitch, T. C., & Knafo-Noam, A. (2015). Synchronous rhythmic interaction enhances children's perceived similarity and closeness towards each other. *PLoS One*, *10*(4), e0120878. doi:10.1371/journal.pone.0120878

Revelle, W. (1979). Hierarchical cluster analysis and the internal structure of tests. *Multivariate Behavioral Research*, *14*(1), 57–74.

Revelle, W., & Zinbarg, R. E. (2009). Coefficients alpha, beta, omega, and the glb: Comments on Sijtsma. *Psychometrika*, *74*(1), 145.

Saint, S., & Lawson, J. R. (1994). *Rules for reaching consensus: A modern approach to decision making*. San Francisco, CA: Jossey-Bass.

Sevindi, T., & Kumcagiz, H. (2018). The relationship between high school students' levels of alexithymia and communication skills. *Kastamonu Education Journal*, *26*(4), 1335.

Shamay-Tsoory, S. G., Saporta, N., Marton-Alper, I. Z., & Gvirts, H. Z. (2019). Herding brains: A core neural mechanism for social alignment. *Trends in Cognitive Sciences*, *23*(3), 174–186. doi:10.1016/j.tics.2019.01.002

Sifneos, P. E. (1973). The prevalence of 'alexithymic' characteristics in psychosomatic patients. *Psychotherapy and Psychosomatics*, *22*(2–6), 255–262.

Sonnby-Borgström, M. (2009). Alexithymia as related to facial imitation, mentalization, empathy, and internal working models-of-self and -others. *Neuropsychoanalysis*, *11*(1), 111–128. doi:10.1080/15294145.2009.10773602

Stamper, R. L. (1985). Haste makes waste. *Ophthalmology*, *92*, 39A. doi:10.1016/S0161-6420(85)80006-3

Sylos-Labini, F., d'Avella, A., Lacquaniti, F., & Ivanenko, Y. (2018). Human-human interaction forces and interlimb coordination during side-by-side walking with hand contact. *Frontiers in Physiology*, *9*(Mar), 179. doi:10.3389/fphys.2018.00179

Tarr, B., Launay, J., & Dunbar, R. I. (2016). Silent disco: Dancing in synchrony leads to elevated pain thresholds and social closeness. *Evolution and Human Behavior*, *37*(5), doi:10.1016/j.evolhumbehav.2016.02.004

Taylor, G. J., & Bagby, R. M. (2000). An overview of the alexithymia construct. In R. Bar-On & J. D. Parker (Eds.), *Handbook of emotional intelligence: Theory, development, assessment, and application at home, school, and in the workplace* (pp. 41–67). San Francisco, CA: Jossey-Bass.

Taylor, G. J., Parker, J. D., Bagby, R. M., & Bourke, M. P. (1996). Relationships between alexithymia and psychological characteristics associated with eating disorders. *Journal of Psychosomatic Research*, *41*(6), 561–568. doi:10.1016/S0022-3999(96)00224-3

Vanheule, S., Desmet, M., Meganck, R., & Bogaerts, S. (2007). Alexithymia and interpersonal problems. *Journal of Clinical Psychology*, *63*(1), 109–117. doi:10.1002/jclp.20324

Vanheule, S., Meganck, R., & Desmet, M. (2011). Alexithymia, social detachment and cognitive processing. *Psychiatry Research*, *190*(1), 49–51. doi:10.1016/j.psychres.2010.06.032

Vorst, H. C., & Bermond, B. (2001). Validity and reliability of the Bermond–Vorst Alexithymia Questionnaire. *Personality and Individual Differences*, *30*(3), 413–434. doi:10.1016/S0191-8869(00)00033-7

Wallbott, H. G. (1991). Recognition of emotion from facial expression via imitation? Some indirect evidence for an old theory. *British Journal of Social Psychology*, *30*(3), 207–219. doi:10.1111/j.2044-8309.1991.tb00939.x

Yosef, D. B., Naamani-Dery, L., Obraztsova, S., Rabinovich, Z., & Bannikova, M. (2017). Haste makes waste: A case to favour voting bots. In *Proceedings of the international conference on Web Intelligence* (pp. 419–425). Leipzig, Germany: ACM. doi:10.1145/3106426.3106532

Zackheim, L. (2007). Alexithymia: The expanding realm of research. *Journal of Psychosomatic Research*, *63*(4), 345–347. doi:10.1016/j.jpsychores.2007.08.011

Zinbarg, R. E., Revelle, W., Yovel, I., & Li, W. (2005). Cronbach's α, Revelle's β, and McDonald's ω H: Their relations with each other and two alternative conceptualizations of reliability. *Psychometrika*, *70*(1), 123–133.

The role of alexithymia in memory and executive functioning across the lifespan

Anthony N. Correro II, Elizabeth R. Paitel, Steven J. Byers and Kristy A. Nielson

ABSTRACT

Alexithymia is a personality trait characterised by difficulties identifying feelings (DIF), describing feelings (DDF), and externally oriented thinking (EOT). Alexithymia has been associated with poorer memory, at least for emotive materials, and recently, with executive and neural dysfunction. Aging is also accompanied by poorer memory and executive functioning (EF), neural dysfunction, and increasing alexithymia. Thus, the hypothesis of a general cognitive impairment in alexithymia, particularly in elders, needs investigation. Three large, independent, cross-sectional experiments ($n = 296$, 139 and 121, respectively) investigated memory and EF in healthy adults, ranging from young to old adulthood, with age, sex, and the three Toronto Alexithymia Scale-20 subscales (DIF, DDF, EOT) as predictors in hierarchical regressions. Across studies, alexithymia contributed to poorer memory (via EOT) and EF (via DIF), in younger and older adults. Additionally, these effects occurred in non-emotive contexts with neutral stimuli. Moreover, although memory was worse with greater age and poor EF contributed to poor memory, those who had both high EOT and poor EF had particularly poor memory. Thus, alexithymia (particularly via high DIF or high EOT) is a risk factor for age-related cognitive decline. Further research should clarify the direction and nature of these complex relationships.

Alexithymia is a personality trait associated with difficulties identifying feelings (DIF), difficulties describing feelings (DDF), and externally oriented thinking (EOT) (Bagby, Parker, & Taylor, 1994; Bagby, Taylor, & Parker, 1994; Nemiah, 1977; Sifneos, 1973; Taylor, 2000). People with high alexithymia scores (HA) have deficits in both the cognitive processing and regulation of emotions (Lane et al., 1996; Swart, Kortekaas, & Aleman, 2009), likely via poor emotional awareness, recognition, and differentiation (da Silva, Vasco, & Watson, 2017); and slower, less accurate emotion identification, suggesting poorer automatic attentional processing (Vermeulen, Luminet, & Corneille, 2006) versus people with low alexithymia scores (LA). Typically, attentional resources are directed toward salient content in the environment, such as negative or arousing stimuli, which enhances memory for the salient content (Mather & Sutherland, 2011; Nielson & Correro, 2017). However, HA cannot as readily process emotional information, exhibiting impairment in perception, attention allocation, and regulation related to emotion (Aftanas, Varlamov, Reva, & Pavlov, 2003; da Silva et al., 2017; Luminet, Vermeulen, Demaret, Taylor, & Bagby, 2006; Swart et al., 2009; van der Velde et al., 2015; Vermeulen et al., 2006), and interpreting emotions at a behavioural or physiological level (Kano & Fukudo, 2013; Moriguchi & Komaki, 2013).

Evidence is accumulating that alexithymia contributes to deficits in learning and memory specifically for emotional information and contexts (Dressaire et al., 2015; Jacob & Hautekeete, 1998; Luminet et al., 2006; Meltzer & Nielson, 2010; Suslow, Kersting, & Arolt, 2003; Vermeulen & Luminet, 2009; Vermeulen, Domachowska, & Nielson, 2018; Vermeulen, Toussaint, & Luminet, 2010), while memory for neutral memoranda appears intact. Yet, such studies typically examined neutral material in the context of emotion. At least one study of young adults ($n = 85$) showed evidence of poorer memory in HA for neutral memoranda in a neutral context (Nielson & Meltzer, 2009). Story and complex figure recall have also been negatively correlated with alexithymia in a sample of 20 older adults (Onor, Trevisiol, Spano, Aguglia, & Paradiso, 2010), and poorer short- and long-term memory in HA was reported for pictures of people in social situations, despite comparable verbal ability across groups and samples of only 12 per group (DiStefano & Koven, 2012). These studies hint at a general memory impairment in alexithymia. Considering alexithymia facets, DIF has been implicated in impaired memory for emotional material (Luminet et al., 2006; Vermeulen & Luminet, 2009), though inconsistently (Dressaire et al., 2015). Similarly, EOT has been related to poorer memory for emotive words (Dressaire et al., 2015; Meltzer & Nielson, 2010) but better memory for neutral words within an emotive context (Meltzer & Nielson, 2010; Vermeulen & Luminet, 2009). Yet, in neutral context, there is evidence EOT associates with impairment, particularly in elders (Onor et al., 2010). Given the paucity of studies, the typically small samples, and little study of specific alexithymia facets, further research is needed in neutral contexts to examine whether a more general memory deficit exists in alexithymia.

Executive functions are the higher-order cognitive processes involved in goal-directed behaviour, such as inhibition, fluency, set-shifting, and performance monitoring (Diamond, 2013). Importantly, executive functioning (EF) impacts the utilisation and effectiveness of other cognitive abilities, including learning and memory (Duff, Schoenberg, Scott, & Adams, 2005; Hill, Alosco, Bauer, & Tremont, 2012). A growing literature suggests executive dysfunction in HA, shown on measures ranging from fluency (Henry, Phillips, Crawford, Theodorou, & Summers, 2006; Santorelli & Ready, 2015; Wood & Williams, 2007) to problem solving (Onor et al., 2010); sequencing, set-shifting, and conflict processing (Wood & Williams, 2007); inhibition (Zhang et al., 2011; Zhang et al., 2012); and self-report (Koven & Thomas, 2010). Ultimately, executive dysfunction may contribute to emotion processing difficulties and related memory deficits in alexithymia. Moreover, most studies of EF employ non-emotive, neutral stimuli (except Zhang et al., 2012), hinting at a general cognitive deficit in alexithymia. However, this literature is small, using small samples and varied measures and approaches; some examined neurologically-induced alexithymia (e.g. Henry et al., 2006; Wood & Williams, 2007). Results are mixed, even across relatively comparable tasks (e.g. Henry et al., 2006; Lamberty & Holt, 1995; Santorelli & Ready, 2015). Finally, few studies have directly examined the facets of alexithymia as related to EF. The limited existing work suggests DIF and DDF are associated with executive dysfunction (Correro, Marra, Reiter, Byers, & Nielson, 2016; Henry et al., 2006; Koven & Thomas, 2010; Santorelli & Ready, 2015). More research examining EF with larger samples and examining the specific facets of EF are particularly needed.

Cognitive dysfunction in alexithymia is apparent across the lifespan (e.g. Correro et al., 2016; Lamberty & Holt, 1995; Onor et al., 2010; Santorelli & Ready, 2015). Yet, after age 30, increasing age is associated with increasing alexithymia (Mattila, Salminen, Nummi, & Joukamaa, 2006; Onor et al., 2010), as well as with neural dysfunction, particularly involving frontal lobe function and circuits, that results in declining EF and memory over time (Charlton et al., 2008; Goerlich & Aleman, 2018; Vermeulen et al., 2018). Thus, it is essential to delineate the unique contributions of alexithymia and age to cognitive functioning, and to better isolate the facets of alexithymia that result in cognitive deficits, to help clarify and address the underlying mechanisms of cognitive effects of alexithymia.

The primary objective of the current experiments was to evaluate the relationships between alexithymia, memory and EF in relatively large young and older adult samples, focusing on general cognitive functioning rather than using emotive contexts or memoranda. We used separate, non-overlapping samples for three experiments; each was a secondary analysis of data from prior protocols.[1] Using non-emotive stimuli and measuring alexithymia with a standard and frequently used measure (the Toronto Alexithymia Scale—20 [TAS-20], Bagby, Parker, et al., 1994; Bagby, Taylor, et al., 1994), we first examined whether a laboratory word memory task would be predicted by alexithymia after accounting for age and sex in a large normative sample of young adults (Experiment 1). In Experiment 2 we examined whether executive functioning, using standardised neuropsychological tests, would be predicted by alexithymia in a large sample including young and older adults. Finally, in Experiment 3 we examined whether alexithymia would predict memory and EF, using standardised neuropsychological tests in young and older adults, and the contribution of alexithymia to the memory-EF relationship.

Experiment 1

Memory is altered by alexithymia in emotional contexts (see Vermeulen et al., 2018). However, studies with larger samples are needed to verify whether memory alterations in alexithymia might be apparent for neutral memoranda, particularly in neutral contexts, and to further probe specific facet(s) of alexithymia. In Experiment 1, young adults completed a verbal, non-emotive memory task that used nouns as memoranda, with long-term retention assessed 60 minutes later. Based on very limited prior research we hypothesised that, after accounting for age and sex, memory for neutral words in a neutral context would be impaired by alexithymia (DiStefano & Koven, 2012; Nielson & Meltzer, 2009; Onor et al., 2010), speculating that EOT might be responsible (Onor et al., 2010) due to its more cognitive role in alexithymia (Vermeulen & Luminet, 2009).

Method

Participants

Young adults ($n = 297$) were recruited from university classes; those ≥18 years and with English as first language (EFL) were included. One subject had incomplete TAS-20 data, leaving a final sample of 296 (214 female). Descriptive statistics are shown in Table 1.

Materials

The memory task used 30 high-imagery nouns (>6.0 on a scale of 1–7; Paivio, Yuille, & Madigan, 1968; e.g. "butterfly", "queen", "house") presented at three-second intervals (white on blue) with instructions to remember the words. Free recall was tested immediately to ensure encoding. Delayed retention was tested by recognition using 140 quasi-randomly ordered prompts; 30 targets, 110 distracters (Nielson, Yee, & Erickson, 2005). A 60-min delay targeted long-term memory and helped prevent recognition ceiling effects. Table 1 provides raw recognition metrics (hits, false alarms), sensitivity (i.e. degree of overlap between signal and noise distributions, $d' = z(\text{false alarms}) - z(\text{hits})$, and response bias, $C = -(z(\text{hits}) + z(\text{false alarms}))/2$; negative = liberal (yes), positive = conservative (no) (Stanislaw & Todorov, 1999)).

Table 1. Experiment 1 ($n = 296$, 214 female), Descriptive statistics.

	Mean	SD
Age (years)	19.68	1.93
BSI-Depression	0.84	0.64
BSI-Anxiety	0.91	0.62
TAS-20 Total	44.85	11.06
Difficulty Identifying Feelings	13.50	5.27
Difficulty Describing Feelings	12.63	4.80
Externally Oriented Thinking	18.80	4.78
Immediate Recall (of 30)	13.58	3.80
Delayed Recognition Hits (%)	67.90	15.80
Delayed Recognition False Alarms (%)	5.50	6.10
Delayed Recognition Sensitivity (d')	2.58	1.33
Delayed Recognition Response Bias (C)	0.71	0.36

Notes: BSI = Brief Symptom Inventory; TAS-20 Total = Toronto Alexithymia Scale-20.

Alexithymia was measured using the 20-item Toronto Alexithymia Scale (TAS-20; Bagby, Parker, et al., 1994; Bagby, Taylor, et al., 1994), using a five-point scale (possible scores = 20–100). Three non-orthogonal subscales include Difficulty Identifying Feelings (DIF; range = 7–35), Difficulty Describing Feelings (DDF; range = 5–25), and Externally Oriented Thinking (EOT; range = 8–40). TAS-20 has good reliability, convergent/concurrent and criterion validity (e.g. Parker, Taylor, & Bagby, 2003; Taylor, Bagby, & Luminet, 2000; Taylor, Bagby, & Parker, 2003). Internal consistency (IC) is typically ≥0.70 with EOT lowest (Parker et al., 2003); current study IC: Total = 0.834, DIF = 0.827, DDF = 0.821, EOT = 0.668. Due to relevance to alexithymia, the depression and anxiety subscales of the Brief Symptom Inventory (BSI) are shown (Table 1). The 53-item BSI measures nine symptom categories (depression and anxiety raw scores = average of 6 items, on scale of 0 (none) to 4 (severe)); it has acceptable reliability, convergent/concurrent and criterion validity, and IC > 0.70 (Derogatis & Melisaratos, 1983).[2]

Design and Procedure

Participants were tested individually, completing a demographic survey followed by the memory task. After encoding and immediate free recall, a delay of 60 minutes was filled with multiple surveys, including the TAS-20, followed by recognition testing (see note 1). Correlations were examined with Pearson *r*, or Spearman's *rho* where non-normality existed. Hierarchical regressions were performed predicting delayed memory measures using age (years) and sex in Step 1, and all three TAS-20 subscales in Step 2 as predictors (SPSS v.24). Given the correlations amongst the variables of interest and the non-orthogonal TAS-20 subscales, multicollinearity (tolerance, variance inflation factor) prevented adding all interaction terms to these models; only targeted interactions were explored. *A priori* power analysis for hierarchical regression (2 + 3 predictors; medium effect (.15), power ≥ 0.80, $p < 0.05$) indicated a sample of 78; adding two predictors (i.e. interactions) suggested a sample of 90 (Soper, 2019).

Results and discussion

Bivariate correlations are shown in Table 2. Outcomes (memory) did not correlate significantly with age, depression or anxiety in this sample. Regarding alexithymia, only EOT correlated significantly with memory (hits and d'), while depression and anxiety correlated with DIF and DDF. The TAS-20 subscores in this large but age-restricted sample were log-transformed prior to regression to improve normality.

Hierarchical regression (see Table 3) produced a significant model predicting memory (d') with sex significant in Step 1; sex, DIF and EOT were significant in Step 2. Similar but weaker models resulted for uncorrected hits and immediate recall. None of the study variables predicted false alarms ($p > .13$) or C ($p > .17$). Thus, men and those with higher DIF and EOT had poorer delayed memory, via sensitivity, for neutral words. Although depression and anxiety did not correlate with memory, including either added no significant prediction in any model ($ps > .54$), nor did they supplant TAS-20 predictors. Although immediate recall was significantly correlated with d', including it in the model did not alter the relationship of TAS-20 to d'. Last, the interaction of sex and EOT as Step 3 was not significant ($p = .54$); other terms were unchanged by this addition. Thus, although females had better memory performance than males, EOT was associated with poorer memory for neutral words in both men and women.

The contribution of both EOT and DIF to the model predicting d', despite the lack of correlation of DIF with d', warranted interrogation with bootstrapped mediation analysis (PROCESS 3.0; Hayes, 2018). Figure 1 demonstrates that EOT mediated the relationship of DIF to memory. Consistent with the lack of bivariate correlation, the direct effect of DIF on d' was not significant (B=-.33, SE = .20, $p = .11$). Thus, DIF did not contribute to predicting d' independently from EOT. Instead, the shared variance of DIF with EOT appeared to cause the significance of DIF in the model. Thus, the relationship of alexithymia to memory was primarily contributed by EOT.

Experiment 1 sought to examine the contribution of alexithymia to long-term memory in young adults for non-emotive memoranda. Through EOT, alexithymia contributed to reduced ability to retrieve neutral words after one hour. The proportion of variance captured by age and alexithymia is small but significant in this young sample. Alexithymia specifically contributed to sensitivity not attributable to depression, anxiety, or encoding. This is a novel finding. Previous studies have shown alexithymia results in poorer memory for emotive memoranda, attributing the effects to stimulus relevance (Luminet et al., 2006; Meltzer & Nielson, 2010) and emotional context (Nielson & Meltzer, 2009; Vermeulen et al., 2010; Vermeulen & Luminet, 2009). Our results, using a larger than typical sample, suggest that EOT contributes to general difficulty distinguishing targets ("signal") from foils ("noise"); contextual and personal salience effects in alexithymia may be *additive* rather than exclusive in memory processing and retrieval.

Table 2. Experiment 1, Bivariate correlations.

	Age	Sex	BSID	BSIA	DIF	DDF	EOT	IR	Hits	FA	d'	C
Age	–											
Sex	0.00	–										
BSID	**−0.15**	**0.15**	–									
BSIA	−0.09	**0.15**	**0.61**	–								
TAS DIF	**−0.18**	0.00	**0.51**	**0.50**	–							
TAS DDF	**−0.22**	0.00	**0.37**	**0.32**	**0.52**	–						
TAS EOT	**−0.17**	−0.10	0.01	−0.03	0.12	**0.37**	–					
IR	−0.08	−0.14	0.06	0.04	0.06	−0.01	−0.13	–				
Hits	0.03	**0.24**	0.09	0.06	0.04	0.03	−0.14	**0.54**	–			
FA	0.05	−0.11	0.01	0.03	0.06	0.01	0.08	**−0.37**	**−0.22**	–		
d'	−0.05	**0.23**	0.06	0.02	0.01	0.01	**−0.15**	**0.55**	**0.82**	**−0.74**	–	
C	−0.01	−0.11	−0.09	−0.07	−0.08	−0.03	0.0	0.07	**−0.70**	**−0.55**	**−0.16**	–

Notes: ≤.05; **<.01**; Pearson *r* except with sex (Spearman's *rho*); TAS = Toronto Alexithymia Scale-20; DIF = Difficulty Identifying Feelings; DDF = Difficulty Describing Feelings; EOT = Externally Oriented Thinking; BSI = Brief Symptom Inventory (D = Depression, A = Anxiety); IR: Immediate recall; FA = False Alarms; d'=sensitivity; C = response bias.

Table 3. Experiment 1, Hierarchical regression predicting delayed recognition memory sensitivity.

		Model summary of each step				Contribution of each variable in last step				
		R^2	DR^2	*F*	*p*	B	SE	b	*t*	*p*
Hits										
Step 1		0.051	–	7.82	**<0.01**					
	Age					−0.011	0.015	−0.041	−0.70	0.48
	Sex					0.236	0.065	0.209	3.65	**<0.01**
Step 2		0.073	0.021	2.22	0.09					
	DIF					0.017	0.090	0.012	0.18	0.86
	DDF					0.079	0.088	0.065	0.90	0.37
	EOT					−0.305	0.121	−0.156	−2.52	**0.01**
False Alarms										
Step 1		0.014	–	2.05	0.13					
	Age					0.011	0.013	0.052	0.86	0.39
	Sex					−0.099	0.056	−0.102	−1.75	0.08
Step 2		0.027	0.013	1.67	0.16					
	DIF					0.100	0.079	0.087	1.27	0.21
	DDF					−0.069	0.077	−0.066	−0.90	0.37
	EOT					0.172	0.106	0.103	1.63	0.11
d′ (sensitivity)										
Step 1		0.022	–	3.24	0.04					
	Age					0.091	0.911	0.006	0.10	0.92
	Sex					0.434	0.171	0.147	2.54	**0.01**
Step 2		0.064	0.042	3.92	**<0.01**					
	DIF					−0.512	0.236	−0.146	−2.17	0.03
	DDF					0.434	0.231	0.135	1.88	0.06
	EOT					−0.969	0.315	−0.191	−3.07	**<0.01**
C (response bias)										
Step 1		0.012	–	1.75	0.18					
	Age					0.000	0.009	−0.002	−0.04	0.97
	Sex					−0.068	0.039	−0.104	−1.77	0.08
Step 2		0.020	0.008	1.18	0.32					
	DIF					−0.058	0.054	−0.074	−1.08	0.28
	DDF					−0.005	0.053	−0.007	−0.10	0.92
	EOT					0.066	0.072	0.059	0.92	0.36

Notes: ≤.05; **<.01**; Toronto Alexithymia Scale-20: DIF = Difficulty Identifying Feelings, DDF = Difficulty Describing Feelings, EOT = Externally Oriented Thinking.

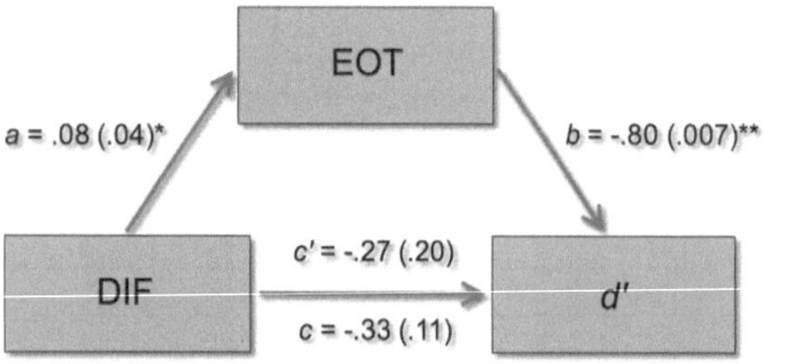

Figure 1. In Experiment 1, both Difficulty Identifying Feelings (DIF) and Externally Oriented Thinking (EOT) were significant predictors of recognition memory (*d′*) after accounting for age and sex. In this *post-hoc* mediation model (showing coefficient (*p*) for each path), the total effect of DIF on *d′* (path *c*) is not significant (consistent with the lack of bivariate correlation between them; see Table 2). Instead, there is a significant relationship between DIF and EOT (path *a*) and between EOT and *d′* (path *b*), which results in a weaker direct effect than total effect of DIF on *d′* (i.e. path *c′*). This demonstrates mediation. That is, the effect of DIF on *d′* did not occur independently from the effect of EOT on *d′*. Instead, EOT mediated the relationship between DIF and *d′*; EOT was the primary contributor to reduced memory in alexithymia.

Experiment 2

Executive functioning declines (e.g. Charlton et al., 2008) while alexithymia increases during older age (Mattila et al., 2006), making aging an important context for evaluating cognitive relationships with alexithymia. A deficit in EF, with specific tasks varying by study, has been shown in a handful of alexithymia studies of neurologically altered and normative samples of younger and older adults (Henry et al., 2006; Koven & Thomas, 2010; Santorelli & Ready, 2015; Zhang et al., 2011; Zhang et al., 2012). Experiment 2 therefore sought to examine alexithymia and EF in a large, normative, cognitively intact sample including young to old adults. We hypothesised that a general executive factor, computed from multiple standard tasks of EF, would be predicted by both age and alexithymia. Based on Experiment 1, this small literature, and a small preliminary study (Correro et al., 2016), we hypothesised that DIF and DDF would specifically predict EF.

Method

Participants

Participants (144 (97 female)) were healthy, EFL, and cognitively intact adults: 40 young adults (18–35 years), and 104 older adults (48–86 years; these drawn from two different samples, targeting healthy adults ≥45 years, although no one 45–47 years volunteered). Participants reported no history of medical, neurological, psychiatric, or substance abuse conditions; hypertension was controlled. Older adults were screened for intact cognition (Mini-Mental State Exam (MMSE), Folstein, Folstein, & McHugh, 1975, ≥26/30). Five participants were missing EF score(s) due to data or record errors, leaving a final sample of 139. Descriptive statistics are in Table 4.

Materials

Alexithymia was assessed using the TAS-20 (IC: Total = 0.838, DIF = 0.839, DDF = 0.726, EOT = 0.652). Depression and anxiety were measured using BSI subscales, as in Experiment 1 (Derogatis & Melisaratos, 1983) (see note 2). EF was measured using standardised tests commonly included in neuropsychological assessment: the Trail-making Tests (TMT, A and B; Reitan, 1955), written Symbol-Digit Modalities Test (SDMT; Smith, 1991), and category fluency (animals; CF). TMT requires connecting numbered circles in order (TMT-A) and connecting lettered and numbered circles in alternation (TMT-B) as quickly as possible; it measures visual search, attention, processing speed, sequencing, and switching/mental flexibility. SDMT requires providing digits corresponding to symbols, as indicated by a key, as quickly as possible; it measures visual search, attention, processing speed, and switching/mental flexibility. Category fluency requires providing as many unique exemplars of a category as possible in one minute; it measures semantic access and search, speed, retrieval strategies, and flexibility. Each of these further requires a degree of inhibitory control (see Lezak, Howieson, Loring, & Fischer, 2004). Principal components analysis (PCA) was used to extract a single EF factor, capturing the EF commonalities across the various tests (eigenvalue = 2.4); it accounted for 60% of variance (loadings .62 (CF) to .88 (TMT-A); positive scores reflect poorer performance).

Design and Procedure

Participants were tested individually, completing a demographic survey, EF tests and surveys, including the TAS-20 (see note 1). Hierarchical regression was performed as in Experiment 1, but with EF as the dependent variable (power analysis: n needed = 78; see Experiment 1).

Results and discussion

Bivariate correlations are shown in Table 5. All TAS-20 subscales were inter-correlated. Age correlated only with EOT. Notably, no alexithymia facets correlated with age within young subjects, but all facets correlated with age within older adults (DIF = 0.22, DDF = 0.38, EOT = 0.22, all *ps* < .025). Depression and anxiety correlated with TAS-20 DIF and DDF, but not with EF. EF tests correlated significantly with age, DIF

Table 4. Experiment 2, Descriptive statistics.

	All (n = 139)		Young (n = 38)		Older (n = 101)		
	Mean	SD	Mean	SD	Mean	SD	*p*
Age (yrs)	57.53	24.95	19.89	2.79	71.69	10.75	**<0.001**
Age range (yrs)			18–35		48–89		
Sex (M/F)	45/94		11/27		34/67		0.60
Education (yrs)	14.91	2.29	13.74	1.08	15.34	2.47	**<0.001**
BSI-Depression	0.40	0.47	0.50	0.54	0.36	0.44	0.10
BSI-Anxiety	0.48	0.46	0.69	0.63	0.40	0.36	**0.01**
Mini-Mental State Exam	–	–	–	–	29.06	1.14	–
TAS-20 Total	43.26	9.76	43.66	9.42	43.11	9.93	0.77
Difficulty Identifying Feelings	12.64	4.39	13.26	4.93	12.41	4.18	0.31
Difficulty Describing Feelings	11.47	3.71	12.55	3.97	11.07	3.52	0.05
Externally Oriented Thinking	19.14	4.42	17.84	3.98	19.63	4.49	0.03
Trail-making A (sec)	28.31	10.29	20.29	5.01	31.31	10.18	**<0.001**
Trail-making B (sec)	68.89	26.15	59.55	19.95	72.41	27.41	**0.003**
Symbol-digit Modalities	52.08	11.88	64.16	9.21	47.53	9.32	**<0.001**
Category Fluency	20.77	4.65	22.66	3.95	20.06	4.71	**0.002**

Notes: ≤.05; **<.01**; TAS-20 Total = Toronto Alexithymia Scale-20 total score; BSI = Brief Symptom Inventory; *p* values correspond to between-group *t*-tests except sex (X2).

Table 5. Experiment 2, Bivariate correlations.

	Age	Sex	BSI-D	BSI-A	DIF	DDF	EOT	EF
Age	–							
Sex	0.05	–						
BSI-D	−0.12	0.05	–					
BSI-A	**−0.25**	0.01	**0.63**	–				
DIF	−0.02	0.05	**0.34**	**0.35**	–			
DDF	−0.04	0.13	0.18	**0.27**	**0.60**	–		
EOT	**0.24**	**0.28**	−0.06	0.05	**0.23**	**0.41**	–	–
TMT-A	**0.58**	0.16	−0.01	−0.03	0.18	0.11	**0.31**	**0.86**
TMT-B	**0.36**	0.07	−0.01	−0.03	**0.22**	0.19	0.13	**0.80**
SDMT	**−0.66**	**−0.22**	0.05	0.10	0.03	0.04	−0.15	**−0.78**
CF	**−0.31**	−0.01	−0.01	0.02	−0.18	−0.07	−0.11	**−0.63**
EF	**0.64**	0.15	0.01	−0.04	0.17	0.10	**0.24**	-

Notes: ≤.05; **<.01**; Pearson r except with sex (Spearman's rho); BSI = Brief Symptom Inventory (D = depression; A = anxiety); DIF = Difficulty Identifying Feelings; DDF = Difficulty Describing Feelings; EOT = Externally Oriented Thinking; TMT = Trail-making Tests; SDMT = Symbol-digit Modalities Test; CF = Category fluency (animals); EF = executive functioning factor score.

(SDMT excepted), and EOT (TMT-A, overall only), but only TMT-B correlated with DDF.

Hierarchical regression (see Table 6) resulted in a significant model predicting executive functioning with age (years) and sex in Step 1. Age, sex and DIF were each significant predictors in Step 2. Age-X-DIF and sex-X-DIF interactions were not significant ($R^2 = .29$, $p < .001$; age $p < .01$, sex $p = .06$, DIF $p = .04$, interaction *ps* .21–.79). Anxiety and depression did not add prediction or reduce DIF effects when included in the model (*ps* > .22). Thus, poorer executive functioning was apparent in older age, male sex, and in those with higher DIF, with none of these contributions dependent on the value of the others.

Experiment 2 is consistent with the few prior studies indicating reduced executive functioning ability in those with higher alexithymia. Specifically, prior studies suggest that HA have poorer ability to attend to, manipulate, and quickly respond to stimuli and abstract information (Correro et al., 2016; Santorelli & Ready, 2015; Zhang et al., 2011). For example, in one study, alexithymia did not impact basic attentional processes (e.g. alerting, orienting) during a flanker-type task, yet HA were significantly slower and less accurate in deciding whether one arrow in an array of other arrows was pointing in the same or opposite direction (Zhang et al., 2011). This, as with our findings, occurred with neutral stimuli, suggesting alexithymia is associated with a generalised EF deficit. Earlier study of participants with traumatic brain injuries also found a unique association between DIF and executive function deficits as indexed by fluency tasks (Henry et al., 2006). The current large, normative sample spanning the adult age spectrum showed that greater DIF (but not DDF) was specifically associated with poorer general EF; fluency was included in this factor. Both age and alexithymia (DIF) were independently related to EF. A previous study reported that worse verbal EF predicted alexithymia in a sample of young and older adults, but the effect was exclusive to older adults (Santorelli & Ready, 2015). Follow-up analysis of our data supported the previous study: DIF contributed to executive dysfunction at all adult ages, but its effects were greater in older age. Thus, DIF and poor EF are particularly important to

Table 6. Experiment 2, Hierarchical regression predicting executive functioning.

		Model summary of each step				Contribution of each variable in last step				
		R^2	DR^2	*F*	*p*	B	SE	b	*t*	*p*
EF Factor										
Step 1		0.39	–	43.15	**<.001**					
	Age					0.03	0.00	0.60	8.64	**<.001**
	Sex					0.29	0.15	0.14	2.01	0.05
Step 2		0.43	0.04	3.29	0.02					
	DIF					0.04	0.02	0.19	2.22	0.03
	DDF					0.00	0.03	0.01	0.12	0.91
	EOT					0.01	0.02	0.03	0.37	0.71

Notes: ≤.05; **<.01**; Toronto Alexithymia Scale-20: DIF = Difficulty Identifying Feelings, DDF = Difficulty Describing Feelings, EOT = Externally Oriented Thinking; EF = Executive Functioning.

consider as risk factors for age-related cognitive decline.

Experiment 3

Our first two experiments indicated that EF and memory are each impacted by aging and alexithymia (i.e. DIF and EOT, respectively). Experiment 3 sought to build upon these experiments. Regarding memory, delayed narrative recall was assessed instead of word recognition. Stories assess "everyday memory", affording greater ecological validity than word lists and retrieval with less cuing than recognition (e.g. Wang, Daselaar, & Cabeza, 2017). Yet, narratives provide more contextual support than word lists, lessening the EF load during retrieval (Rubin, 2006), which could be assistive to older adults with higher alexithymia. The task also allowed standardised neuropsychological testing to be used for both memory and EF assessment. We hypothesised that Experiment 3 would replicate Experiments 1 and 2. We further explored the relationship of EF to memory performance and the role of alexithymia in that relationship.

Method

Participants

Participants (121 (81 female)) were healthy, EFL, and cognitively intact adults (34 young, 18–22 years; 87 older, 50–92 years, targeting healthy adults ≥ 45 years) drawn from two different samples within the university's metropolitan area. Participants were screened as in Experiment 2. All participants completed the EF tests, while only one of the older samples (*n* = 42, 50–87 years) completed memory testing. Descriptive statistics are in Table 7.

Materials

Alexithymia was assessed using the TAS-20 (IC: Total = 0.820, DIF = 0.833, DDF = 0.655, and EOT = 0.716). Depression and anxiety were measured using the Beck Depression and Anxiety Inventories (BDI, BAI; raw score sum of 21 items, scale of 0 (none) to 3 (severe)), which have good reliability, convergent/concurrent and criterion validity, and IC (Beck & Steer, 1990; Beck, Steer, & Brown, 1996) (see note 2).

EF was measured using the TMT-A/B (Reitan, 1955); PCA extracted commonalities into a single EF factor (77% of variance; loadings = .88; positive standard score = poorer EF). Memory was assessed using the Rivermead Behavioural Memory Test (RBMT) story subtest, a standardised test of everyday memory with strong reliability and construct, clinical and ecological validity (Wilson, Cockburn, Baddeley, & Hiorns, 1989). Immediate recall assessed attention/encoding, while 30-minute delayed recall (standardised delay) examined long-term memory.

Design and Procedure

Participants were tested individually, completing a demographic survey, followed by the RBMT and TMT. Surveys, including the TAS-20 were administered

Table 7. Experiment 3, Descriptive statistics.

	All (*n* = 121)		Young (*n* = 34)		Older (*n* = 87)		
	Mean	SD	Mean	SD	Mean	SD	*p*
Age (yrs)	53.25	22.9	19.24	0.99	66.55	9.80	0.10
Age range (yrs)	18–92		18–22		50–92		
Sex (M/F)	40/81		15/19		25/62		0.11
Education (yrs)	15.03	2.77	12.72	1.01	15.93	2.71	**0.01**
Mini-Mental State Exam	–	–	–	–	28.93	1.37	–
Beck Depression Inventory	4.03	4.21	5.65	5.40	3.40	3.48	0.03
Beck Anxiety Inventory	4.23	5.02	7.94	7.31	2.83	2.78	**<0.01**
TAS-20 Total Score	41.37	10.91	45.18	11.26	39.78	10.42	0.04
Difficulty Identifying Feelings	11.79	5.02	13.32	5.13	11.19	4.87	**<0.01**
Difficulty Describing Feelings	11.00	3.68	12.56	3.74	10.38	3.44	0.31
Externally Oriented Thinking	18.58	4.81	19.29	5.36	18.30	4.57	0.33
Trail-making A (sec)	30.14	12.04	28.41	11.63	30.82	12.19	**<0.01**
Trail-making B (sec)	70.41	29.12	58.58	17.66	75.02	31.41	0.03
Executive Factor	0.00	1.00	−0.31	0.80	0.12	1.05	**<0.01**
RBMT IR (raw)	9.58	3.52	10.97	3.02	8.63	3.59	**<0.01**
RMBT DR (raw)	8.38	3.2	9.52	2.96	7.46	3.12	**<0.01**

Notes: ≤.05; **<.01**; TAS-20 = Toronto Alexithymia Scale: DIF = Difficulty Identifying Feelings, DDF = Difficulty Describing Feelings, EOT = Externally Oriented Thinking; Trails = Trail-making Tests; RBMT = Rivermead Behavioural Memory Test, IR = immediate recall; DR = 30-min delayed recall; *p* values correspond to between-group *t*-tests except sex (X^2); *RBMT *n* = 42.

during the delay (see note 1). Hierarchical regression was used, with the EF component score or memory score as the dependent variable (power analysis: n needed = 78, see Experiment 1). The Johnson-Neyman procedure was used (CAHOST, Carden, Holtzman, & Strube, 2017) to examine interaction effects.

Results and discussion

Bivariate correlations among the study variables are shown in Table 8. EF significantly correlated with age, sex, and DIF. Memory significantly correlated with age, sex, and EF. Although age did not correlate with alexithymia total score across the full sample or in young alone ($r = .17$, $p = .33$), age and alexithymia significantly correlated in older adults alone ($r = .25$, $p < .02$).

Hierarchical regression produced a significant model in which age and sex predicted EF in Step 1, with DIF adding significant variance in Step 2 (see Table 9). A *post-hoc* hierarchical regression analysis added the DIF interaction terms with age and sex in subsequent steps. Neither interaction term was significant ($ps > .12$), while age, sex and DIF remained significant as independent predictors. Anxiety and depression did not correlate with EF; adding either to the model had no effect ($ps > .35$). Thus, older age, male sex, and greater DIF each contributed to poorer executive functioning.

Hierarchical regression produced a significant model in which delayed memory was predicted by age and sex in Step 1, with EOT (only) adding significant variance in Step 2 (see Table 9). Anxiety and depression, not correlated with memory, provided no prediction when included ($ps > .31$). Addition of the age-X-EOT and sex-X-EOT interaction terms also produced no significant prediction ($ps > .09$); age and EOT remained significant. The EOT contribution was particularly notable when examined solely in older adults (while sex lost significance; see Table 9). Indeed, restricted to older adults, simple bivariate correlations of immediate and delayed recall were significant with EOT (but not DIF or DDF; $n = 42$, StoryIR = −.353, $p = .022$, StoryDR = −.395, $p = .010$).

Given the expected correlations between memory and EF, and amongst age, EF and memory, follow-up analyses were conducted to examine potential interactions. EF moderated the relationship between age and memory ($R^2 = .28$, $p < .001$, interaction $p = .04$). That is, memory showed little variance in young adults and EF did not distinguish it, but the greater variance in memory of older subjects showed that those with poorer EF were particularly impaired (see Figure 2). We further interrogated whether alexithymia, specifically EOT, contributed to this model. The age-X-EOT, EF-X-EOT, and age-X-EF-X-EOT interaction terms were added in successive subsequent steps. No interactions were significant prior to the final step. The final model remained significant ($R^2 = .37$, $p < .001$) with memory predicted by age (B = −.05, $p = .003$), EF (B = −.79, $p = .06$), and the 3-way interaction (B = −.81, $p = .04$; $R^2_{change} = .04$). Figure 3 demonstrates that although memory was poorer at advanced age, poorer executive functions were predictive of poor memory specifically in those who also had high EOT.

Experiment 3 supports Experiments 1 and 2, indicating alexithymia is associated with poorer EF via DIF and poorer memory via EOT. Furthermore, poor EF substantively contributed to poorer memory, which was specific to those with high EOT. Thus, memory deficits for neutral memoranda were, at least in part, due to generally poorer EF in older

Table 8. Experiment 3, Bivariate correlations.

	Age	Sex	BDI	BAI	DIF	DDF	EOT	Exec	IR	DR
Age	–									
Sex	.001	–								
BDI	−0.16	−0.02	–							
BAI	**−0.41**	0.13	**0.36**	–						
DIF	−0.08	−0.13	**0.44**	**0.45**	–					
DDF	−0.20	**−0.24**	**0.37**	0.22	**0.64**	–				
EOT	−0.06	**−0.37**	0.22	0.10	**0.36**	**0.47**	–			
Exec	**0.37**	−0.22	0.10	−0.07	**0.24**	0.14	0.10	–		
IR	**−0.43**	0.23	0.20	0.20	0.15	0.18	−0.13	**−0.40**	–	
DR	**−0.43**	0.25	0.17	0.21	0.09	0.09	−0.19	**−0.38**	**0.84**	–

Notes: ≤.05; **<.01**; Pearson r except sex (rho); $N = 121$ (except IR, DR: $N = 76$); BDI = Beck Depression Inventory; BAI = Beck Anxiety Inventory; Toronto Alexithymia Scale-20: DIF = Difficulty Identifying Feelings, DDF = Difficulty Describing Feelings, EOT = Externally Oriented Thinking; Exec = factor score of Trail-making Tests A and B; IR = immediate, DR = delayed recall on the Rivermead Behavioural Memory Tests (story subtest).

Table 9. Experiment 3, Hierarchical Regression Predicting Executive Functioning.

	Model Summary of Each Step				Contribution of Each Variable in Last Step				
	R^2	DR^2	F	p	B	SE	b	t	p
Executive function									
Step 1	0.20	–	14.99	**<.001**					
Age					0.02	0.00	0.41	5.02	**<.001**
Sex					−0.57	0.18	−0.27	−3.15	**<.01**
Step 2	0.27	0.07	3.60	0.02					
DIF					0.05	0.02	0.25	2.39	0.02
DDF					0.01	0.03	0.05	0.45	0.65
EOT					−0.02	0.02	−0.09	−0.92	0.36
Immediate recall									
Step 1	0.26	–	12.54	**<.001**					
Age					−0.02	0.01	−0.43	−4.17	**<.001**
Sex					−0.47	0.23	−0.22	−2.04	**0.05**
Step 2	0.31	0.05	1.81	0.15					
DIF					0.02	0.03	0.08	0.56	0.58
DDF					0.05	0.04	0.18	1.25	0.22
EOT					−0.05	0.03	−0.22	−1.87	0.07
Delayed memory (all)									
Step 1	0.28	–	13.86	**<.001**					
Age					−0.02	0.00	−0.46	−4.52	**<.001**
Sex					0.45	0.23	0.21	1.97	0.05
Step 2	0.33	0.05	1.82	0.15					
DIF					0.02	0.03	0.09	0.69	0.50
DDF					0.04	0.04	0.13	0.93	0.36
EOT					−0.05	0.03	−0.25	−2.12	0.04
Delayed memory (Older only)									
Step 1	0.36	–	10.72	**<.001**					
Age					−0.05	0.01	−0.52	−3.75	**<.001**
Sex					0.33	0.34	0.15	0.96	0.34
Step 2	0.50	0.14	3.34	0.03					
DIF					0.01	0.04	0.06	0.34	0.74
DDF					0.11	0.06	0.33	1.81	0.08
EOT					−0.12	0.04	−0.47	−3.04	**<.01**

Notes: ≤.05; **<.01**; Toronto Alexithymia Scale-20: DIF = Difficulty Identifying Feelings, DDF = Difficulty Describing Feelings, EOT = Externally Oriented Thinking.

adults, and alexithymia. As Experiments 2 and 3 showed that high DIF contributes specifically to executive dysfunction, these results suggest that elevated DIF and EOT may both be risk factors for age-related cognitive decline.

General discussion

Three independent experiments suggest alexithymia contributes to generally poorer memory and EF in younger and older adults. Specifically, one-hour delayed memory for neutral words was poorer in young adults with high EOT (Exp. 1), and young and older adults with HA via DIF had poorer EF, as measured by a composite of non-emotive standardised tests (Exp. 2). Furthermore, DIF had greater prediction of EF at older age. In Experiment 3, young and older adults with high EOT had poorer 30-min delayed memory for neutral narratives, and those with higher DIF had poorer EF. Moreover, poorer memory was explained by those with poor EF, and specifically those who also had high EOT (see Figure 3).

Importantly, poorer memory and EF were associated with alexithymia using neutral stimuli. This is novel; prior studies show poorer memory only for emotive material (DiStefano & Koven, 2012; Dressaire et al., 2015; Luminet et al., 2006; Meltzer & Nielson, 2010; Vermeulen & Luminet, 2009) or contexts (Nielson & Meltzer, 2009; Vermeulen et al., 2010). Stimulus relevance may partially explain prior studies. Attentional resources are typically directed toward salient information, which subsequently modulates memory (Mather & Sutherland, 2011; Nielson & Correro, 2017). Alexithymia is fundamentally a difficulty of processing emotive content (Vermeulen et al., 2006). Thus, emotion words receive less boost from salience (Luminet et al., 2006), making encoding and retrieval of emotive information particularly difficult (Vermeulen et al., 2018). Conversely, alexithymia is frequently associated with functional somatic

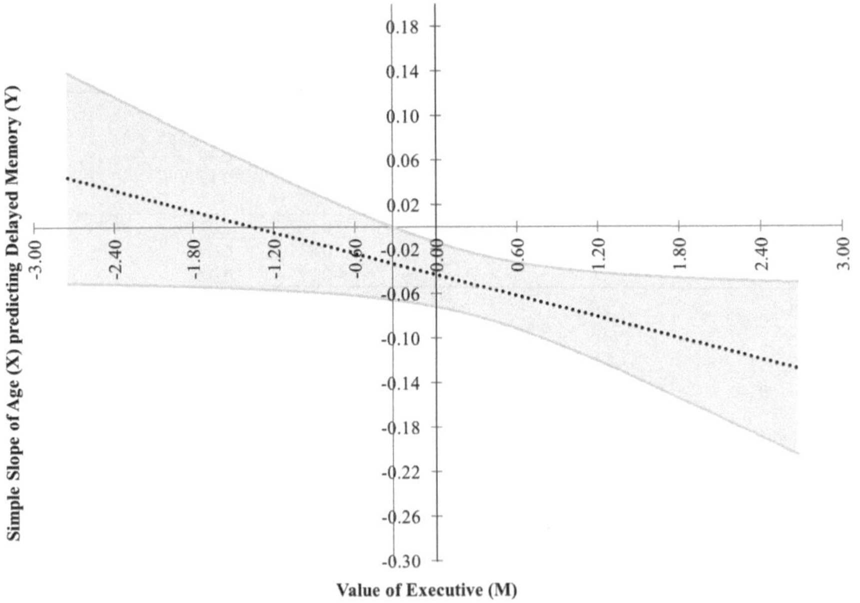

Figure 2. Experiment 3 data plotted using the Johnson-Neyman technique for moderation. The simple slope of age (X) predicting delayed narrative recall (Y) is plotted against the moderator (M), executive functioning (EF). These are shown with the slope (dotted line) and 95% confidence interval (grey band). The vertical black line (left of the Y axis) indicates the significance region where the slope crosses zero (−0.317); greater values, where the grey band does not include 0, were statistically significant. That is, EF from this point and greater (i.e. poorer performance) significantly moderated the relationship between age and memory. Thus, although memory was poorer in older than young adulthood, poor EF was highly detrimental to memory, especially in older age.

symptoms (Taylor, Parker, Bagby, & Acklin, 1992), making illness-related information more salient and better remembered (Meltzer & Nielson, 2010). Salience of neutral memoranda in HA is unclear. Nevertheless, EOT predicted worse memory for neutral word lists and stories, suggesting salience effects may be *additive* to generalised memory effects in alexithymia, rather than exclusive. Prior studies may have missed this due to small sample sizes and examining neutral material in emotional contexts.

EOT was influential to neutral memory (Experiments 1, 3). Although DIF also predicted memory (Exp. 1), EOT mediated that relationship. These findings extend one prior aging study (Onor et al., 2010) to encompass a broader range of age and context. Prior studies indicated DIF contributed to poorer emotional memory (Luminet et al., 2006; Vermeulen & Luminet, 2009), while EOT contributed to better neutral memory (Meltzer & Nielson, 2010; Vermeulen & Luminet, 2009). Yet, salience may have influenced those findings (Ferre, Fraga, Comesana, & Sanchez-Casas, 2015), consistent with the emotion processing deficits typifying alexithymia (Luminet et al., 2006), as these studies examined neutral materials alongside emotional material or in emotive contexts. Some suggest memory effects in alexithymia may depend on separate emotive (i.e. DIF) and cognitive (i.e. EOT) mechanisms and brain regions that, respectively, influence encoding and retrieval (Vermeulen & Luminet, 2009). With non-emotive memoranda, DIF and DDF would play lesser roles, while an externally oriented style may contribute to difficulty limiting distraction during encoding and retrieval. Indeed, for words and stories, high EOT was detrimental to memory performance, across variations in age, sample size, retention interval and memory type (i.e. recall, recognition).

The words used in Experiment 1 were highly imageable, which can assist learning. As EOT can impede the utilisation of such encoding resources, poor encoding might be responsible for the memory results. Nevertheless, delayed memory was better predicted by alexithymia than immediate memory. Some also suggest alexithymia influences decision criteria (Jacob & Hautekeete, 1998) or promotes guessing (Vermeulen & Luminet, 2009). Yet, the results were specific to sensitivity rather than guessing. These issues warrant further investigation, but the findings indicate that memory influence of alexithymia extends beyond encoding.

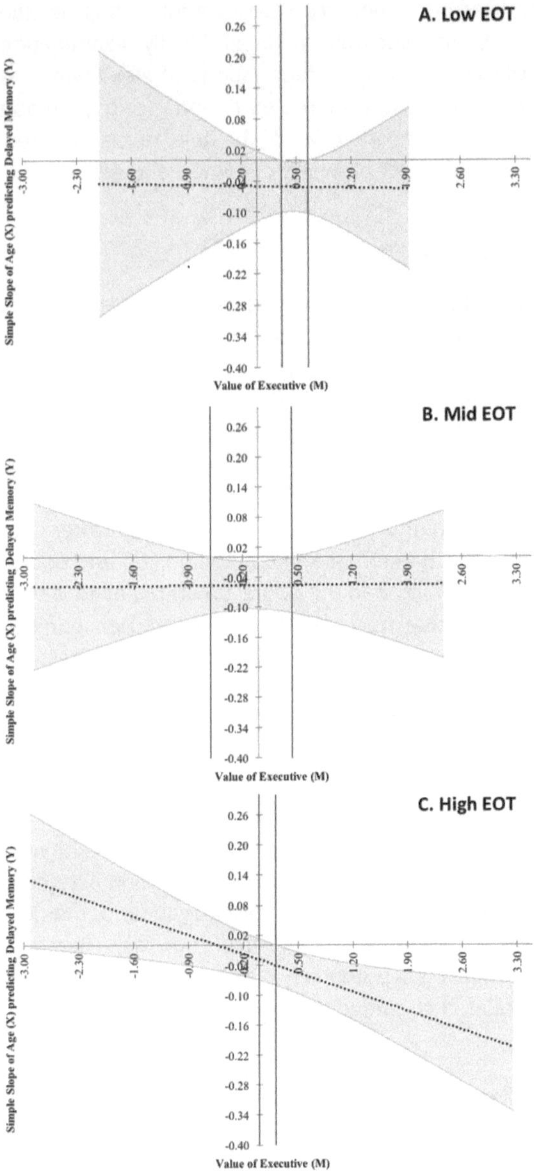

Figure 3. Experiment 3 data, plotted using the Johnson-Neyman procedure, to examine whether alexithymia (via Externally Oriented Thinking (EOT)) moderated the model shown in Figure 2 (i.e. moderated moderation). The simple slope (dotted line; grey band = 95% confidence interval (CI)) of age (X) predicting delayed narrative recall (Y) is plotted against the moderator (M), executive functioning (EF, positive score = poorer EF), split by EOT tertile: A. Low EOT (≤15), B. Mid EOT (16–19), and C. High EOT (≥20). Vertical black lines show significance regions where the slope crosses zero and beyond which, where CI does not include 0, constitutes statistically significant moderation (A: ≥0.32, ≤0.65; B: ≥−0.61, ≤0.43; C: ≥0.21). However, only panel C showed a significant slope for moderation. These plots confirm the 3-way interaction (i.e. moderated moderation) indicating that although EF moderated the relationship between age and memory (see Figure 2), EOT moderated that moderation. That is, poor EF predicted poor memory with greater age, but it did so specifically in those who also had high EOT (panel C), indicating that alexithymia is a risk factor for cognitive dysfunction in older age.

DIF was particularly impactful on EF, supporting previous demonstrations of verbal fluency deficits in alexithymia (e.g. Henry et al., 2006) and more general EF findings undifferentiated by TAS-20 subscale (Koven & Thomas, 2010; Wood & Williams, 2007; Zhang et al., 2011). Other studies, especially those emphasising EF via fluency, instead reported DDF correlated with EF (Correro et al., 2016; Santorelli & Ready, 2015), which we did not replicate. The EF variable in the current study was a composite of EF tasks including attentional control, sequencing, switching, semantic control, and processing speed. While DIF and DDF are highly correlated, our factor perhaps biased findings toward the ability to interpret internal experience (DIF) rather than capacity to effectively communicate emotion state (DDF), as fluency alone might tap. Overall, the present experiments extend previous findings suggesting a generalised EF deficit in alexithymia. Moreover, Experiments 2 and 3 suggest that the contribution of alexithymia, specifically DIF, to executive dysfunction increases with advancing age, highlighting DIF as a risk factor for age-related cognitive decline.

Higher-order cognitive processes are essential to allocating cognitive resources toward other complex abilities, such as memory (Duff et al., 2005), perception and interpretation of cognitive, emotional (i.e. mentalisation, Aboulafia-Brakha, Christe, Martory, & Annoni, 2011), and bodily states (i.e. interoception, Menon & Uddin, 2010). Both mentalisation and interoception require internal awareness to interpret ones' own state and what others may be experiencing. Indeed, the social and emotional dysfunction common in alexithymia is often characterised by difficulty with mentalising (Moriguchi et al., 2006; Wastell & Taylor, 2002); interoception (Murphy, Catmur, & Bird, 2017); an external cognitive style; and difficulty with abstraction, which is essential for emotion identification and regulation (Rinaldi, Radian, Rossignol, Arachchige, & Lefebvre, 2017; Wotschack & Klann-Delius, 2013). Internal representations are not readily accessible in HA (Rinaldi et al., 2017), leading to ineffective application of a "primitive" and physiological level of emotional awareness (Bermond, Vorst, & Moormann, 2006; Kano & Fukudo, 2013; Lane et al., 1996). Similarly, poorer EF is associated with DIF – a feature at the intersection of bottom-up emotional awareness and top-down interpretation of social and emotive content and situations (Bar-On, Tranel, Denburg, & Bechara, 2003; Frawley & Smith, 2001). This appears to describe alexithymia, where instrumental relationships are manageable but more expressive and complex relationships are impeded (Wastell & Taylor, 2002). Our findings further reinforce these characterisations.

Although alexithymia did not correlate with age in our full samples, it did significantly correlate with age within older samples, consistent with previous research (Gunzelmann, Kupfer, & Brahler, 2002; Mattila et al., 2006; Salminen, Saarijarvi, Aarela, Toikka, & Kauhanen, 1999). Indeed, some suggest alexithymia may be better understood as a reflection of generalised neurocognitive functioning (Messina, Beadle, & Paradiso, 2014; Sturm & Levenson, 2011) and that it may reflect a neuropsychiatric consequence of normal aging (Santorelli & Ready, 2015). Despite deficits in cognitive control that are typical with aging (e.g. Gutchess, 2019; Nielson, Langenecker, & Garavan, 2002), our results support previous findings of exacerbated deficits in alexithymia. Indeed, young and older adults with high EOT have shown difficulty intentionally inhibiting the recall of negative information, suggesting alexithymia may contribute more to impairment in cognitive control than does age (Dressaire et al., 2015). In the current study, age and alexithymia (DIF) both predicted EF, with some indication that DIF is increasingly impactful at older age, and in Experiment 3, poorer memory in older age was characterised by those with poor EF and high EOT. Thus, alexithymia added significant predictive value beyond and in interaction with aging effects to understanding memory performance in older adults. This complex interplay of age, EF, memory and alexithymia is consistent with the accumulating neuroimaging studies in alexithymia showing reduced grey matter volume and deficits in interhemispheric and cortical–subcortical transfer and cortical networks (see Goerlich & Aleman, 2018).

This study had limitations. The samples were large compared with most relevant studies, but smaller in Experiment 3, which could affect generalisability. This study reflected a secondary analysis of previous experiments; differences across samples (e.g. measures, tasks, exclusion/inclusion criteria, retention interval, what filled the interval) and representation of middle adulthood could be improved upon in future work. Our EF factor results are generally consistent with verbal fluency (Henry et al., 2006; Santorelli & Ready, 2015) and attentional control (Wood & Williams, 2007; Zhang et al., 2011) deficits in HA, but future work disentangling the role of discrete executive abilities in alexithymia is important. As EOT has low IC, future memory studies might consider the items of this subscale in detail. Finally, examination of the possible neural foundations of alexithymia, as well as interventions directed at enhancing cognition or reducing alexithymia, might help to clarify directionality of effect between cognition and alexithymia.

Conclusion

Across three independent experiments, alexithymia was associated with poorer delayed memory for neutral memoranda and poorer general EF. An external cognitive style (i.e. EOT) was responsible for the role of alexithymia in memory, and difficulty with emotion perception (i.e. DIF) was responsible for executive dysfunction. Critically, poor EF contributed to poorer memory at older age, and EOT further contributed such that those who had high EOT and poorer executive ability had the poorest memory at advanced age. EOT likely precludes the use of internal cognitive control that facilitates memory processes (Dressaire et al., 2015), suggesting memory and executive dysfunction in alexithymia may be understood by the inefficient use of or ineffective access to internal awareness (Moriguchi & Komaki, 2013). Based on the present results, we posit that executive functions are generally impaired in those with higher alexithymia via DIF, and the tendency to view the world externally (i.e. EOT) hinders internal monitoring and memory functions, even in non-emotive contexts. Therefore, alexithymia is a potentially substantive contributor to age-related cognitive dysfunction.

Notes

1. Multiple measures collected for these protocols (i.e. original purposes, hypothesis) masking are not shown. The corresponding author can provide a complete list. Validated test ordering was used to avoid contamination (e.g. no verbal/memory tests during memory retention). All subjects with valid data were included. All procedures were approved by the Institutional Review Board (IRB).
2. Normal range was exceeded if: both depression and anxiety *T*-scores > 63 ($n = 15$ Experiment 1, $n = 15$, Experiment 2, $n = 9$ (7 young)); or BDI > 13 and/or BAI > 15 (mild) (Experiment 3, $n = 5$, all young). Removal of these subjects from models did not alter study results.

Acknowledgements

For assistance with various aspects of these experiments, the authors gratefully acknowledge the contributions of Drs. Kathleen Hazlett Elverman, Shaun English, Christina Figueroa,

Stephanie Potts, and Katherine Reiter; and David Amy, Crystal Becker, Jessica Burkard, Megan Fabisch, Emily Gaber, Zachary Grese, Abigail Helbling, Joshua Krueger, Sarah Lentes, Riley Marinelli, Cara Macchia, Carolyn Madry, David Marra, Marie Mejaki, Emma Murry, Holly Robertson, Stephanie Ocwieja, Kara Pierce, Angela Preston, Stephenie, Quirke, Kristen Skells, Olivia Speeter, Megan Spoo, Aubrey Tschanz, Janel Wasisco, and Alex Zurek.

Disclosure statement

No potential conflict of interest was reported by the authors.

Funding

The work was supported by a grant from the Clinical and Translational Science Award (CTSA) program of the National Center for Research Resources and the National Center for Advancing Translational Science [8UL1TR000055], a Way-Klingler Sabbatical Fellowship award from Marquette University, a National Science Foundation Graduate Research Fellowship [#1452781] and grants from the Scientific Research Network on Decision Neuroscience and Aging (Stanford University Center on Longevity), National Center for Advancing Translational Sciences, and the National Institutes of Health [UL1TR001436 and TL1TR001437].

ORCID

Kristy A. Nielson http://orcid.org/0000-0001-8977-3138

References

Aboulafia-Brakha, T., Christe, B., Martory, M. D., & Annoni, J. M. (2011). Theory of mind tasks and executive functions: A systematic review of group studies in neurology. *Journal of Neuropsychology*, *5*(Pt 1), 39–55. doi:10.1348/174866410X533660

Aftanas, L. I., Varlamov, A. A., Reva, N. V., & Pavlov, S. V. (2003). Disruption of early event-related theta synchronization of human EEG in alexithymics viewing affective pictures. *Neuroscience Letters*, *340*(1), 57–60. doi:10.1016/S0304-3940(03)00070-3

Bagby, R. M., Parker, J. D., & Taylor, G. J. (1994). The twenty-item Toronto Alexithymia Scale–I. Item selection and cross-validation of the factor structure. *Journal of Psychosomatic Research*, *38*(1), 23–32. doi:10.1016/0022-3999(94)90005-1

Bagby, R. M., Taylor, G. J., & Parker, J. D. (1994). The twenty-item Toronto Alexithymia Scale–II. Convergent, discriminant, and concurrent validity. *Journal of Psychosomatic Research*, *38*(1), 33–40. doi:10.1016/0022-3999(94)90006-X

Bar-On, R., Tranel, D., Denburg, N. L., & Bechara, A. (2003). Exploring the neurological substrate of emotional and social intelligence. *Brain*, *126*(Pt 8), 1790–1800. doi:10.1093/brain/awg177

Beck, A. T., & Steer, R. A. (1990). *Manual for the Beck Anxiety Inventory*. San Antonio, TX: Psychological Corporation.

Beck, A. T., Steer, R. A., & Brown, G. K. (1996). *Beck Depression Inventory-II (BDI-II)*. San Antonio, TX: Psychological Corporation.

Bermond, B., Vorst, H. C., & Moormann, P. P. (2006). Cognitive neuropsychology of alexithymia: Implications for personality typology. *Cognitive Neuropsychiatry*, *11*(3), 332–360. doi:10.1080/13546800500368607

Carden, S. W., Holtzman, N. S., & Strube, M. J. (2017). CAHOST: An excel workbook for facilitating the Johnson-Neyman technique for two-way interactions in multiple regression. *Frontiers in Psychology*, *8*(1293), 1–7. doi:10.3389/fpsyg.2017.01293

Charlton, R. A., Landau, S., Schiavone, F., Barrick, T. R., Clark, C. A., Markus, H. S., & Morris, R. G. (2008). A structural equation modeling investigation of age-related variance in executive function and DTI measured white matter damage. *Neurobiology of Aging*, *29*(10), 1547–1555. doi:10.1016/j.neurobiolaging.2007.03.017

Correro, A. N., Marra, D. E., Reiter, K., Byers, S. J., & Nielson, K. A. (2016). Executive functioning and verbal memory are predictive of alexithymia across the lifespan [Abstract]. *The Clinical Neuropsychologist*, *30*(3), 425.

da Silva, A. N., Vasco, A. B., & Watson, J. C. (2017). Alexithymia and Emotional Processing: A Mediation Model. *Journal of Clinical Psychology*, *73*(9), 1196–1205. doi:10.1002/jclp.22422

Derogatis, L. R., & Melisaratos, N. (1983). The Brief Symptom Inventory: An introductory report. *Psychological Medicine*, *13*, 595–605.

Diamond, A. (2013). Executive functions. *Annual Review of Psychology*, *64*(64), 135–168. doi:10.1146/annurev-psych-113011-143750

DiStefano, R. A., & Koven, N. S. (2012). Dysfunctional emotion processing may explain visual memory deficits in alexithymia. *Personality and Individual Differences*, *52*(5), 611–615. doi:10.1016/j.paid.2011.12.007

Dressaire, D., Stone, C. B., Nielson, K. A., Guerdoux, E., Martin, S., Brouillet, D., & Luminet, O. (2015). Alexithymia impairs the cognitive control of negative material while facilitating the recall of neutral material in both younger and older adults. *Cognition and Emotion*, *29*(3), 442–459. doi:10.1080/02699931.2014.919898

Duff, K., Schoenberg, M. R., Scott, J. G., & Adams, R. L. (2005). The relationship between executive functioning and verbal and visual learning and memory. *Archives of Clinical Neuropsychology*, *20*(1), 111–122. doi:10.1016/j.acn.2004.03.003

Ferre, P., Fraga, I., Comesana, M., & Sanchez-Casas, R. (2015). Memory for emotional words: The role of semantic relatedness, encoding task and affective valence. *Cognition and Emotion*, *29*(8), 1401–1410. doi:10.1080/02699931.2014.982515

Folstein, M. F., Folstein, S. E., & McHugh, P. R. (1975). "Mini-mental state". *Journal of Psychiatric Research*, *12*(3), 189–198.

Frawley, W., & Smith, R. N. (2001). A processing theory of alexithymia. *Cognitive Systems Research*, *2*(3), 189–206. doi:10.1016/S1389-0417(01)00029-8

Goerlich, K. S., & Aleman, A. (2018). Neuroimaging studies of alexithymia. In O. Luminet, R. M. Bagby, & G. J. Taylor (Eds.), *Alexithymia: Advances in research, theory and clinical practice* (pp. 207–249). Cambridge: Cambridge University Press.

Gunzelmann, T., Kupfer, J., & Brahler, E. (2002). Alexithymia in the elderly general population. *Comprehensive Psychiatry*, *43*(1), 74–80. doi:10.1053/comp.2002.29855

Gutchess, A. (2019). *Cognitive and social neuroscience of aging*. Cambridge: Cambridge University Press.

Hayes, A. F. (2018). *Introduction to mediation, moderation, and conditional process analysis: A regression-based approach* (2nd ed.). New York: Guilford Press.

Henry, J. D., Phillips, L. H., Crawford, J. R., Theodorou, G., & Summers, F. (2006). Cognitive and psychosocial correlates of alexithymia following traumatic brain injury. *Neuropsychologia*, *44*(1), 62–72. doi:10.1016/j.neuropsychologia.2005.04.011

Hill, B. D., Alosco, M., Bauer, L., & Tremont, G. (2012). The relation of executive functioning to CVLT-II learning, memory, and process indexes. *Applied Neuropsychology: Adult*, *19*(3), 198–206. doi:10.1080/09084282.2011.643960

Jacob, S., & Hautekeete, M. (1998). Alexithymia and memory: A more rigorous criterion for acceptance in recognition tasks? *Encephale-Revue De Psychiatrie Clinique Biologique Et Therapeutique*, *24*(3), 199–204.

Kano, M., & Fukudo, S. (2013). The alexithymic brain: The neural pathways linking alexithymia to physical disorders. *BioPsychoSocial Medicine*, *7*(1), 1. doi:10.1186/1751-0759-7-1

Koven, N. S., & Thomas, W. (2010). Mapping facets of alexithymia to executive dysfunction in daily life. *Personality and Individual Differences*, *49*, 24–28. doi:10.1016/j.paid.2010.02.034

Lamberty, G. J., & Holt, C. S. (1995). Evidence for a verbal deficit in alexithymia. *The Journal of Neuropsychiatry and Clinical Neurosciences*, *7*(3), 320–324. doi:10.1176/jnp.7.3.320

Lane, R. D., Sechrest, L., Reidel, R., Weldon, V., Kaszniak, A., & Schwartz, G. E. (1996). Impaired verbal and nonverbal emotion recognition in alexithymia. *Psychosomatic Medicine*, *58*(3), 203–210.

Lezak, M. D., Howieson, D. B., Loring, D. W., & Fischer, J. S. (2004). *Neuropsychological assessment*. New York, NY: Oxford University Press.

Luminet, O., Vermeulen, N., Demaret, C., Taylor, G. J., & Bagby, R. M. (2006). Alexithymia and levels of processing: Evidence for an overall deficit in remembering emotion words. *Journal of Research in Personality*, *40*(5), 713–733. doi:10.1016/j.jrp.2005.09.001

Mather, M., & Sutherland, M. R. (2011). Arousal-biased competition in perception and memory. *Perspectives on Psychological Science*, *6*(2), 114–133. doi:10.1177/1745691611400234

Mattila, A. K., Salminen, J. K., Nummi, T., & Joukamaa, M. (2006). Age is strongly associated with alexithymia in the general population. *Journal of Psychosomatic Research*, *61*(5), 629–635. doi:10.1016/j.jpsychores.2006.04.013

Meltzer, M. A., & Nielson, K. A. (2010). Memory for emotionally provocative words in alexithymia: A role for stimulus relevance. *Consciousness and Cognition*, *19*(4), 1062–1068. doi:10.1016/j.concog.2010.05.008

Menon, V., & Uddin, L. Q. (2010). Saliency, switching, attention and control: A network model of insula function. *Brain Structure and Function*, *214*(5-6), 655–667. doi:10.1007/s00429-010-0262-0

Messina, A., Beadle, J. N., & Paradiso, S. (2014). Towards a classification of alexithymia: Primary, secondary and organic. *Journal of Psychopathology*, *20*(1), 38–49.

Moriguchi, Y., & Komaki, G. (2013). Neuroimaging studies of alexithymia: Physical, affective, and social perspectives. *BioPsychoSocial Medicine*, *7*(1), 8. doi:10.1186/1751-0759-7-8

Moriguchi, Y., Ohnishi, T., Lane, R. D., Maeda, M., Mori, T., Nemoto, K., … Komaki, G. (2006). Impaired self-awareness and theory of mind: An fMRI study of mentalizing in alexithymia. *Neuroimage*, *32*(3), 1472–1482. doi:10.1016/j.neuroimage.2006.04.186

Murphy, J., Catmur, C., & Bird, G. (2017). Alexithymia is associated with a multidomain, multidimensional failure of interoception: Evidence from novel tests. *Journal of Experimental Psychology: General*. doi:10.1037/xge0000366

Nemiah, J. C. (1977). Alexithymia. Theoretical considerations. *Psychotherapy and Psychosomatics*, *28*(1-4), 199–206. doi:10.1159/000287064

Nielson, K. A., & Correro, A. N., 2nd (2017). Post-learning arousal enhances veridical memory and reduces false memory in the Deese-Roediger-McDermott paradigm. *Neurobiology of Learning and Memory*, *144*, 198–207. doi:10.1016/j.nlm.2017.07.009

Nielson, K. A., Langenecker, S. A., & Garavan, H. (2002). Differences in the functional neuroanatomy of inhibitory control across the adult life span. *Psychology and Aging*, *17*(1), 56–71. doi:10.1037/0882-7974.17.1.56

Nielson, K. A., & Meltzer, M. A. (2009). Modulation of long-term memory by arousal in alexithymia: The role of interpretation. *Consciousness and Cognition*, *18*(3), 786–793. doi:10.1016/j.concog.2009.06.001

Nielson, K. A., Yee, D., & Erickson, K. I. (2005). Memory enhancement by a semantically unrelated emotional arousal source induced after learning. *Neurobiology of Learning and Memory*, *84*, 49–56. doi:10.1016/j.nlm.2005.04.001

Onor, M., Trevisiol, M., Spano, M., Aguglia, E., & Paradiso, S. (2010). Alexithymia and aging: A neuropsychological perspective. *The Journal of Nervous and Mental Disease*, *198*(12), 891–895. doi:10.1097/NMD.0b013e3181fe743e

Paivio, A., Yuille, J. C., & Madigan, S. A. (1968). Concreteness, imagery, and meaningfulness values for 925 nouns. *Journal of Experimental Psychology*, *76*(Suppl.), 1–25. doi:10.1037/h0025327

Parker, J. D., Taylor, G. J., & Bagby, R. M. (2003). The 20-item Toronto Alexithymia Scale. III. Reliability and factorial validity in a community population. *Journal of Psychosomatic Research*, *55*(3), 269–275. doi:10.1016/S0022-3999(02)00578-0

Reitan, R. M. (1955). The relation of the trail making test to organic brain damage. *Journal of Consulting Psychology*, *19*(5), 393–394.

Rinaldi, R., Radian, V., Rossignol, M., Arachchige, K. G. K., & Lefebvre, L. (2017). Thinking about one's feelings association between Alexithymia and cognitive styles in a nonclinical population. *The Journal of Nervous and Mental Disease*, *205*(10), 812–815. doi:10.1097/Nmd.0000000000000721

Rubin, D. C. (2006). The basic-systems model of episodic memory. *Perspectives on Psychological Science*, *1*(4), 277–311. doi:10.1111/j.1745-6916.2006.00017.x

Salminen, J. K., Saarijarvi, S., Aarela, E., Toikka, T., & Kauhanen, J. (1999). Prevalence of alexithymia and its association with sociodemographic variables in the general population of Finland. *Journal of Psychosomatic Research*, *46*(1), 75–82. doi:10.1016/S0022-3999(98)00053-1

Santorelli, G. D., & Ready, R. E. (2015). Alexithymia and executive function in younger and older adults. *The Clinical Neuropsychologist*, *29*(7), 938–955. doi:10.1080/13854046.2015.1123296

Sifneos, P. E. (1973). The prevalence of 'alexithymic' characteristics in psychosomatic patients. *Psychotherapy and Psychosomatics*, *22*(2), 255–262. doi:10.1159/000286529

Smith, A. (1991). *Symbol digit modalities test*. Los Angeles, CA: Western Psychological Services.

Soper, D. S. (2019). A-priori sample size calculator for multiple regression [Software]. Retrieved from http://www.danielsoper.com/statcalc.

Stanislaw, H., & Todorov, N. (1999). Calculation of signal detection theory measures. *Behavior Research Methods, Instruments, & Computers, 31*(1), 137–149.

Sturm, V. E., & Levenson, R. W. (2011). Alexithymia in neurodegenerative disease. *Neurocase, 17*(3), 242–250. doi:10.1080/13554794.2010.532503

Suslow, T., Kersting, A., & Arolt, V. (2003). Alexithymia and incidental learning of emotional words. *Psychological Reports, 93* (3 Pt 2), 1003–1012. doi:10.2466/pr0.2003.93.3f.1003

Swart, M., Kortekaas, R., & Aleman, A. (2009). Dealing with feelings: Characterization of trait alexithymia on emotion regulation strategies and cognitive-emotional processing. *PLoS One, 4*(6), e5751. doi:10.1371/journal.pone.0005751

Taylor, G. J. (2000). Recent developments in alexithymia theory and research. *The Canadian Journal of Psychiatry, 45*(2), 134–142. doi:10.1177/070674370004500203

Taylor, G. J., Bagby, R. M., & Luminet, O. (2000). Assessment of alexithymia: Self-report and observer-rated measures. In J. D. A. Parker & R. Bar-On (Eds.), *The handbook of emotional intelligence* (pp. 301–319). San Francisco, CA: Jossey Bass.

Taylor, G. J., Bagby, R. M., & Parker, J. D. (2003). The 20-item Toronto Alexithymia Scale. IV. Reliability and factorial validity in different languages and cultures. *Journal of Psychosomatic Research, 55*(3), 277–283. doi:10.1016/S0022-3999(02)00601-3

Taylor, G. J., Parker, J. D., Bagby, R. M., & Acklin, M. W. (1992). Alexithymia and somatic complaints in psychiatric outpatients. *Journal of Psychosomatic Research, 36*(5), 417–424. doi:10.1016/0022-3999(92)90002-J

van der Velde, J., Gromann, P. M., Swart, M., Wiersma, D., de Haan, L., Bruggeman, R., … Aleman, A. (2015). Alexithymia influences brain activation during emotion perception but not regulation. *Social Cognitive and Affective Neuroscience, 10*(2), 285–293. doi:10.1093/scan/nsu056

Vermeulen, N., Domachowska, I., & Nielson, K. A. (2018). Memory and executive functions in alexithymia. In O. Luminet, R. M. Bagby, & G. J. Taylor (Eds.), *Alexithymia: Advances in research, theory, and clinical practice* (pp. 78–89). Cambridge, UK: Cambridge University Press.

Vermeulen, N., & Luminet, O. (2009). Alexithymia factors and memory performances for neutral and emotional words. *Personality and Individual Differences, 47*, 305–309. doi:10.1016/j.paid.2009.03.018

Vermeulen, N., Luminet, O., & Corneille, O. (2006). Alexithymia and the automatic processing of affective information: Evidence from the affective priming paradigm. *Cognition & Emotion, 20*(1), 64–91. doi:10.1080/02699930500304654

Vermeulen, N., Toussaint, J., & Luminet, O. (2010). The influence of alexithymia and music on the incidental memory for emotion words. *European Journal of Personality, 24*(6), 551–568. doi:10.1002/per.758

Wang, W. C., Daselaar, S. M., & Cabeza, R. (2017). Episodic memory decline and healthy aging. In J. Stein (Ed.), *Reference module in neuroscience and biobehavioral psychology* (pp. 476–492). Nijmegen: Radboud University.

Wastell, C. A., & Taylor, A. J. (2002). Alexithymic mentalising: Theory of mind and social adaptation. *Social Behavior and Personality: an International Journal, 30*(2), 141–148. doi:10.2224/sbp.2002.30.2.141

Wilson, B., Cockburn, J., Baddeley, A., & Hiorns, R. (1989). The development and validation of a test battery for detecting and monitoring everyday memory problems. *Journal of Clinical and Experimental Neuropsychology, 11*(6), 855–870. doi:10.1080/01688638908400940

Wood, R. L., & Williams, C. (2007). Neuropsychological correlates of organic alexithymia. *Journal of the International Neuropsychological Society, 13*(3), 471–479. doi:10.1017/S1355617707070518

Wotschack, C., & Klann-Delius, G. (2013). Alexithymia and the conceptualization of emotions: A study of language use and semantic knowledge. *Journal of Research in Personality, 47* (5), 514–523. doi:10.1016/j.jrp.2013.01.011

Zhang, L., Ye, R., Yu, F., Cao, Z., Zhu, C., Cai, Z., … Wang, K. (2012). How does emotional context modulate response inhibition in alexithymia: Electrophysiological evidence from an ERP study. *PLoS One, 7*(12), e51110. doi:10.1371/journal.pone.0051110

Zhang, L., Zhu, C., Ye, R., Cao, Z., Tian, Y., Yang, P., … Wang, K. (2011). Impairment of conflict processing in alexithymic individuals. *Neuroscience Letters, 504*(3), 261–264. doi:10.1016/j.neulet.2011.09.043

The influence of alexithymia on memory for emotional faces and realistic social interactions

Nathan Ridout, Jade Smith and Holly Hawkins

ABSTRACT

High levels of alexithymia are typically associated with impaired memory for emotional, but not neutral words. We conducted two experimental studies to establish if this effect generalises to non-verbal socially relevant stimuli. Thirty-nine female undergraduates (Study 1) viewed faces with different expressions (neutral, angry, happy or sad) and 38 female students (Study 2) viewed videos of realistic social interactions (featuring anger, happiness, sadness or neutral affect). Participants were asked to identify the emotion portrayed and were subsequently given an intentional recognition memory test for the stimuli. They also completed self-report measures of alexithymia and mood (depression & anxiety). In Study 1, memory for emotional (especially angry), but not neutral faces was negatively related to the "difficulty describing feelings" facet of alexithymia. In Study 2, memory for emotional (particularly those featuring anger), but not neutral videos was negatively related to the "difficulty identifying feelings" and "externally oriented thinking" facets of alexithymia. In both studies, these memory deficits were independent of the effects of age and mood. Furthermore, the deficits appear to be most evident in the conscious recollection of the emotional stimuli. Our findings confirm that the memory deficit for emotional words in alexithymia generalises to important non-verbal socially relevant stimuli.

Alexithymia (ALX) is a multifaceted construct that is associated with difficulties identifying and describing one's feelings, problems differentiating between bodily sensations (e.g. hunger) and affect, a lack of imagination or fantasies, and an externally oriented cognitive style (Taylor et al., 1997). The Toronto Alexithymia Scale (TAS-20; Bagby et al., 1994a, 1994b) is the most widely used self-report measure of alexithymia, which assesses the three core facets of the alexithymia construct, *difficulty identifying feelings (DIF)*, *difficulty describing feelings (DDF)* and *externally oriented thinking (EOT)*. DIF concerns the ability to identify one's feelings (e.g. *"I am often confused about what emotion I am feeling")*, DDF refers to the ability to put one's feelings into words (e.g. *"It is difficult for me to find the right words for my feelings"*), whereas EOT concerns a focus on external as opposed to internal aspects of a person's experience (e.g. *"I prefer to speak to people about their daily activities rather than their emotions")*. Scores on the three subscales are combined to provide an overall measure of alexithymia (total TAS-20 score). Using the recommended cut off (a total TAS-20 score of 62 or greater), Mason et al. (2005) reported a prevalence rate of 17.92% for alexithymia in a sample of UK students. However, it should be noted that alexithymia scores tend to be higher in participants exhibiting symptoms of psychological distress, notably depression and anxiety (Honkalampi et al., 2000).

Suslow et al. (2003) characterised alexithymia as a deficit in the cognitive processing of affect. In line with this conception, there is a growing body of evidence that alexithymia is associated with marked changes in memory function. For example, alexithymia appears to undermine the memory advantage for emotional material that has been well-established in the literature (see reviews in LaBar & Cabeza, 2006; Talmi, 2013). Suslow et al. (2003) reported that memory for emotional words was negatively associated with scores on the DIF subscale of the TAS-20. Similarly, Luminet et al. (2006) reported that participants exhibiting high levels of alexithymia (total TAS-20 score) recalled fewer positive and negative words in comparison to individuals with low levels of alexithymia. Notably, both of these studies demonstrated that memory for neutral words was unaffected by alexithymia. Luminet et al. (2006) utilised the Remember-know paradigm (Gardiner, 1988) and reported that the memory deficit for emotional words in high alexithymia scorers was only evident in the *Remember* and not the *Know* responses. *Remember* responses are where the participant consciously recollects seeing the item during encoding, including details of the context (e.g. what they were thinking at the time). *Know* responses, on the other hand, are where the participant only experiences a feeling of familiarity about the item, without a conscious recollection of the context in which it was experienced. With this in mind, the findings of Luminet et al. (2006) suggest that alexithymia is associated with impaired conscious recollection of emotional words. Vermeulen and Luminet (2009) extended this work by examining the influence of alexithymia on memory for specific categories of words denoting joy, anger, disgust and neutral affect. Their findings also demonstrated that memory for emotional, but not neutral words was negatively related to alexithymia (DIF scores) and this relationship was stronger for *Remember* than *Know* responses. It has been suggested that the recollective advantage for emotional material over neutral is due to the emotional material being encoded more distinctively than the neutral material (Ochsner, 2000). Further, it has been proposed that alexithymia is associated with problems in the symbolic representation of emotions (i.e. using words or images), thus it is argued that individuals exhibiting elevated levels of alexithymia have less elaborated/ integrated emotional schema (Luminet et al., 2006; Suslow et al., 2003). With this in mind, one potential explanation for impaired memory for emotional material in alexithymia is that valence may be less conceptually salient for individuals with high alexithymia.

Vermeulen et al. (2010) confirmed the finding that alexithymia is associated with impaired memory for emotional words. However, this relationship varied as a function of the emotional context (manipulated using background music). In the context of angry music, memory for joy words was negatively associated with DIF and DDF scores, DDF scores were also negatively associated with memory for angry words. When the background music was happy, memory for joy words was positively associated with DIF scores and memory for angry words was negatively related to EOT scores, which strongly suggests that the relationships between alexithymia and memory for emotional stimuli are context dependent. One possible explanation is that the emotional context created by the music may have altered the relative salience of the different affective words. Interestingly, Meltzer and Nielson (2010) demonstrated that although individuals with high alexithymia (total TAS-20 score) recalled fewer negative words (e.g. "hatred"), they recalled a greater number of illness-related words (e.g. "pain"), which confirms that individuals with high alexithymia can remember emotional words when they are personally salient.

Although the memory deficit for emotional words in high alexithymia scorers would appear to be robust, some studies have failed to find any effect of alexithymia on memory function (Jacob & Hautekeete, 1998; Lundh et al., 2002). This could be due to variations in the experimental methods employed in the different studies. For example, Lundh et al. (2002) examined retrieval times on the autobiographical memory test (AMT; Williams & Broadbent, 1986), whereas studies reporting a memory deficit in alexithymia have tended to examine memory content. Furthermore, although studies have tended show intact memory for neutral material in high alexithymia scorers (Luminet et al., 2006; Suslow et al., 2003; Vermeulen & Luminet, 2009), Correro et al. (2019) provided evidence of impaired memory for neutral material in participants with elevated alexithymia scores.

To date, work investigating the relationship between memory and alexithymia has focused on changes in memory for verbal material. A notable exception is a study conducted by DiStefano and Koven (2012) who examined the influence of alexithymia on intentional memory for non-emotional (neutral) faces and images of people in social scenes. They reported that individuals with high TAS-20 scores exhibited impaired memory for people in social scenes relative to low scorers. However, the two groups did not differ in their memory for neutral faces. This is important, as it confirms that the effects of alexithymia on memory are not confined to verbal stimuli. Given that there was an emotional dimension to the social images it could be argued that these findings are consistent with the memory deficit that has been observed in verbal material (i.e. impaired memory for emotional but not neutral material). However, as the social images differed from the neutral faces on several factors in addition to the emotional content (e.g. the images were more complex), it is difficult to draw firm conclusions from these data. It remains unclear if alexithymia would influence memory for individual faces featuring emotional expressions. Takahashi et al. (2015) examined short-term memory for emotional faces in alexithymia using a change detection paradigm. They demonstrated that alexithymia was associated with impaired visual short-term memory for faces with happy, but not angry expressions. However, as their study examined short-term memory and did not include neutral faces as a comparison, it has yet to be determined if the pattern of long-term memory deficits exhibited by high alexithymia scorers generalise from verbal to non-verbal stimuli. Therefore, the aim of the current study was to investigate if variations in alexithymia influenced recognition memory for faces. Specifically, we examined if high levels of alexithymia were associated with reduced memory for emotional, but not neutral faces.

It is notable that alexithymia is associated with high levels of depression and anxiety (Honkalampi et al., 2000) factors that have been shown to influence memory for emotional material, including faces (Mayer et al., 1995; Noreen & Ridout, 2010; Ridout et al., 2003; 2009a, 2009b). With this in mind, it is important to control for the presence of these mood variables when examining the influence of alexithymia on memory for faces. Similarly, as there is evidence of a relationship between age and alexithymia scores in student samples (Bagby et al., 1994a) there is a need to control for the potential influence of this factor when analysing the current data.

Study 1

Overview and predictions

The aim of Study 1 was to determine if alexithymia is associated with variations in memory for emotional and neutral faces. To this end, a group of female undergraduates was presented with a series of emotional and neutral faces and asked to identify the emotion portrayed by each face (a forced choice from happy, sad, angry or neutral). Following a 5-minute filled delay, the faces were presented again, intermingled with a set of novel "foils", and participants were invited to make "old/ new" and "remember/ know/ guess" judgements. They also completed the 20-item Toronto Alexithymic Scale (TAS-20; Bagby et al., 1994a, 1994b) and the Hospital Anxiety and Depression Scale (HADS; Zigmond & Snaith, 1983). Based on previous research (e.g. Grynberg et al., 2012), it was predicted that the percentage of facial expressions correctly labelled would be negatively related to scores on the subscales of TAS-20. In line with Vermeulen and Luminet (2009) and DiStefano and Koven (2012), it was expected that memory for faces would be negatively related to scores on the subscales of the TAS-20. However, it was expected that this relationship would only be evident for emotional and not neutral faces. Furthermore, in line with Vermeulen and Luminet (2009), it was expected that the relationship between alexithymia and memory for emotional faces would only be evident in the *Remember* responses and not in the *Know* responses. Importantly, these relationships were expected to be independent from the influence of age and mood (depression and anxiety).

Method

Participants

Thirty-nine[1] female[2] undergraduate students took part in the study in exchange for course credit. The mean age of the sample was 19.5 years (SD = 1.1). Individuals with a history of psychiatric illness were requested not to take part in study. The study was approved by Aston University's Research Ethics Committee and full written informed consent was gained from all participants prior to taking part in the study.

Measures and tasks

The 20-item Toronto alexithymia scale (TAS-20; Bagby et al., 1994a) is the most widely used measure of alexithymia, which has been shown to be both valid and reliable. For example, Parker et al. (2003) reported an internal reliability coefficient of .86. Each item consists of a statement, e.g. *"I am often confused about what emotion I am feeling"*, which is then rated using a 5-point Likert scale ranging from 1 *"Strongly disagree"* to 5 *"Strongly agree"*, thus the total score on the TAS-20 ranges between 20 and 100, with higher scores indicating more severe alexithymia. The items on the TAS-20 are split into three factors that relate to different aspects of alexithymia: *"difficulty identifying feelings"* (DIF), *"difficulty describing feelings"* (DDF) and *"externally oriented thinking"* (EOT).

The Hospital Anxiety and Depression Scale (HADS; Zigmond & Snaith, 1983) is a 14-item self-report measure of depression and anxiety; seven items relate to symptoms of depression and seven to symptoms of anxiety. Each item consists of a statement, e.g. *"I feel cheerful"* followed by four possible responses indicating the extent of agreement with the statement. The range of scores on each item are 0–3, thus the range of scores on each subscale is 0–21 with higher scores indicating greater depression and anxiety. Both subscales have been shown to have good reliability (.7) and validity, as they have been shown to correlate positively (.7) with clinicians' ratings of the severity of symptoms (Zigmond & Snaith, 1983).

The Digit Symbol Substitution Task and the Digit Span Task, both of which are from the WAIS-R IQ test (Wechsler, 1981), were used as a distraction during the 5-minute filled delay period between the encoding and recognition memory phases.

Emotional faces

Three hundred and twenty photographic images were drawn from the Karolinska (Lundqvist et al., 1998) and Nimstim (Tottenham et al., 2009) face sets. These images featured forty males and forty females each portraying four different emotional facial expressions (happiness, sadness, anger and neutral affect). The faces were pseudo-randomly assigned to subsets (each containing 10 happy, 10 sad, 10 angry and 10 neutral faces, with each emotion being portrayed by five different males and females). The external features (e.g. hair) was digitally removed from each face, to ensure that participants could not use variations in external facial features to make their recognition memory judgements, and then all images were transformed to greyscale. Faces differed slightly in size due to differences in the original image sizes but were all approximately 380 pixels x 400 pixels. These faces have been shown to have good face validity, with an average recognition rate for these four emotions of 88% (range 83–92) for the NIMSTIM (Tottenham et al., 2009) and 79% (range 62–92) for the KDEF (Goeleven et al., 2008). They are also reliable with a Kappa of .84 for the NIMSTIM. Average Test re-test matches for labelling of the KDEF faces was 91% (ranging from 84 to 97). For both face-sets it has consistently been shown that angry, happy and sad expressions are matched for arousal levels, with neutral faces being rated as significantly less arousing (Adolph & Alpers, 2010; Czerwon et al., 2011; Goeleven et al., 2008).

Procedure

During the encoding phase, participants were presented with a random sequence of forty faces (10 happy, 10 sad, 10 angry and 10 neutral), via a computer with a 19" monitor, and were asked to identify the emotion portrayed by each face – a forced choice from happiness, sadness, anger or neutral affect. They were also informed that they their memory for these faces would be tested later in the study (in line with DiStefano & Koven, 2012). Superlab Pro 2.0.4 was used to present the stimuli and to record the participants' accuracy and response times (in milliseconds). Each trial began with a fixation cross (presented centrally for 500 milliseconds), followed by a face (presented centrally) and four emotional labels (presented horizontally across the screen below the face in a new random order for each trial), which remained on screen until a response was made. Participants were asked to press the key (*z*, *v*, *m*, or */*) that corresponded to the location of the label that matched the emotion shown by the face. Once all faces had been presented there was a five-minute delay, during which time the participants were asked to complete the Digit Symbol Substitution Task and Digit Span Task. Participants were subsequently given an intentional recognition memory test for the faces. During this task, participants were presented with the forty faces they had previously viewed intermingled with forty "foils" - consisting of 10 happy, 10 sad, 10 angry and 10 neutral faces[3] – and were asked to make old/new and remember/ know/ guess decisions for each face. Each trial began with a centrally presented fixation cross (for 500 ms), followed by a face which remained in the centre of the screen until a response was made. Participants pressed *"z"* for "old" faces they recognised from the encoding phase and *"v"* for "new" faces that they did not recognise. They were also asked to make *"Remember"*, *"Know"* or *"Guess"* judgements about any faces that they recognised. *Remember* was defined to the participants as *"having a specific memory of the time the face appeared on the screen, such as a particular image or thought associated with the face, or the feeling state experienced when viewing the face"*. A *Know* response was defined as *"knowing the face was part of the original set but not being able to retrieve more memories"* and a *Guess* response as *"a situation where you think* *it was plausible that the face was presented in the original set but you do not have any degree of certainty".* Finally, participants were asked to complete the HADS and TAS-20.

Data analysis

The percentage of correctly recognised emotional expressions and the mean emotion recognition times (in milliseconds) were calculated for each type of emotional expression. Recognition memory was examined using signal detection analysis, with proportion of correctly recognised faces "hits" and proportion of incorrectly recognised "novel" faces (false positives) used to calculate measures of memory sensitivity (d') and response bias (C) for emotional and neutral faces. The advantage of using signal detection analysis in recognition memory is that it provides a measure (d') of "pure" memory sensitivity that is uncontaminated by the participants' response bias (Parks, 1966). In addition, the number of *Remember*, *Know* and *Guess* responses were recorded for emotional and neutral faces. Differences in these metrics between emotional and neutral faces were assessed using a series of paired samples t-tests (or Wilcoxon tests where parametric assumptions were not met). The influence of alexithymia, controlling for age and mood, on emotion recognition and recognition memory performance was established using a series of hierarchical multiple regressions with age and mood (depression and anxiety) at Step 1 and alexithymia (the three subscales of the TAS-20) at Step 2.

Results

Participant characteristics

Mean age of the participants in Study 1 and their alexithymia, depression and anxiety scores are presented in Table 1.

Table 1. Mean age, depression, anxiety and alexithymia scores of the participants in study 1 (Standard deviations are presented in parentheses).

n = 39	Mean (SD)	Range
Age	19.50 (1.1)	18–22
Alexithymia (TAS-20)	39.69 (8.0)	25–60
Difficulty identifying feelings (TAS-DIF)	11.59 (3.5)	7–22
Difficulty describing feelings (TAS-DDF)	10.97 (4.4)	5–21
Externally oriented thinking (TAS-EOT)	17.23 (3.3)	8–24
Anxiety (HADS)	5.64 (3.0)	0–11
Depression (HADS)	2.08 (1.8)	0–7

TAS-20 = Toronto Alexithymia Scale; HADS = Hospital Anxiety and Depression Scale.

Facial emotion recognition

Analysis of emotion recognition accuracy revealed a significant main effect of emotion, $F(2.3, 86.5) = 7.87$, $p < .001$; $\eta_p^2 = .17$ (Greenhouse Geisser), with happy expressions being recognised more accurately (Mean = 97.43, SD = 5.5) than angry (M = 90, SD = 10), neutral (M = 86.15, SD = 16.3) and sad faces (M = 88.21, SD = 10.5), all tests $p < .001$(Bonferroni corrected). Analysis of reactions times for emotion recognition judgements revealed a significant main effect of emotion; $F(1.7, 63.7) = 3.41$, $p < .05$; $\eta_p^2 = .08$ (Greenhouse Geisser), with happy expressions being recognised more quickly (M = 2206.18 ms, SD = 562) than angry (M = 2569.13 ms, SD = 674), neutral (M = 2499.31 ms, SD = 658) and sad faces (M = 2523 ms, SD = 1059), all tests $p < .01$ (Bonferroni corrected).

After controlling for age and mood, none of the facets of alexithymia predicted emotion recognition accuracy or latencies, all tests $p > .05$. However, these analyses did reveal that depression significantly predicted emotion recognition latencies for angry ($\beta = .47$, $p = .016$), happy ($\beta = .54$, $p = .002$), Sad ($\beta = .54$, $p = .001$) and neutral expressions ($\beta = .64$, $p = .001$).

Memory for emotional faces[4]

Analysis of the recognition memory metrics (see Table 2) revealed no significant differences between emotional and neutral faces on all memory scores, all tests $p > .05$.

The results of a hierarchical regression revealed that age and mood combined explained around about 12% of the variance in d' scores for emotional

Table 2. Mean recognition memory performance indices (Study 1) as a function of emotional and neutral faces (standard deviations are presented in parentheses).

	Emotional	Neutral	Significance
Correct recognitions (max 10)	6.22 (1.4)	5.97 (2.1)	$t(38) = .72$, $p > .05$
False positives (max 10)	2.8 (1.3)	3.08 (1.8)	$t(38) = 1.18$, $p > .05$
d' (sensitivity)	1.04 (.36)	.86 (.44)	$t(38) = 1.42$, $p > .05$
C (response bias)	.15 (.38)	.14 (.44)	$t(38) = .14$, $p > .05$
Remember (max 10)	3.12 (1.4)	2.77 (2.1)	$T(39) = 1.35$, $p > .05$
Know (max 10)	1.66 (1.1)	1.87 (1.5)	$T(39) = 1.1$, $p > .05$
Guess (max 10)	1.41 (1.41)	1.41 (1.0)	$T(39) = .29$, $p >$ 05

T = Wilcoxon tests and t = paired samples t-tests

Table 3. Hierarchical regression to predict d′ and hits for emotional faces with alexithymia subscales as predictor variables (controlling for age and mood).

DV = d′ emotion		Model Summary				Contribution of Each Factor at Step 2				
		R^2	$R^2\Delta$	F	*p*	B	SE	b	t	*p*
Step 1		.12	-	1.53	.22					
	Age					−.04	.05	−.22	−.78	.44
	HADS-D					−.01	.03	−.04	−.27	.79
	HADS-A					−.03	.02	−.27	−1.56	.13
Step 2		.44	.32	5.93	**.003**					
	DIF					.06	.02	.60	3.52	**.001**
	DDF					−.04	.02	−.53	−2.8	**.009**
	EOT					−.01	.02	−.11	−.63	.53
DV = Hits emotion		Model Summary				Contribution of Each Factor at Step 2				
		R^2	$R^2\Delta$	F	*p*	B	SE	b	t	*p*
Step 1		.003	-	.99						
	Age					.002	.02	.02	.08	.93
	HADS-D					−.01	.02	−.13	−.64	.53
	HADS-A					.003	.01	.06	.28	.78
Step 2		.13	.13	1.5	.23					
	DIF					.02	.01	.42	**1.96**	**.06**
	DDF					−.01	.01	−.37	−1.54	.13
	EOT					.002	.01	.29	.29	.78

faces (see Table 3); R^2=.12, F(1, 36) = 1.53, *p* = .22. At Step 2, alexithymia explained an additional 32% of the variance in d′ scores for emotional faces, which was significant; $R^2\Delta$=.32, F(3, 31) = 5.93, *p* = .003. DIF and DDF scores both entered as significant predictors; such that higher DIF scores were associated with better memory for emotional faces (d′ scores); β=.60, *p* = .001 and higher DDF scores were associated with poorer memory (d′) for emotional faces; β=−.53, *p* = .009. Further analysis using partial correlations (controlling for age and mood) revealed that d′ values for angry faces were negatively associated with DDF scores; r(33)=−.44, *p* = .008 and d′ values for sad faces were positively related to DIF scores; r(33) = .25, *p* = .07. There were no other significant relationships, all tests *p* > .3. Analysis of the number of recognition memory hits for emotional faces (see Table 3) revealed that age and mood explained a negligible amount (<1%) of the variance in the number of hits for emotional faces, F < 1. At step 2, alexithymia explained an additional 13% of the variance in the number of hits; $R^2\Delta$=.32, F(3, 31) = 1.5, *p* = .21. Follow up analyses using partial correlations, controlling for age and mood, revealed that DDF scores were negatively associated with the number of hits for angry faces; r(33)=−.39, *p* = .02, but DDF scores were not significantly related to the number of hits for happy, sad of neutral faces, all tests *p* > .05. After controlling for age and mood, none of the facets of alexithymia significantly predicted d′, *remember*, *know*, or *guess* scores for neutral faces, and *know* or *guess* scores for emotional faces, all tests *p* > .05. However, after controlling for mood, there was a non-significant trend towards a negative relationship between DDF and *remember* scores for emotional faces, r(35)=−.26, *p* = .057. Follow up analyses confirmed that *remember* scores for angry faces were negatively related to DDF scores, r(36)= −.24, *p* = .07, but remember scores for happy, sad or neutral faces were not related to DDF scores, all tests *p* > .05.

Discussion

Facial emotion recognition

It was predicted that emotion recognition accuracy would be negatively associated with scores on the TAS-20 and emotion recognition latencies would be positively related to alexithymia. These predictions were not supported by our data, as neither emotion recognition accuracy nor latencies were related to alexithymia. These findings are inconsistent with previous evidence showing impaired facial emotion recognition in alexithymia (Grynberg et al., 2012). However, our results are congruent with findings from several clinical and healthy samples showing no emotion recognition deficits in participants with elevated alexithymia scores (Kessler et al., 2006; Prkachin et al., 2009; Ridout et al., 2012; Sharpe et al., 2016; Wallis et al., 2018). The variation in findings might be a consequence of differences in the emotion recognition tasks used in the respective studies. For example, Parker et al. (2005) reported that emotion recognition deficits in alexithymia were more evident when participants were put under time pressure (i.e. by presenting the faces for only a short duration). Furthermore, Kätsyri et al. (2008) demonstrated that high alexithymia scorers exhibited emotion recognition deficits when faces were spatially degraded, but not when non-degraded images were used. Starita et al. (2018) reported that emotion recognition deficits in alexithymia were more evident for low intensity emotional expressions. With this in mind, it would seem likely that the current task may not have been sufficiently challenging to result in emotion recognition deficits in those with higher alexithymia scores. It should also be noted that the use of a forced choice paradigm may not be ideal for revealing of the kind of emotion recognition difficulties that occur in everyday social situations (Russell, 1993).

Memory for faces

It was expected that memory for faces would be negatively related to alexithymia. However, this relationship was only expected for emotional and not neutral faces. The current findings for neutral faces were congruent with these predictions, as none of the memory metrics for neutral faces were associated with alexithymia. This is consistent with previous studies using words (Luminet et al., 2006; Suslow et al., 2003; Vermeulen & Luminet, 2009) and neutral faces (DiStefano & Koven, 2012), but differs from Correro et al. (2019), who reported evidence of impaired memory for neutral words and stories in high alexithymia scorers. Memory performance for emotional faces was also consistent with our predictions, as d' scores and the number of hits for emotional faces were negatively related to scores on the DDF subscale of the TAS-20. Interestingly, follow-up analyses revealed that these relationships were limited to angry faces and not sad or happy. Importantly, DDF scores were associated with lower *Remember* scores for angry faces, which suggests that alexithymia is linked to impaired conscious recollection of the angry faces. The current findings suggest that the memory deficit for affective words reported in previous studies (Luminet et al., 2006; Suslow et al., 2003; Vermeulen & Luminet, 2009) generalises to the processing of emotional faces in alexithymia. However, it would appear that there is some variability in the facet(s) of alexithymia that is (are) associated with memory deficits for emotional material. In some previous studies (Suslow et al., 2003; Vermeulen & Luminet, 2009) memory for emotional words was negatively associated with DIF scores, whereas in Luminet et al. (2006) memory for emotional words was negatively related to total TAS-20 scores, and in the current study, memory for emotional faces was negatively related to DDF scores. The current findings also represent an important development of the recent work examining memory for non-verbal stimuli in alexithymia (DiStefano & Koven, 2012; Takahashi et al., 2015). DiStefano and Koven (2012) reported that high alexithymia scorers exhibited impaired memory for people in social scenes, but as the emotional expressions featured in these images were not varied systematically it was not possible to ascertain if alexithymia impaired memory for specific emotional expressions. The current findings extend this work by confirming that alexithymia specifically impairs conscious memory for angry faces. There would also appear to be a difference in the pattern of deficits exhibited by high alexithymia scorers in short- and long-term memory. In the current study, deficits in long-term memory were most evident for angry faces, whereas participants with elevated alexithymia scores exhibited impaired short-term memory for happy faces (Takahashi et al., 2015). However, this might also relate to differences in the facial stimuli used in the two studies; Takahashi and colleagues used schematic representations of facial expressions, whereas we used validated photographs of facial expressions.

As it has been proposed that individuals with high levels of alexithymia have less elaborated/ integrated emotional schema (Luminet et al., 2006; Suslow et al., 2003), it is plausible that angry faces might have been perceived as less conceptually salient by participants with high alexithymia (DDF) scores. This is a particularly relevant for the findings relating to *Remember* scores, as conceptual salience has been identified as a critical factor in the remembering experience (Rajaram, 1998). However, if emotional faces were less salient to individuals with high alexithymia scores then we would have expected to see differences in the processing of these stimuli during encoding, yet these differences were not evident in the emotion recognition latencies or accuracy scores. Nevertheless, it is plausible that alexithymia could have influenced processing of the faces at encoding in ways that did not influence response times and performance; for example, individuals with high DDF scores might have spent less time looking at the eyes than did low scorers. In line with this suggestion, Fujiwara (2018) used an eye tracker and demonstrated that individuals with high levels of alexithymia tended to avoid looking at eyes, which led the author to conclude that eye contact might be emotionally challenging for individuals with high alexithymia – hence they avoid looking at eyes. This is notable, as reduced eye movements when viewing faces has been shown to influence memory for angry faces (Wells et al., 2010).

In contrast to studies showing a negative relationship between DIF scores and memory for affective words (e.g. Suslow et al., 2003; Vermeulen & Luminet, 2009), current findings revealed that DIF scores were positively related to memory for sad faces. This finding might also be a consequence of alexithymia-related differences in the perceived salience of the faces. For example, the sad faces might have been considered as more salient by those with high DIF scores. In line with this proposal, Meltzer and Nielson (2010) reported that whilst high alexithymia scorers demonstrated impaired memory for emotional words, they actually exhibited a memory advantage for words connoting illness, which the authors concluded was due to differences in the relative salience of the material.

Methodological considerations

It is notable that participants in the current study were informed that their memory was going to be tested for the faces (in line with DiStefano & Koven, 2012), whereas studies examining memory for emotional and neutral words have tended to use an incidental learning paradigm, where participants were not prior warned about the memory test. This is likely to have influenced how the participants processed the faces at encoding, as in addition to making emotion recognition judgements they might also have been looking for distinctive elements of each face that could aid their memory at later testing. It is also notable that the delay (of five minutes) between encoding and retrieval was relatively short in comparison to some previous studies (e.g. DiStefano and Koven (2012) who used 45 min, and Nielson and Meltzer (2009) who used 24 h). Nevertheless, the current delay period is consistent with other studies (e.g. Luminet et al., 2006; Ridout et al., 2003; Ridout et al., 2009ab). A further limitation of the study was that we did not pilot test the faces for valence and arousal. Neither did we get participants to rate their level of arousal in response to the stimuli. However, several studies using the NIMSTIM and KDEF face sets have demonstrated that angry, sad, and happy faces differ in valence ratings but not in arousal. Moreover, all three emotions were rated as more arousing that neutral faces (Adolph & Alpers, 2010; Czerwon et al., 2011; Goeleven et al., 2008).

In sum, the findings of Study 1 revealed that alexithymia (DDF) scores were negatively associated with memory (hits and d' scores) for emotional, but not neutral faces, particularly when the faces expressed anger. This pattern was evident for *Remember* but not *Know* scores, which suggests that alexithymia impaired conscious recollection of angry faces. It is plausible that the angry faces may have been less conceptually salient for the high alexithymia scorers in comparison to the low scorers, which would have reduced the distinctiveness of these faces at encoding. On the other hand, sad faces may have been perceived as more salient, which might account for the finding of a positive relationship between DIF scores and memory for sad faces. The current findings are important, as they extend previous work examining memory for non-verbal material in alexithymia and demonstrate that the memory deficit observed for affective words generalises to the processing of important non-verbal socially relevant stimuli (i.e. emotional faces). As noted by Takahashi et al. (2015) biased memory for faces in alexithymia might impair normal social functioning, which in turn might undermine key social bonds. This is important, as social support has shown to be vital in protecting against psychological distress.

Study 2

The findings of Study 1 demonstrated that DDF scores were negatively associated with memory (d', hits, and *remember* scores) for emotional, but not neutral faces. This suggests that the memory deficit shown in high alexithymia scorers for affective words generalises to non-verbal socially relevant stimuli. This is the first study to directly test this, although the findings of DiStefano and Koven (2012) could also be interpreted as evidence of impaired memory for emotional but not neutral non-verbal stimuli. In their study, individuals with high levels of alexithymia exhibited impaired memory for images of people in social scenarios (which included some emotional content), but intact memory for neutral faces. This is important, as this memory deficit for important social stimuli could have implications for social functioning of individuals with high levels of alexithymia (Takahashi et al., 2015). However, there were several limitations to their study. Firstly, the two types of stimuli varied on factors other than emotional content (e.g. the social images were more complex), which makes it difficult to draw firm conclusions from their findings. Furthermore, they did not systematically manipulate the emotional content of the social interactions. Finally, in line with the faces from Study 1 their stimuli were static, whereas in everyday interactions the social signals are dynamic and rapidly changing. With this in mind, it is important to determine if alexithymia influences memory for dynamic social interactions.

The Awareness of Social Inference Test (TASIT; McDonald et al., 2002) features short video clips of individuals in realistic social interactions and includes protagonists displaying different emotions, as well as neutral affect. It is also notable, that McDonald et al. (2006) reported that performance on this task in healthy participants was positively related to memory for faces (.69) and to measures of facial emotion processing (Ekman faces task) both recognition (.69) and matching (.7). Thus, these stimuli would seem to be ideal for the purposes of the proposed study. Given that previous work from our group has shown that alexithymia was negatively associated with the recognition of emotion from these realistic social displays (Ridout et al., 2010) and given the findings of Study 1 regarding static faces, it would be expected that alexithymia would also influence memory for these complex social stimuli.

Overview and predictions

The aim of Study 2 was to determine if variations in alexithymia were associated with differences in memory for videos of realistic social interactions. To address this question a different sample of female undergraduates was presented with a series of short video clips of social interactions and were asked to identify the emotion portrayed by the central (or lone) protagonist in each video clip (forced choice from angry, happy, neutral or sad). After a 5-minute filled delay, participants were given an intentional recognition memory test for the video clips they had viewed at encoding. Participants also completed the TAS-20 and HADS questionnaires.

In line with Ridout et al. (2010), it was expected that the percentage of correctly recognised emotional displays would be negatively related to alexithymia. In line with previous findings using non-verbal stimuli (DiStefano & Koven, 2012) and the results of Study 1, it was expected that memory for emotional, but not neutral video clips would be negatively related to alexithymia. The relationship was expected to be more evident in the *Remember* than *Know* responses. **Note:** these findings were expected to be independent of the influence of age and mood (depression and anxiety).

Method

Participants

Thirty-eight[5] female undergraduates took part in exchange for course credit.[6] The mean age of the sample was 19.63 years (SD = 2.7). Individuals with a history of psychiatric illness were requested not to take part in study. Participants provided full-written informed consent before taking part. The study was approved by the Psychology Subcommittee of Aston University's Research Ethics Committee.

Measures and tasks

Alexithymia was measured using the 20-item Toronto Alexithymia Scale (TAS-20; Bagby et al., 1994b) and mood was assessed using the Hospital Anxiety and Depression Scale (HADS; Zigmond & Snaith, 1983). As in study 1, the Digit Symbol Substitution Task and the Digit Span Task from the WAIS-R (Wechsler, 1981) were included as distractor tasks during the filled delay between encoding and recognition memory testing.

Video clips

Thirty-two video clips were drawn from the Emotion Evaluation phase of The Awareness of Social Inference Test (TASIT; McDonald et al., 2002). Each clip featured either a social interaction between two protagonists or a single speaker - on the phone or directly addressing the viewer. During each clip the central (or lone) protagonist expresses one of four emotions (sadness, happiness, anger or neutral affect). Each emotion was featured in eight video clips, four featuring a male protagonist and four featuring a female. The social interactions were performed by professional actors and the average percentage agreement, obtained from a large community sample (n > 250) was 82% for the different emotions. Furthermore, McDonald et al. (2006) reported that emotion recognition from these videos correlated positively with performance on the Ekman task, both emotion matching (.7) and emotion recognition (.69) – all of which suggests that the emotions portrayed in the videos are valid. Given that video clips in TASIT varied in length, each clip was edited to 15 s (containing the most relevant emotional components) in order to reduce inter stimulus differences, which may have influenced memory performance. Twenty clips (five each of the neutral, sad, angry & happy videos), ten featuring a male and ten featuring a female protagonist were pseudo-randomly selected to be presented during the encoding stage. The remaining 12 clips (three each of the neutral, sad, angry & happy videos) were used as novel "foils" during the recognition memory task.[7]

Procedure

During the encoding phase, participants were shown a PowerPoint presentation featuring the twenty video clips in a fixed randomised order and were asked to identify the emotion portrayed by the central (or lone) protagonist in each clip, by choosing the most appropriate emotion label from a choice of four (happiness, sadness, anger or neutral affect), which were presented in a random order for each trial. They were given unlimited time to select the appropriate emotion and were able to control the onset of the next clip. The label chosen for each trial was recorded by the experimenter using a modified version of the TASIT scoresheet. Participants were also informed that their memory for the video clips would be tested later in the study. Once all clips had been presented, there was a 5-minute filled delay during which time the participants were invited to complete the Digit Symbol Substitution Task and the Digit Span Task. Participants were subsequently given an intentional recognition memory test for the video clips they had viewed at encoding, during which they were shown a PowerPoint presentation featuring the twenty clips they had previously viewed intermingled with twelve novel "foils" and were asked to make an old/new judgement for each clip. For every clip that the participant recognised they were asked to make remember/ know/ guess judgements. Finally, they were invited to complete the TAS-20 and the HADS.

Data analysis

The percentage of correctly identified emotional displays was calculated for each type of social interaction (angry, happy, neutral and sad), which were analysed using a one-way repeated measures ANOVA, with emotion entered as the within subjects' factor. Pairwise comparisons were conducted using Bonferroni tests (to adjust alpha for multiple comparisons). The mean number of correctly recognised video clips (hits)[8], the number of falsely recognised clips (false positives), and the number of *Remember* and *Know* responses for emotional and neutral clips were compared using paired t-tests (or Wilcoxon tests where parametric assumptions were not met). Hierarchical multiple regression, with age entered at Step 1, mood (depression and anxiety) entered at Step 2 and alexithymia (scores on the three subscales of the TAS-20) entered at Step 3, was used to determine the influence of alexithymia on emotion recognition and recognition memory performance.

Results

Participant characteristics

Mean age of the participants in Study 2 and their alexithymia, depression and anxiety scores are presented in Table 4.

Emotion recognition

Analysis of emotion recognition scores revealed a significant main effect of type of emotion ($F(2.4, 88.8) = 38.5$, $p < .001$, $\eta_p^2 = .51$ (Greenhouse Geisser)), with fewer neutral interactions being correctly identified (M = 77.37, SD = 14.1) than happy (M = 96.3, SD = 7.9), angry (M = 97.90, SD = 6.2) or sad (M = 95.26, SD = 8.6), all tests $p < .001$ (Bonferroni corrected).

Table 4. Mean age, mood and alexithymia scores of the participants in Study 2 (Standard deviation are presented in parentheses).

n = 38	Mean (SD)	Range
Age	19.63 (2.7)	18–34
Alexithymia (TAS-20)	42.00 (12.8)	23–71
Difficulty identifying feelings (TAS-DIF)	12.89 (6.1)	7–27
Difficulty describing feelings (TAS-DDF)	11.58 (5.3)	5–23
Externally oriented thinking (TAS-EOT)	17.26 (4.1)	11–30
Anxiety (HADS)	6.97 (3.1)	3–14
Depression (HADS)	3.05 (2.3)	0–9

TAS-20 = Toronto Alexithymia Scale; HADS = Hospital Anxiety and Depression Scale.

Table 5. Hierarchical regression to predict correct emotion recognition of angry video clips with alexithymia subscales as predictor variables (controlling for age and mood).

DV = ER angry		Model Summary				Contribution of Each Factor at Step 2				
		R^2	$R^2\Delta$	F	*p*	B	SE	b	t	*p*
Step 1		.06	-	.66	.58					
	Age					.27	.41	.12	.66	.51
	HADS-D					−.57	.63	−.21	1.0	.37
	HADS-A					.4	.37	.12	1.1	.30
Step 2		.20	.14	1.8	.16					
	DIF					−.50	.22	−.49	2.3	**.031**
	DDF					.39	.31	.33	1.3	.22
	EOT					−.01	.28	−.1	.04	.97

The influence of alexithymia on emotion recognition

Hierarchical regression (see Table 5) revealed that age and mood had a negligible influence on the recognition of anger; $R^2 = .06$; $F(2, 34) = .66$, $p = .58$. The addition of alexithymia at Step 2 resulted in a non-significant increase in variance explained; $R^2\ \Delta = .14$; $F(3, 31) = 1.8$, $p = .16$. Nevertheless, DIF entered as a significant predictor of emotion recognition scores for angry videos; $\beta = -.49$, $p = .031$ but alexithymia did not influence the recognition of happiness, sadness or neutral affect from the video clips; all tests $p > .05$.

Memory for video clips

Analysis of the recognition memory data (see Table 6) revealed that participants made a greater number of correct recognitions (hits) for neutral clips than emotional. Similarly, participants made a greater number of *Remember* judgements for neutral clips compared to emotional. However, participants made a greater number of false recognitions of emotional foils than neutral. Participants did not differ in the number of *Know* judgements they made for emotional and neutral clips.

Table 6. Mean recognition memory performance indices (Study 2), as a function of emotional and neutral video clips (standard deviations are presented in parentheses).

	Emotional	Neutral	Significance
Correct recognitions (max 5)	4.49 (.58)	4.79 (.47)	T(38) = 329.5, *p* < .05
False positives (max 3)	.27 (.30)	.11 (.31)	T(38) = 73.5, *p* < .05
Remember (max 5)	3.68 (.96)	4.13 (1.1)	T(38) = 455, *p* < .01
Know (max 5)	.75 (.67)	.55 (1.0)	T(38) = 319.5, *p* > .05

T = Wilcoxon tests

The influence of alexithymia on memory for video clips

Hierarchical regression (see Table 7) revealed that age and mood explained about 20% of the variance in the number of hits for emotional videos; $R^2 = .21$, $F(2, 34) = 2.96$, $p = .04$. Depression entered as the only significant predictor, $\beta = -.49$, $p = .006$. The addition of alexithymia at Step 2 explained an additional 23% of the variance in the number of emotional video clips that were correctly recognised at memory testing, which was significant; $R^2\ \Delta = .23$, $F(3, 31) = 4.18$, $p = .014$. At Step 2, the influence of depression was no longer significant, $\beta = -.35$, $p = .08$ but DIF and EOT both entered as significant predictors of memory for emotional interactions, $\beta = -.41$, $p = .03$ and $\beta = -.33$, $p = .044$.

Hierarchical regression (see Table 7) revealed that age and mood explained 9% of the variance in the *Remember* scores for emotional video clips; $R^2 = .09$, $F(2, 34) = 1.1$, $p = .38$. The addition of the alexithymia scores at step 2 explained an additional 18% of the *Remember* scores for emotional video clips, but this did not represent a significant increase in variance; $R^2\ \Delta = .18$, $F(3, 31) = 2.54$, $p = .075$. At Step 2, no factors entered as significant predictors, but there was a trend for a negative relationship between DIF and *Remember* scores for emotional clips; $\beta = -.39$, $p = .07$. Follow up analyses using partial correlations, controlling for age and mood, revealed that DIF scores were negatively associated with *Remember* scores for happy and angry videos; $r(33) = -.36$, $p = .032$ and $r(33) = -40$, $p = .019$, but not sad; $r(33) = -.21$, $p = .27$.

After controlling for age and mood, alexithymia did not significantly influence the number of hits for neutral videos, false positives for emotional or neutral clips, *Remember* scores for neutral videos, or *Know* scores for emotional scenes, all tests $p > .05$. However, alexithymia did influence the number of *Know* responses for neutral videos (see Table 8). Age and

Table 7. Hierarchical regression to predict recognition memory "hits" and remember scores for emotional video clips with alexithymia subscales as predictor variables (controlling for age and mood).

DV = Hits emotion		Model Summary				Contribution of Each Factor at Step 2				
		R^2	$R^2\Delta$	F	*p*	B	SE	b	t	*p*
Step 1		.21	-	2.96	**.046**					
	Age					–.04	.03	–.16	–1.1	.27
	HADS-D					–.09	.05	–.35	–1.8	.08
	HADS-A					.03	.03	.20	1.35	.33
Step 2		.44	.23	4.18	**.014**					
	DIF					–.04	.02	–.41	–2.26	**.03**
	DDF					.018	.02	.16	.74	.47
	EOT					–.05	.02	–.33	–2.1	**.04**
DV = remember emotion		Model Summary				Contribution of Each Factor at Step 2				
		R^2	$R^2\Delta$	F	*p*	B	SE	b	t	*p*
Step 1		.09	-	1.1	.38					
	Age					–.05	.06	–.39	.8	.40
	HADS-D					–.07	.09	–.16	.72	.48
	HADS-A					.05	.05	.14	.84	.41
Step 2		.27	.18	2.5	**.08**					
	DIF					–.06	.03	–.39	1.88	**.07**
	DDF					.02	.05	.09	.38	.72
	EOT					–.06	.04	–.25	1.41	.17

Table 8. Hierarchical regression to predict recognition memory know scores for neutral video clips with alexithymia subscales as predictor variables (controlling for age and mood).

DV = know neutral		Model Summary				Contribution of Each Factor at Step 2				
		R^2	$R^2\Delta$	F	*p*	B	SE	b	t	*p*
Step 1		.09	-	1.1	.37					
	Age					–.07	.06	–.18	1.1	.30
	HADS-D					.16	.10	.38	1.7	.096
	HADS-A					–.06	.06	–.19	1.1	.27
Step 2		.29	.21	3.0	**.043**					
	DIF					.09	.03	.54	2.67	**.012**
	DDF					–.08	.05	–.42	1.72	.096
	EOT					–.04	.04	–.18	1.0	.31

mood explained 9% of the variance in *Know* scores for neutral videos; $R^2 = .09$, $F(2, 34) = 1.1$, $p = .37$. The addition of alexithymia at Step 2 explained an additional 29% of the variance; $R^2\ \Delta = .29$; $F(3, 31) = 3.0$, $p = .043$. At Step 2, DIF scores entered as the only significant predictor of *Know* scores for neutral videos; $\beta = .54$, $p = .012$.

Relationship between emotion recognition and memory performance

The total emotion recognition score was positively related to the number of hits for emotional, but not neutral videos; $r(38) = .44$, $p = .006$ and $r(38) = -.07$, $p = .66$ respectively. Total emotion recognition score was also positively related to the *Remember* scores for both emotional and neutral videos; $r(38) = .34$, $p = .03$ and $r(38) = .36$, $p = .025$. Separate analyses by valence revealed that the percentage of angry videos correctly labelled at encoding was positively related to the number of *Remember* scores for angry videos; $r(38) = .33$, $p = .04$. Similarly, the number of neutral video clips that were correctly labelled was positively related to the *Remember* scores for neutral videos, $r(38) = .35$, $p = .033$.

Discussion

Emotion recognition

It was expected that the percentage of correctly recognised emotional displays would be negatively related to alexithymia. Our findings were only partially consistent with this expectation, as alexithymia (DIF) scores were only negatively related to the recognition of anger and not happiness, sadness or neutral affect. This differs from our previous finding that alexithymia was associated with a general deficit in the recognition of emotion from these videos (Ridout et al., 2010). One possible explanation concerns the fact that the video clips were shortened for the current study. When editing the videos we focused on the most relevant emotional elements, which might have made the emotion recognition task easier by removing some of the distracting information. In line with this argument, Ridout et al. (2007) reported that emotion recognition performance from the full-length video clips was positively associated with on scores on inhibitory executive tasks (Stroop and Hayling's tests). This was thought to reflect the need to inhibit the task irrelevant elements of these complex social interactions in order to make the correct emotion recognition judgements. With this in mind it is notable that facets of alexithymia have been associated with deficits in executive function, including inhibition and conflict processing (Correro et al., 2019; Koven & Thomas, 2010; Zhang et al., 2011), thus the observed deficit in anger recognition might plausibly be a consequence of impaired executive function in those with high alexithymia.

Another possibility is that high DIF scorers may have allocated fewer attentional resources to the processing of the angry videos. In line with this argument, Vermeulen et al. (2008) reported that participants with high alexithymia scores exhibited lower activity in the attentional components of the event related potential (N2b and P3a) in response to angry faces, which the authors interpreted as evidence of abnormal attentional processing of anger in alexithymia. Furthermore, Vermeulen et al. (2006) reported reduced affective priming from angry faces in participants with high alexithymia, which suggests angry expressions were not automatically processed by these individuals. Thus, the current findings support the growing body of work showing a deficit in anger processing in participants with high levels of alexithymia.

Memory for social interactions

It was predicted that alexithymia would be negatively associated with memory for emotional, but not neutral video clips. In line with these predictions, none of the memory metrics for neutral scenarios were related to alexithymia, with the exception of a positive relationship with *Know* responses (see below). These findings are consistent with Study 1 and with studies examining memory for neutral faces (DiStefano & Koven, 2012) and words (Luminet et al., 2006; Suslow et al., 2003; Vermeulen & Luminet, 2009). However, they differ from recent evidence of an alexithymia-related deficit in memory for neutral stimuli (Correro et al., 2019). The finding that higher alexithymia scores (DIF and EOT) were associated with poorer memory (hits) for emotional videos also supports our hypotheses. Furthermore, the findings that higher DIF scores were related to lower *Remember* scores for happy and angry videos are consistent with the prediction that the negative relationship between alexithymia and memory for emotional videos would be more evident in the *Remember* than *Know* responses. However, the lack of relationship between alexithymia and *Remember* scores for sad videos is inconsistent with this prediction. Taken together, our findings are congruent with previous work examining memory for words (Luminet et al., 2006; Suslow et al., 2003; Vermeulen & Luminet, 2009). Furthermore, the current findings expand upon the work of DiStefano and Koven (2012) and Study 1 by demonstrating that higher alexithymia scores are associated with poorer memory for dynamic social stimuli, but only when they feature emotional content.

In line with the findings of Study 1, memory deficits for the emotional video clips associated with elevated alexithymia scores might plausibly relate to differences in the perceived salience of the emotional videos. This explanation is particularly pertinent for the findings of lower *Remember* scores for happy and angry videos, given that conceptual salience is considered a key factor underpinning remember experiences (Rajaram, 1998). In line with this proposal, Aaron et al. (2018) reported that individuals with high levels of alexithymia reported lower affective responses to emotive video clips in comparison to low scorers, with high scorers often reporting "no emotional response" to the videos. Furthermore, in the current study we observed that the ability to correctly label emotions (a conceptual processing task) during encoding was positively related to memory performance (hits and *Remember* scores). Specifically, the ability to correctly label angry and neutral videos was positively associated with the *Remember* scores for these stimuli. Thus, individuals with low DIF would have been able to correctly label the angry videos, presumably as their anger schema was more integrated than the high scorers, enabling them to make use of the conceptually salient aspects to encode the angry videos more distinctly. However, the finding that emotion recognition of happy videos and subsequent memory for these stimuli were not related is not consistent with this explanation. Nevertheless, evidence demonstrating reduced emotional response to appetitive words and images (Koven, 2014) suggests that lower perceived salience might still be a viable explanation for the current finding of poor memory (Remember scores) for happy videos in those with elevated DIF scores.

The current finding that DIF was positively associated with *Know* responses for neutral videos was not expected. Given that processing fluency is thought to underpin *Know* but not *Remember* responses (Rajaram, 1998), it would appear that individuals exhibiting elevated DIF scores were processing the neutral clips more fluently than were low scorers, perhaps due to the lack of emotional content in these stimuli.

Methodological considerations

There are a number of limitations to Study 2 that need to be considered. Firstly, the number of stimuli was quite low, which meant the initial memory set was small and the number of distractors at memory testing was even smaller. Although it is not a necessity that there are equal numbers of targets and foils, having a greater number of foils would have potentially reduced the number of hits (which was close to ceiling in the current study) and increased the number of false positives (which was close to floor in the current study). Unfortunately, this was unavoidable given the limited number of available videos from the TASIT. Future work using a larger set of videos and with an increased delay between encoding and retrieval would be expected to produce stronger findings. Another limitation is that we did not pilot test the images for valence and arousal ratings. In terms of valence, the reported participant agreement from a large community sample (n > 250) was >82%, which suggests that the emotions portrayed were valid (McDonald et al., 2002). Furthermore, performance of a group of participants on emotion recognition from the videos correlated highly (.7) with Ekman test of emotion recognition (McDonald et al., 2006). Nevertheless, it would have been useful to ensure the emotional videos were matched for arousal and these videos were more arousing than the neutral clips. Future work examining memory for emotional videos should confirm the valence and arousal ratings to enable these factors to be included in the analysis.

In sum, the findings of Study 2 revealed that alexithymia (DIF scores) was associated with a deficit in the recognition of anger from videos of social interactions. Furthermore, memory (number of hits) for the emotional, but not neutral videos was negatively related to alexithymia (DIF and EOT) and DIF scores were negatively linked to *Remember* scores for angry and happy videos, which suggests that alexithymia is linked to impaired conscious recollection of these emotional videos. This represents an important extension to the previous work on memory for important socially relevant stimuli in alexithymia (e.g. DiStefano & Koven, 2012; Takahashi et al., 2015). In line with Takahashi et al. (2015) it is plausible that deficits in the processing of these important social stimuli could have a negative impact on the social functioning of individuals with elevated alexithymia scores.

General discussion

We conducted two experimental studies to determine if alexithymia influenced memory for emotional faces (Study 1) and realistic social interactions (Study 2). Our key findings were that, in both studies, facets of alexithymia were associated with impaired recognition memory for emotional but not neutral stimuli. Furthermore, in both studies, participants with elevated alexithymia exhibited impaired conscious recollection of the emotional stimuli, particularly when they featured anger. Taken together these findings are consistent with studies examining memory deficits for verbal material in alexithymia (Luminet et al., 2006; Suslow et al., 2003; Vermeulen & Luminet, 2009). A plausible explanation for these memory deficits is that individuals with elevated alexithymia might not have perceived the emotional stimuli as more conceptually salient than the neutral material. Thus, for these individuals the emotional material would not have been considered as more distinctive than the neutral stimuli. This is particularly relevant when considering the negative relationship between alexithymia and *Remember* responses for the emotional stimuli. This explanation is also consistent with studies examining memory deficits for emotional words in alexithymia (Luminet et al., 2006; Vermeulen & Luminet, 2009). However, there were a number of inconsistencies in the findings of our two studies that need to be considered. Notably, whilst memory for emotional faces (Study 1) was negatively related to DDF scores, memory for emotional videos (Study 2) was negatively related to DIF and EOT. Furthermore, DIF scores were positively related to memory for sad faces (Study 1) but negatively related to memory for emotional videos (Study 2).

As noted in the discussion of Study 1, the finding of a positive relationship between DIF scores and memory for sad faces could also be explained by salience, as previous studies have demonstrated participants with elevated alexithymia can show enhanced memory for emotional material, when these stimuli were personally relevant (Meltzer & Nielson, 2010). With this in mind, it is possible that the type of stimuli used in two studies might account for the different pattern of memory in participants with high DIF scores. The emotional expressions portrayed by the faces (Study 1) were directed towards the participant, whereas in the majority of the video clips (Study 2) the affect was directed at another protagonist either seen or unseen (e.g. on the other end of a phone). Thus, it is conceivable that when the sad expressions were directed at the participants those with high DIF scores may have perceived them as more personally relevant than when sadness was directed at another person. Salience can also account for the influence of EOT on memory for emotional videos, as a recent study reported that this factor was associated with "no emotional response" to affective video clips (Aaron et al., 2018). However, salience cannot explain the lack of a negative relationship between DIF scores and memory for happy and angry faces, as would have been expected from the studies examining memory for verbal material (Suslow et al., 2003; Vermeulen & Luminet, 2009) and as was observed for happy and angry videos in Study 2.

Differences in the stimuli used in the two studies might also account for why DDF scores were negatively associated with memory for emotional faces (Study 1), but not video clips (Study 2). Fujiwara (2018) reported that high alexithymia scorers avoid looking at the eye regions of angry faces. The authors proposed that direct eye contact is emotionally challenging for those with high alexithymia. Therefore, as the faces (Study 1) featured direct gaze towards the participants, they would arguably have been more emotionally challenging for the high alexithymia scorers than would the videos (Study 2), where gaze was averted. Furthermore, faces featuring threat (e.g. angry expressions) would have been expected to be particularly challenging for high alexithymia scorers. For example, it has been proposed that appraising threatening faces (fear and anger) depletes attentional resources in those with high alexithymia, due to these individuals allocating resources to regulate the negative affective impact of these stimuli (Grynberg et al., 2014; Pouga et al., 2010). In line with this notion, Vermeulen et al. (2008) reported that higher levels of alexithymia were associated with reduced attentional processing of angry faces, indexed by lower activity in the N2b/P3a components of the EEG signal. Taken together these findings suggest that participants with high alexithymia scores would have had fewer available resources to encode the faces, which would explain the poorer memory for angry faces. However, this does not explain why it was DDF and not DIF or EOT that was related to poorer memory for angry faces. Although the studies demonstrating biased attentional processing of angry faces have tended to use the total TAS-20 scores rather than the subscales, there is evidence that DDF is associated with impaired processing of negative faces (Grynberg et al., 2014; Parker et al., 2005). Thus, it is plausible that the previous findings relating to reduced attentional processing of anger faces could have been due to DDF rather than the other facets of alexithymia. This would explain the current findings, as DDF would have been linked to reduced attentional processing of the faces, and subsequent poorer recognition memory of these stimuli but this factor would not have been expected to influence the processing of the videos, as the gaze was averted. This could be tested using eye tracking technology to examine if there variations in viewing of faces and videos linked to facets of alexithymia and whether the pattern of eye movements predicted later memory for the stimuli. This also highlights the importance of considering the individual facets of alexithymia rather than, or in addition to, the total score.

As noted above, the negative relationship between DIF scores and memory for emotional videos, particularly those featuring anger, could feasibly be a consequence of reduced perceived salience of these stimuli for those with high DIF scores. However, another factor that might explain this finding is executive function. Importantly, this factor might also account for the variation in the findings of the two studies. Although the videos used in Study 2 were shortened and simplified, they were still more complex than the static faces used in Study 1. For example, they often involved more than one speaker, or required participants to infer the other side of a conversation (e.g. when the protagonist is speaking on the phone) and contained more task irrelevant content. Thus, appraising the videos would have made greater demands on the executive functions than would the faces. For example, Ridout et al. (2007) demonstrated that emotion recognition from these videos was related to performance on measures of inhibitory function. This is notable, as recent evidence (Correro et al., 2019) confirmed that DIF, and not DDF, scores were negatively associated with scores on an executive factor (extracted from a battery of executive tasks). Therefore, assuming that individuals with high DIF scores also exhibit impaired executive function, this would explain the observed negative relationship between DIF scores and emotion recognition from the videos (in line with Ridout et al., 2007) and the negative association between DIF scores and memory for the videos, as these individuals would have had fewer resources to allocate to the encoding of the videos.

Alternative explanations and other considerations

Another factor that might account for the differential effects of alexithymia on memory for emotional and neutral material is arousal. Arousal is proposed to play a key role in the long-term consolidation of emotional memories (Sharot et al., 2004). This factor is also thought to exert an influence at the time of memory encoding by modifying cognitive processes, such as attention (Talmi et al., 2007), which is thought to explain the advantage for emotional material over neutral at immediate memory testing. With this in mind, it is notable that there is evidence of reduced physiological arousal in alexithymia from studies using skin conductance (e.g. Constantinou et al., 2014; Franz et al., 2003), heart rate (e.g. Franz et al., 2003) and facial electromyography (EMG) (e.g. Scarpazza, 2015). However, this also some evidence of hyperarousal (e.g. Davydov et al., 2013; Luminet et al., 2004) and other studies showing no arousal differences between high and low alexithymia scorers (e.g. Gilbert, 2008; Stone & Nielson, 2001). In a recent review, Panayiotou et al. (2018) concluded that, although there are several contradictory findings, the weight of evidence supports there being no difference in physiological arousal between high and low alexithymia scorers. Nevertheless, they concluded that hypo-arousal was often found when tasks were emotional in nature (e.g. appraising images or films). With this mind, future work could examine the role that arousal plays in these alexithymia-related memory deficits using physiological measurements of arousal such as galvanic skin response, heart rate or facial EMG.

In summary, the findings of two experimental studies demonstrate that elevated levels of alexithymia are associated with poorer memory for emotional non-verbal socially relevant stimuli, whereas memory for neutral stimuli was unaffected. These deficits were particularly evident in the conscious recollection of emotional stimuli, especially those featuring anger. However, the findings of the two studies were related to different facets of alexithymia, as high DDF scores were associated with impaired memory for emotional faces (Study 1) and high DIF scores were linked to lower memory for emotional videos (Study 2). These differences are thought to be related to the nature of the emotional stimuli. Finally, in line with Takahashi et al. (2015), it is proposed that impaired memory for these important social stimuli could have a negative impact on the social functioning of individuals with elevated alexithymia.

Notes

1. Based on the observed effect size reported in a previous study examining the influence of alexithymia on memory for faces (DiStefano & Koven, 2012) a large effect size (f^2=.35) was expected. The results of a power calculation using G*Power to determine the required sample size for a multiple regression to detect a significant change in R^2 with 3 tested predictors and a total of 6 predictors revealed that a minimum of 36 participants would be required to detect a large effect size with a power of .8 and an alpha level of .05. Therefore, this study was sufficiently powered.
2. Five male participants were also recruited. However, given that males and females differ in face processing (Sullivan et al., 2015) and alexithymia (Levant et al., 2009), and that there was an insufficient number of males to allow for a reliable group comparison we chose to exclude these participants from the analysis of the data from Study 1.
3. The faces presented at encoding and as "foils' during the recognition memory test were counterbalanced to ensure that each individual poser appeared equally often as a "target' and "foil' and equally often with a sad, happy, angry or neutral expression.
4. Memory for faces was not related to facial emotion recognition performance (% correct or response times) at encoding, all tests p>.05.
5. Based on the observed effect sizes reported in Study 1 and in a previous study examining the influence of alexithymia on memory for faces (DiStefano & Koven, 2012) a large effect size (f^2=.35) was expected. The results of a power calculation using G*Power to determine the

required sample size to detect a significant change in R^2 on a multiple regression with three tested predictors and a total of six predictors revealed that a minimum of 36 participants would be required to detect a large effect size with a power of .8 and an alpha level of .05. Therefore, this study was sufficiently powered.
6. Two male participants were also recruited. However, given that males and females differ in face processing (Sullivan et al., 2015) and alexithymia (Levant et al., 2009), and that there were an insufficient number of males to allow for a reliable group comparison we chose to exclude these participants from the analysis of the data from Study2.
7. The video clips presented at encoding and as 'foils' during the recognition memory test were counterbalanced across participants to ensure that, as far as possible, each individual actor appeared equally often as a 'target' and 'foil' and equally often when expressing sadness, happiness, anger or neutral affect.
8. We had planned to conduct signal detection analysis on the data from Study 2, but initial inspection of the data revealed that hits were close to ceiling and false positives close to floor, thus signal detection analysis would have been unreliable. Therefore, we analysed the hits and false positives separately. Furthermore, the number of *guess* responses was extremely low, therefore these data are not reported or analysed.

Disclosure statement

No potential conflict of interest was reported by the author(s).

ORCID

Nathan Ridout http://orcid.org/0000-0002-7111-2996

References

Aaron, R. V., Snodgress, M. A., Blain, S. D., & Park, S. (2018). Affect labeling and other aspects of emotional experiences in relation to alexithymia following standardized emotion inductions. *Psychiatry Research*, *262*, 115–123. https://doi.org/10.1016/j.psychres.2018.02.014

Adolph, D., & Alpers, G. W. (2010). Valence and arousal: A comparison of two sets of emotional facial expressions. *American Journal of Psychology*, *123*(2), 209–219. https://doi.org/10.5406/amerjpsyc.123.2.0209

Bagby, R. M., Parker, J. D. A., & Taylor, G. J. (1994a). The 20-item Toronto-alexithymia-scale. 1. Item selection and cross-validation of the factor structure. *Journal of Psychosomatic Research*, *38*(2), 3–32. https://doi.org/10.1016/0022-3999.(94)90005-1

Bagby, R. M., Taylor, G. J., & Parker, J. D. A. (1994b). The 20-item Toronto-alexithymia-scale. 2. Convergent, discriminant, and concurrent validity. *Journal of Psychosomatic Research*, *38*(3), 3–40. https://doi.org/10.1016/0022-3999.(94)90006-X

Constantinou, E., Panayiotou, G., & Theodorou, M. (2014). Emotion processing deficits in alexithymia and response to a depth of processing intervention. *Biological Psychology*, *103*, 212–222. https://doi.org/10.1016/j.biopsycho.2014.09.011

Correro IIA. N., Paitel, E. R., Byers, S. J., & Nielson, K. A. (2019). The role of alexithymia in memory and executive functioning across the lifespan. *Cognition and Emotion*, 1–16. https://doi.org/10.1080/02699931.2019.1659232

Czerwon, B., Lüttke, S., & Werheid, K. (2011). Age differences in valence judgments of emotional faces: The influence of personality traits and current mood. *Experimental Aging Research*, *37*(5), 503–515. https://doi.org/10.1080/0361073X.2011.619468

Davydov, D. M., Luminet, O., & Zech, E. (2013). An externally oriented style of thinking as a moderator of responses to affective films in women. *International Journal of Psychophysiology*, *87*(2), 152–164. https://doi.org/10.1016/j.ijpsycho.2012.12.003

DiStefano, R. A., & Koven, N. S. (2012). Dysfunctional emotion processing may explain visual memory deficits in alexithymia. *Personality and Individual Differences*, *52*(5), 611–615. https://doi.org/10.1016/j.paid.2011.12.007

Franz, M., Schaefer, R., & Schneider, C. (2003). Psychophysiological response patterns of high and low alexithymics under mental and emotional load conditions. *Journal of Psychophysiology*, *17*(4), 203–213. https://doi.org/10.1027/0269-8803.17.4.203

Fujiwara, E. (2018). Looking at the eyes interferes with facial emotion recognition in alexithymia. *Journal of Abnormal Psychology*, *127*(6), 571–577. https://doi.org/10.1037/abn0000361

Gardiner, J. M. (1988). Functional aspects of recollective experience. *Memory & Cognition*, *16*(4), 309–313. https://doi.org/10.3758/BF03197041

Gilbert, A. M. (2008). The physiological response to implicit and explicit fear faces in alexithymia (Doctoral dissertation, University of Pittsburgh).

Goeleven, E., De Raedt, R., Leyman, L., & Verschuere, B. (2008). The Karolinska directed emotional faces: A validation study. *Cognition and Emotion*, *22*(6), 1094–1118. https://doi.org/10.1080/02699930701626582

Grynberg, D., Chang, B., Corneille, O., Maurage, P., Vermeulen, N., & Luminet, O. (2012). Alexithymia and the processing of emotional facial expressions (EFEs): Systematic review, unanswered questions and further perspectives. *PLoS ONE*, *7*(8), Article e42429. https://doi.org/10.1371/journal.pone.0042429

Grynberg, D., Vermeulen, N., & Luminet, O. (2014). Amplification of attentional blink by distress related facial expressions: Relationships with alexithymia and affectivity. *International Journal of Psychology*, *49*(5), 371–380. https://doi.org/10.1002/ijop.12006

Honkalampi, K., Hintikka, J., Tanskanen, A., Lehtonen, J., & Viinamäki, H. (2000). Depression is strongly associated with alexithymia in the general population. *Journal of Psychosomatic Research*, *48*(1), 99–104. https://doi.org/10.1016/S0022-3999(99)00083-5

Jacob, S., & Hautekeete, M. (1998). Alexithymia and memory: A more rigorous criterion for acceptance in recognition tasks? *Encephale-Revue De Psychiatrie Clinique Biologique Et Therapeutique*, *24*, 199–204.

Kätsyri, J., Saalasti, S., Tiippana, K., von Wendt, L., & Sams, M. (2008). Impaired recognition of facial emotions from low-spatial frequencies in Asperger syndrome. *Neuropsychologia*,

46(7), 1888–1897. https://doi.org/10.1016/j.neuropsychologia.2008.01.005
Kessler, H., Schwarze, M., Filipic, S., Traue, H. C., & von Wietersheim, J. (2006). Alexithymia and facial emotion recognition in patients with eating disorders. *International Journal of Eating Disorders*, *39*(3), 245–251. https://doi.org/10.1002/eat.20228
Koven, N. S. (2014). Abnormal valence differentiation in alexithymia. *Personality and Individual Differences*, *68*, 102–106. https://doi.org/10.1016/j.paid.2014.04.007
Koven, N. S., & Thomas, W. (2010). Mapping facets of alexithymia to executive dysfunction in daily life. *Personality and Individual Differences*, *49*(1), 24–28. https://doi.org/10.1016/j.paid.2010.02.034
LaBar, K. S., & Cabeza, R. (2006). Cognitive neuroscience of emotional memory. *Nature Reviews Neuroscience*, *7*(1), 54–64. https://doi.org/10.1038/nrn1825
Levant, R. F., Hall, R. J., Williams, C. M., & Hasan, N. T. (2009). Gender differences in alexithymia. *Psychology of men & Masculinity*, *10*(3), 190–203. https://doi.org/10.1037/a0015652
Luminet, O., Rimé, B., Bagby, R. M., & Taylor, G. (2004). A multimodal investigation of emotional responding in alexithymia. *Cognition and Emotion*, *18*(6), 741–766. https://doi.org/10.1080/02699930341000275
Luminet, O., Vermeulen, N., Demaret, C., Bagby, R. M., & Taylor, G. J. (2006). Alexithymia and levels of processing: Evidence for an overall deficit in remembering emotion words. *Journal of Research in Personality*, *40*(5), 713–733. https://doi.org/10.1016/j.jrp.2005.09.001
Lundh, L. G., Johnsson, A., Sundqvist, K., & Olsson, H. (2002). Alexithymia, memory of emotion, emotional awareness, and perfectionism. *Emotion*, *2*(4), 361–379. https://doi.org/10.1037/1528-3542.2.4.361
Lundqvist, D., Flykt, A., & Ohman, A. (1998). *The Karolinska directed emotional faces (KDEF)*. Department of Neurosciences Karolinska Hospital.
Mason, O., Tyson, M., Jones, C., & Potts, S. (2005). Alexithymia: Its prevalence and correlates in a British undergraduate sample. *Psychology and Psychotherapy: Theory, Research and Practice*, *78*(1), 113–125. https://doi.org/10.1348/147608304X21374
Mayer, J. D., McCormick, L. J., & Strong, S. E. (1995). Mood-congruent memory and natural mood: New evidence. *Personality and Social Psychology Bulletin*, *21*(7), 736–746. https://doi.org/10.1177/0146167295217008
McDonald, S., Bornhofen, C., Shum, D., Long, E., Saunders, C., & Neulinger, K. (2006). Reliability and validity of the awareness of social Inference test (TASIT): A clinical test of social perception. *Disability and Rehabilitation*, *28*(24), 1529–1542. https://doi.org/10.1080/09638280600646185
McDonald, S., Flanagan, S., & Rollins, J. (2002). *The awareness of social inference test. Bury St. Edmonds*. Thames Valley Test Company.
Meltzer, M. A., & Nielson, K. A. (2010). Memory for emotionally provocative words in alexithymia: A role for stimulus relevance. *Consciousness and Cognition*, *19*(4), 1062–1068. https://doi.org/10.1016/j.concog.2010.05.008
Nielson, K. A., & Meltzer, M. A. (2009). Modulation of long-term memory by arousal in alexithymia: The role of interpretation. *Consciousness and Cognition*, *18*(3), 786–793. https://doi.org/10.1016/j.concog.2009.06.001
Noreen, S., & Ridout, N. (2010). Short-term memory for emotional faces in dysphoria. *Memory (Hove, England)*, *18*(5), 486–497. https://doi.org/10.1080/09658211003762092
Ochsner, K. N. (2000). Are aVective events richly recollected or simply familiar. The experience and process of recognizing feelings past. *Journal of Experimental Psychology-General*, *129*(2), 242–261. https://doi.org/10.1037/0096-3445.129.2.242
Panayiotou, G., Panteli, M., & Vlemincx, E. (2018). Processing emotions in alexithymia: A systematic review of physiological Markers. *Alexithymia: Advances in Research, Theory, and Clinical Practice*, *291*, 291–320.
Parker, P. D., Prkachin, K. M., & Prkachin, G. C. (2005). Processing of facial expressions of negative emotion in alexithymia: The influence of temporal constraint. *Journal of Personality*, *73*(4), 1087–1107. https://doi.org/10.1111/j.1467-6494.2005.00339.x
Parker, J. D., Taylor, G. J., & Bagby, R. M. (2003). The 20-item Toronto alexithymia Scale: III. Reliability and factorial validity in a community population. *Journal of Psychosomatic Research*, *55*(3), 269–275. https://doi.org/10.1016/S0022-3999(02)00578-0
Parks, T. E. (1966). Signal-detectability theory of recognition memory. *Psychological Review*, *73*(1), 44–58. https://doi.org/10.1037/h0022662
Pouga, L., Berthoz, S., de Gelder, B., & Grezes, J. (2010). Individual differences in socioaffective skills influence the neural bases of fear processing: The case of alexithymia. *Human Brain Mapping*, *31*(10), 1469–1481. https://doi.org/10.1002/hbm.20953
Prkachin, G. C., Casey, C., & Prkachin, K. M. (2009). Alexithymia and perception of facial expressions of emotion. *Personality and Individual Differences*, *46*(4), 412–417. https://doi.org/10.1016/j.paid.2008.11.010
Rajaram, S. (1998). The effects of conceptual salience and perceptual distinctiveness on conscious recollection. *Psychonomic Bulletin Review*, *5*(1), 71–78. https://doi.org/10.3758/BF03209458
Ridout, N., Astell, A. J., Reid, I. C., Glen, T., & O' Carroll, R. E. (2003). Memory bias for emotional facial expressions in major depression. *Cognition and Emotion*, *17*(1), 101–122. https://doi.org/10.1080/02699930302272
Ridout, N., Dritschel, B., Matthews, K., McVicar, M., Reid, I. C., & O' Carroll, R. E. (2009b). Memory for emotional faces in major depression following judgment of physical facial characteristics at encoding. *Cognition and Emotion*, *23*(4), 739–752. https://doi.org/10.1080/02699930802121137
Ridout, N., Noreen, A., & Johal, J. (2009a). Memory for emotional faces in naturally occurring dysphoria and induced negative mood. *Behaviour, Research & Therapy*, *47*(10), 851–860. https://doi.org/10.1016/j.brat.2009.06.013
Ridout, N., O'Carroll, R. E., Dritschel, B., Christmas, D., Eljamel, M., & Matthews, K. (2007). Emotion recognition from dynamic emotional displays following anterior cingulotomy and anterior capsulotomy for chronic depression. *Neuropsychologia*, *45*(8), 1735–1743. https://doi.org/10.1016/j.neuropsychologia.2006.12.022
Ridout, N., Thom, C., & Wallis, D. J. (2010). Emotion recognition and alexithymia in females with non-clinical disordered eating. *Eating Behaviors*, *11*(1), 1–5. https://doi.org/10.1016/j.eatbeh.2009.07.008

Ridout, N., Wallis, D. J., Autwal, Y., & Sellis, J. (2012). The influence of emotional intensity on facial emotion recognition in disordered eating. *Appetite*, *59*(1), 181–186. https://doi.org/10.1016/j.appet.2012.04.013

Russell, J. A. (1993). Forced-choice response format in the study of facial expression. *Motivation and Emotion*, *17*(1), 41–51. https://doi.org/10.1007/BF00995206

Scarpazza, C. (2015). *Deficit in the Emotional Embodiment in Alexithymia* (Doctoral dissertation, alma).

Sharot, T., Delgado, M. R., & Phelps, E. A. (2004). How emotion enhances the feeling of remembering. *Nature Neuroscience*, *7*(12), 1376–1380. https://doi.org/10.1038/nn1353

Sharpe, E., Wallis, D. J., & Ridout, N. (2016). The influence of variations in eating disorder-related symptoms on processing of emotional faces in a non-clinical female sample: An eye-tracking study. *Psychiatry Research*, *240*, 321–327. https://doi.org/10.1016/j.psychres.2016.04.065

Starita, F., Borhani, K., Bertini, C., & Scarpazza, C. (2018). Alexithymia is related to the need for more emotional intensity to identify static fearful facial expressions. *Frontiers in Psychology*, *9*, 929. https://doi.org/10.3389/fpsyg.2018.00929

Stone, L. A., & Nielson, K. A. (2001). Intact physiological response to arousal with impaired emotional recognition in alexithymia. *Psychotherapy and Psychosomatics*, *70*(2), 92–102. https://doi.org/10.1159/000056232

Sullivan, L., Camic, P. M., & Brown, J. S. (2015). Masculinity, alexithymia, and fear of intimacy as predictors of UK men's attitudes towards seeking professional psychological help. *British Journal of Health Psychology*, *20*(1), 194–211. https://doi.org/10.1111/bjhp.12089

Suslow, T., Kersting, A., & Arolt, V. (2003). Alexithymia and incidental learning of emotional words. *Psychological Reports*, *93* (7), 1003–1012. https://doi.org/10.2466/PR0.93.7.1003-1012

Takahashi, J., Hirano, T., & Gyoba, J. (2015). Effects of facial expressions on visual short-term memory in relation to alexithymia traits. *Personality and Individual Differences*, *83*, 128–135. https://doi.org/10.1016/j.paid.2015.04.010

Talmi, D. (2013). Enhanced emotional memory: Cognitive and neural mechanisms. *Current Directions in Psychological Science*, *22*(6), 430–436. https://doi.org/10.1177/0963721413498893

Talmi, D., Schimmack, U., Paterson, T., & Moscovitch, M. (2007). The role of attention and relatedness in emotionally enhanced memory. *Emotion*, *7*(1), 89. https://doi.org/10.1037/1528-3542.7.1.89

Taylor, G. J., Bagby, R. M., & Parker, J. D. A. (1997). *Disorders of affect regulation: Alexithymia in medical and psychiatric illness*. Cambridge University Press.

Tottenham, N., Tanaka, J. W., Leon, A. C., McCarry, T., Nurse, M., Hare, T. A., Marcus, D. J., Westerlund, A., Casey, B. J., & Nelson, C. (2009). The NimStim set of facial expressions: Judgments from untrained research participants. *Psychiatry Research*, *168*(3), 24–249. https://doi.org/10.1016/j.psychres.2008.05.006

Vermeulen, N., & Luminet, O. (2009). Alexithymia factors and memory performances for neutral and emotional words. *Personality and Individual Differences*, *47*(4), 305–309. https://doi.org/10.1016/j.paid.2009.03.018

Vermeulen, N., Luminet, O., Cordovil de Sousa, M., & Campanella, S. (2008). Attentional processing of emotional facial expressions in alexithymia: A visual ERP study. *Cognition and Emotion*, *22*(6), 1052–1067. https://doi.org/10.1080/02699930701597635

Vermeulen, N., Luminet, O., & Corneille, O. (2006). Alexithymia and the automatic processing of affective information: Evidence from the affective priming paradigm. *Cognition and Emotion*, *20*(1), 64–91. https://doi.org/10.1080/02699930500304654

Vermeulen, N., Toussaint, J., & Luminet, O. (2010). The influence of alexithymia and music on the incidental memory for emotion words. *European Journal of Personality*, *24*(6), 551–568. https://doi.org/10.1002/per.758

Wallis, D. J., Ridout, N., & Sharpe, E. (2018). The influence of non-clinical eating-related psychopathology on the recognition of emotion from static faces and realistic social interactions. *Eating Behaviors*, *29*, 19–24. https://doi.org/10.1016/j.eatbeh.2018.01.004

Wechsler, D. (1981). *Wechsler Adult Intelligence Scale- revised*. Psychological Corporation.

Wells, T. T., Beevers, C. G., Robison, A. E., & Ellis, A. J. (2010). Gaze behavior predicts memory bias for angry facial expressions in stable dysphoria. *Emotion*, *10*(6), 894–902. https://doi.org/10.1037/a0020022

Williams, J. M. G., & Broadbent, K. (1986). Autobiographical memory in attempted suicide patients. *Journal of Abnormal Psychology*, *95*(2), 144–149. https://doi.org/10.1037/0021-843X.95.2.144

Zhang, L., Zhu, C., Ye, R., Cao, Z., Tian, Y., Yang, P., Hu, P., & Wang, K. (2011). Impairment of conflict processing in alexithymic individuals. *Neuroscience Letters*, *504*(3), 261–264. https://doi.org/10.1016/j.neulet.2011.09.043

Zigmond, A. S., & Snaith, R. P. (1983). The Hospital anxiety and depression Scale. *Acta Psychriatica Scandinavia*, *67*(6), 361–370. https://doi.org/10.1111/j.1600-0447.1983.tb09716.x

Alexithymia disrupts verbal short-term memory

Nicolas Vermeulen

ABSTRACT
While some research has now started to suggest that there are long-term memory (LTM) deficits in alexithymia, short-term memory (STM) in alexithymia remained largely unexplored. This study investigated whether the STM trace for emotion and neutral words might also be disrupted by alexithymia. Forty-four participants were randomly assigned to Study 1 in which the to-be-memorised six-word lists were composed of words belonging to the same valence (i.e. pure lists condition, Study 1), and 44 other participants were randomly assigned to Study 2 in which six-word lists were composed of embedded neutral and emotional words (i.e. mixed lists condition). All the participants completed the Toronto-Alexithymia Scale (TAS-20) and a current mood states scale (PANAS). Results showed that the main effect of alexithymia was observed in the pure lists condition while no alexithymia groups effect emerged in the mixed lists condition. In the pure lists condition only correlation analyses confirmed that alexithymia significantly and negatively correlated with recall accuracy. The results are discussed with regard to the influence of alexithymia on the proposed role of (1) semantic organisation of LTM on STM performance in the pure lists condition and (2) attentional capture by emotional words in the mixed lists condition.

Alexithymia encompasses (1) difficulty identifying feelings and distinguishing between feelings and the bodily sensations of emotional arousal; (2) difficulty describing feelings to others and (3) a stimulus-bound, externally oriented cognitive style (Taylor & Bagby, 2000, 2004). Importantly, numerous studies have found that alexithymia impairs the cognitive processing of emotional information. For instance, cognitive processing of visual information-like emotional words or facial expressions (Franz, Schaefer, Schneider, Sitte, & Bachor, 2004; Meriau et al., 2006; Mueller, Alpers, & Reim, 2006; Swart, Kortekaas, & Aleman, 2009; Vermeulen & Luminet, 2009; Vermeulen, Luminet, & Corneille, 2006; Vermeulen, Luminet, De Sousa, & Campanella, 2008), as well as auditory information such as spoken sentences, prosody and even non-verbal vocalisations (Bayot et al., 2014) is hampered in people who score high on alexithymia. Taylor and Bagby (2004) suggest that alexithymia might be related to a deficit in the ability to link somatic sensations of emotional arousal to symbols like words or images. Some research has also started to investigate long-term memory performance in alexithymia. Indeed, it has already been suggested over 20 years ago that people scoring high on alexithymia might be unable to link their feelings with memories (Taylor, Bagby, & Parker, 1997). This proposal fits perfectly with Bucci (1997)'s idea that high alexithymia scorers develop weak links between symbolic and subsymbolic representations of their past affective experiences (see also Taylor & Bagby, 2004). Collectively, there is evidence that a high level of alexithymia, especially the facet that involves the identification of emotion, influences memory performance (i.e. memory accuracy but not processing time) when the to-be-remembered stimuli or the events are emotional, while memory for neutral stimuli remains unaffected (for a review, see, Vermeulen, Domachowska, & Nielson, 2018). Interestingly, Meltzer and Nielson (2010) found preserved or even improved memory for emotionally provocative words (i.e. illness-related words) in high alexithymia scorers, suggesting that personal relevance might capture the attention of high alexithymia scorers.

However, only a few published papers have started to investigate the influence of alexithymia on short-term memory. First, Distefano and Koven (2012) found, using a non-emotional neuropsychological assessment (i.e. the Wechsler Memory Scale-III) of low alexithymia scorers (LA) and high alexithymia scorers (HA), that LA performed better than HA on the immediate and delayed visual memory subscales. Results on verbal subscales (words and stories) were comparable between the alexithymia groups. Even if there were methodological limitations, like a small sample size and no statistical control for mood states or anxiety, the findings emphasised the poor ability of HA to memorise in a short period of time socially oriented stimuli such as neutral faces and pictures of social interactions (i.e. without any emotional content). Second, the other published short-term memory research involving alexithymia used crowds of facial expressions (Takahashi, Hirano, & Gyoba, 2015). The study found that short-term storage of facial expression was hampered in HA. Together, these two studies found deficits in short-term memory for pictorial information, irrespective of whether the information was emotional or not. However, to our knowledge, no published study has examined verbal short-term memory for neutral and emotional words in alexithymia. Therefore, the main aim of the present study is to investigate whether the immediate memory trace for emotion and neutral words might also be disrupted by alexithymia.

The cognitive literature on short-term memory for verbal material emphasised the separated role of attentional capture and long-term memory (LTM) organisation in short-term memory (STM) performance. For instance, Majerus and D'argembeau (2011) examined systematically the effect of emotional content on short-term memory of word lists. They used two different types of six-word lists. The list was composed either of embedded neutral and emotional words (i.e. mixed lists) or of words belonging to the same valence (i.e. pure lists). Majerus and D'argembeau (2011) showed that in mixed lists, an immediate recall was improved for emotion-infrequent lists (i.e. two emotion words embedded among four neutral words). The fact that the mixed lists containing a minority of emotion words led to better recall was interpreted as an attentional grabbing effect of emotion in STM. On the other hand, in pure lists, Majerus and D'argembeau (2011) showed that emotional valence increases STM performance. Hence, in pure lists, the impact of emotional valence on STM performance was discussed as an effect of lexico-semantic long-term memory (LTM) organisation. In other words, LTM and its organisation provide a structural support to STM when all the words belong to the same category.

In the present research, on the one hand, since HA have deficits in LTM for emotion stimuli and because STM depends on LTM organisation and support, we hypothesise that HA would show deficits in STM for pure lists of emotion words. On the other hand, we hypothesise that alexithymia will have little impact on mixed lists condition. Indeed, because LTM research in alexithymia showed preservation of an attention-grabbing effect of emotion due to, for instance, to personal relevance (Meltzer & Nielson, 2010), we hypothesise that alexithymia would not impact STM performance in conditions in which attention is captured or attracted by emotions as in mixed lists (Majerus & D'argembeau, 2011). In the current paper, we present two experiments using the exact same method and the same controlled and validated stimuli as those used in Majerus and D'argembeau (2011; Experiments 1 and 3). The material was directly obtained from the authors.

Materials and methods

Participants were randomly assigned to either the pure list experiment (Study 1; Majerus and D'argembeau (2011; Experiment 1)) or to the mixed list experiment (Study 2; Majerus and D'argembeau (2011; Experiment 3)). In both experiments, participants were tested individually for approximately 75 min. All participants completed a validated French translation of the Toronto-Alexithymia Scale (TAS-20, Loas, Parker, Otmani, Verrier, & Fremaux (1997)). The TAS-20 is the most widely used measure of the alexithymia construct (Bagby, Parker, & Taylor, 1994a; Bagby, Taylor, & Parker, 1994b). It is comprised of 20 items that are rated on five-point Likert scales ranging from 1 (strongly disagree) to 5 (strongly agree). The items load on three factors – difficulty identifying feelings, difficulty describing feelings and externally oriented thinking. Total scores range from 20 to 100 points. Based on Taylor et al. (1997), people are considered as non-alexithymic if their score is below or equal to 51. A score from 52 to 60 represents moderate alexithymia levels. Finally, a score above or equal to 61 represents the clinical threshold of alexithymia.

In order to control for the influence of the current mood states, participants also completed the Positive Affect Negative Affect Schedule (PANAS; Watson, Clark, & Tellegen (1988)). The PANAS is a 20-item scale which assesses the general positive and negative affective states that the participants feel at a particular moment It consists of 10 positive (e.g. interested) and 10 negative (e.g. guilty) affective states rated on five-point Likert-type scales ranging from 1 (not at all) to 5 (extremely). The PANAS is the most widely used scale for the assessment of current affective states. We used the French version in the present study and participants completed the PANAS in order to assess how they felt at the moment, just before starting the memory test (Gaudreau, Sanchez, & Blondin, 2006). Possible scores range from 10 to 50 for each scale (Positive Affect: PA and Negative Affect: NA). Usually, alexithymia correlates with mood states. In the present studies, PA and NA were indeed significantly correlated with alexithymia, $r = -.29$, $p = .005$ and $r = .25$, $p = .02$, respectively, for PA and NA.

In the original experiments of Majerus and D'argembeau (2011; Experiments 1 and 3), there were 15 and 16 participants, respectively, in Experiments 1 and 3. Thus, we envisaged collecting at least 20 participants in each condition for the within-participant effect (type of words). However, as we expected an influence of alexithymia, we decided to increase the sample size in order to conduct valid correlation analyses. We expected to observe medium ($r = .3$) to large ($r = .5$) correlations as defined by Cohen (1988). In order to estimate the appropriate sample size for this type of correlation (medium to large; $r = .4$), we ran a power analysis using a two-sided significance level test ($\alpha = 0.05$) with 80% power ($\beta = 0.2$), the sample size required to detect such an effect was approximately 47 ($n = 47$). We, therefore, proposed 100-time slots (75 min) for a memory study, and 88 unscreened (non-clinical) undergraduate students actually came to the laboratory after signing up. These 88 participants were then randomly assigned to one of the two conditions (pure: $n = 44$ or mixed list: $n = 44$). Descriptive data and group comparisons are illustrated in Table 1.

Study 1: Pure lists. 44 participants took part (29 women and 15 men) in the present pure list study (mean age = 20.84 years; SD = 2.31, range = 18–30).

The stimuli were the same as those used by Majerus and D'argembeau (2011; Experiment 1). For the pure lists, we used six-item lists of French words belonging to three categories: (1) positive lists: triumph–luck–lake–treasure–encouragement–harmony; (2) negative lists: drowning–dagger–horror–migraine–boredom–avalanche and (3) neutral lists: piece–habit–tendency–pawn–estimation–jar. Lists from Majerus and D'argembeau (2011; Experiment 1) were presented in each of the three categories.

Study 2: Mixed lists. 44 new participants took part (33 women and 11 men) in the present mixed list study (mean age = 21.02 years; SD = 2.16, range = 19–28). For the mixed lists, the same words as in pure lists condition were used but they were compiled by Majerus and D'argembeau (2011; Experiment 3) in six-word lists alternating emotional and neural words, in the proportion of two rare and four frequent word types, for instance: meter–assassin–pepper–bankruptcy–camp–secretary. The two rare words were always presented in positions 2 and 4 embedded among four frequent words (i.e. words belonging to the same valence). Four types of lists combining frequent and rare words were used. The four list types were: (a) negative frequent list (4 negative-2 neutral); (b) positive frequent list (4 positive-2 neutral); (c) negative rare list (4 neutral-2 negative); (d) positive rare list (4 neutral-2 positive). Each of the four list types contained 20 instances of six-word lists. Collectively, 80 lists from Majerus and D'argembeau (2011; Experiment 3) containing six words each were presented in the present study.

In both Study 1 and Study 2, participants first signed an informed consent and then completed questionnaires. The six-word lists were prerecorded sound files from Majerus and D'argembeau (2011) presenting auditory words at a rate of one word every 2 s. Participants were then asked to wear headphones. Once each auditory presentation of a list was completed, participants were asked, to repeat aloud the six words accurately and in the same order (order counts). As in Majerus and D'argembeau (2011), the lists were presented in a random order.

Results

In order to analyse the data, we first used a repeated measure ANOVA with the type of words as a within-participant variable and alexithymia group (High vs. Low) as a between-participant variable. In each condition, using a median-split approach, we created

Table 1. Descriptive data for the pure list condition (Study 1), mixed list condition (Study 2) and group comparison.

	Study 1 (pure list)		Study 2 (mixed list)			
Variables	Mean (SD)	Range	Mean (SD)	Range	*t*	*p*
Gender (ratio female/male)	75% female 33/11	–	66% female 29/15	–	1.18	.248
Age (year)	20.84 (2.31)	18–30	21.11 (2.20)	19–28	<1	ns
Alexithymia (total score) – TAS-20	45.34 (9.31)	24–68	47.80 (9.47)	32–68	1.23	.224
TAS-20 DIF	16.39 (3.91)	7–28	17.73 (4.49)	10–28	1.49	.139
TAS-20 DDF	12.55 (3.90)	5–23	13.77 (4.20)	6–23	1.42	.159
TAS-20 EOT	16.41 (4.34)	10–29	16.30 (4.10)	8–28	<1	ns
Negative affect (NA)	14.70 (5.32)	10–32	14.45 (5.14)	10–37	<1	ns
Positive affect (PA)	29.41 (6.71)	12–41	30.70 (5.75)	14–43	<1	ns

Note. TAS-20 DIF: factor difficulty identifying feelings; TAS-20 DDF: factor difficulty describing feelings; TAS-20 EOT: the factor externally oriented thinking.

the two alexithymia groups (High vs. Low). In a second step, in order to understand the relationship between alexithymia, its three subscales and short-term memory performance, we ran hierarchical regression and correlation analyses.

The analyses showed, as illustrated in Table 1, that the 44 participants of the mixed lists did not differ in age ($M = 21.11$ years; SE = 0.33), level of alexithymia ($M = 47.80$; SE = 1.43; Median TAS-20 total score = 46; range: 32–68; six participants ≥ 61 years old), negative affect ($M = 14.45$; SE = 0.78) or positive affect ($M = 30.70$; SE = 0.87) compared to the 44 participants of the pure lists condition (age ($M = 20.84$ years; SE = 0.35), level of alexithymia ($M = 45.34$; SE = 1.40; Median TAS-20 total score = 44; range: 24–68; 4 participants ≥ 61 years old), negative affect ($M = 14.70$; SE = 0.80) or positive affect ($M = 29.41$; SE = 1.01)).

Study 1: Pure lists. As in Majerus and D'argembeau (2011), we computed a score of item accuracy (items errors in a category: omissions, phonological, semantic or unrelated intrusions/total presented items in the same category). In the first analytical step, we ran a repeated-measures ANOVA in order to examine whether we were able to replicate the results of Majerus and D'argembeau (2011; Experiment 1). We, therefore, applied a median-split in order to create two groups of Low alexithymia scorers (LA) and High alexithymia scorers (HA). The median-spilt in the pure lists condition created groups of 20 Low alexithymia (LA) scorers (TAS-20 total score ≤ 43, Mean TAS-20 = 38.05; SE = 1.04) and 24 High alexithymia (HA) scorers (TAS-20 total score > 43, Mean TAS-20 = 51.42; SE = 1.57). In order to examine the combined influence of alexithymia levels and type of words, we ran a repeated measure ANOVA on the accuracy of immediate recall with a 2 (alexithymia level: low vs. high) × 3 (Type of words: Neutral vs. Positive vs. Negative) design, with the level of alexithymia as a between-subject factor. First of all, the results confirmed the main effect of type of words, $F(2, 41) = 21{,}59$, $p < .001$, $\eta^2 = .51$. Replicating Majerus and D'argembeau (2011), Positive words ($M = 0.82$, $SE = 0.01$) were better recalled than Negative ($M = 0.77$, $SE = 0.01$), $t(43) = 6.58$, $p < .001$ and Neutral words ($M = 0.78$, $SE = 0.01$), $t(43) = 4.20$, $p < .001$; and recall of the last two word categories did not differ from each other, $t(43) = 1.86$, $p > .05$. Importantly, as illustrated in Figure 1, we also found the main effect of alexithymia, $F(1, 42) = 6.09$, $p < .02$, $\eta^2 = .13$ showing that LA recalled words more accurately ($M = 0.82$, $SE = 0.02$) than HA ($M = 0.77$, $SE = 0.02$). The interaction between alexithymia and type of words was non-significant, $F(2, 41) < 1$.

In a second step, we ran a series of hierarchical regression analyses for short-term memory performance on positive words, negative words and neutral words separately. A hierarchical multiple regression analysis was conducted to explore the factors that predict better short-term memory performance (See Table 2). We first entered age and gender in a block of predictors. As both PA and NA were significantly correlated with alexithymia, we, therefore, included these variables as covariates in the regression model in a second block. Finally, the Alexithymia total score was introduced in a third block. The hierarchical multiple regressions revealed that at Stage 1, age and gender did not contribute significantly to the regression model, $F(2,41) < 1$, n.s. and accounted for 2.4% of the variation (R^2 change) in memory for positive words, 0.3% for negative words and 4.8% for neutral words. Introducing PA and NA in a second block did not explain an additional significant variation in memory performance, neither for positive words, negative words nor neutral words (R^2 change of, respectively, 3.2%, 0.9% and 1.2%), all $F(2, 39) < 1$, n.s. Finally, adding the Alexithymia total score in a

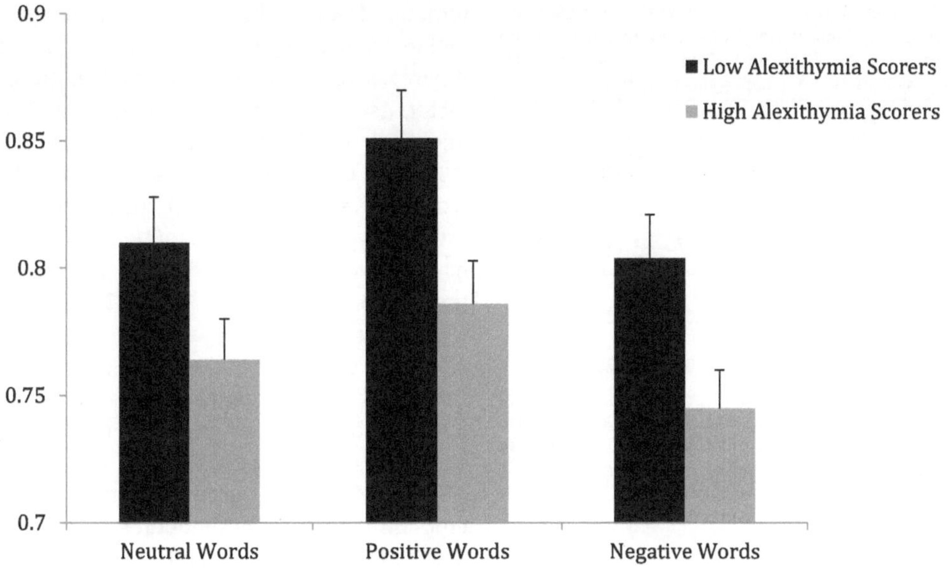

Figure 1. Mean (SE) proportions of words immediately recalled as a function of Alexithymia level (low vs. high) and the type of words (neutral vs. positive vs. negative) in Study 1 (pure lists).

third block to the regression model explained an additional 14.6% of the variation (R^2 change) in memory for positive words and this change in R^2 was significant, $F(1, 38) = 6.94$, $p = .01$. A similar effect appeared for negative words, in which the Alexithymia total score explained an additional 13.1% of the variation (R^2 change) in memory for negative words and this change in R^2 was significant, $F(1, 38) = 5.83$, $p = .02$. For neutral words, the variation in memory due to alexithymia did not reach significance (R^2 change = 7.9%). Collectively, the Alexithymia total score was a significant predictor of short-term memory for positive words ($\beta = -.415$, $p = .01$), negative words ($\beta = -.394$, $p = .02$) and only marginally predicted memory for neutral words ($\beta = -.306$, $p = .07$).

The second series of regressions were conducted, introducing each of the subscales separately in separate steps in the third block. Adding the factor difficulty identifying feelings (DIF) did not explain an additional part of the variance, neither for emotion nor for neutral words. None of the βs was significant (see Table 2). For difficulty describing feelings (DDF), a significant additional 11.3% of the variation (R^2 change) in memory for positive words was observed, $F(1, 38) = 5.16$, $p = .03$. For negative (7.9%) and neutral (7.1%) words, DDF did not significantly predict the variation (R^2 change) in memory. Regarding the factor externally oriented thinking (EOT), a significant additional percentage of the variation (R^2 change) in memory

Table 2. The third step of the hierarchical multiple regressions of the predictors of memory accuracy in the pure list condition (Study 1).

	Pure list (Study 1)			
	R^2 change Step 3[a]	β	t	p-value
Hierarchical regression Models 1b				
TAS-20 (step 3)				
Positive words	.15**	−.415	−2.635	.01**
Negative words	.13*	−.394	−2.414	.02*
Neutral words	.08	−.306	−1.871	.07
Hierarchical regression Models 2, 3 and 4c				
Model 2 – DIF (step 3)				
Positive words	.01	−.119	<1	.52
Negative words	.04	−.223	−1.215	.23
Neutral words	.01	−.119	<1	.52
Model 3 – DDF (step 3)				
Positive words	.11*	−.349	−2.273	.03*
Negative words	.08	−.293	−1.821	.08
Neutral words	.07	−.277	−1.763	.09
Model 4 – EOT (step 3)				
Positive words	.17**	−.440	−2.873	.007**
Negative words	.12*	−.370	−2.286	.03*
Neutral words	.07	−.282	−1.739	.09

Note. DIF: first factor of alexithymia "difficulty identifying feelings"; DDF: second factor of alexithymia "difficulty describing feelings"; EOT: third factor of alexithymia "externally oriented thinking."
[a]Explained additional variation (R^2 change) in memory following the inclusion of the predictors in the third step.
[b]In the first step, gender and age were entered. In the second step, positive and negative affect were entered. None of these predictors played a significant role in memory accuracy.
[c]In Models 2, 3, 4, Alexithymia total score was, respectively, replaced by DIF, DDF and EOT.
*$p \leq .05$; **$p \leq .01$.

Table 3. Partial correlations between short-term memory proportions in pure lists (Study 1) and mixed lists (Study 2) on the one hand and Alexithymia total score, DIF, DDF and EOT on the other hand, after controlling for positive (PA) and negative affectivity (NA).

	Type of words	TAS-20[a]	DIF	DDF	EOT
Pure lists (Study 1)	Neutral	−.305	−.107	−.290	−.294
	Positive	−.376*	−.087	−.336*	−.421**
	Negative	−.341*	−.178	−.267	−.341*
Mixed lists (Study 2)	Rare neutral	−.047	−.013	−.120	.030
	Rare positive	−.105	−.082	−.221	.076
	Rare Negative	−.045	.057	−.126	−.035

Note. DIF: first factor of alexithymia "difficulty identifying feelings"; DDF: second factor of alexithymia "difficulty describing feelings"; EOT: third factor of alexithymia "externally oriented thinking."
[a]Level of significance for the correlations involving TAS-20 and its subscales were determined by a two-tailed test.
*$p < .05$; **$p < .01$.

for positive (16.8%) and negative (12.0%) words was observed, respectively, $F(1, 38) = 8.25$, $p = .007$ for positive words and $F(1, 38) = 5.35$, $p = .03$ for negative words. For neutral words, the variation (R^2 change = 6.9%) due to EOT was not significant. The different βs are illustrated in Table 2.

In the pure lists condition, as illustrated in Table 3, correlation analyses supported this effect by showing that the Alexithymia total score as well as the factors difficulty describing feelings (DDF) and externally oriented thinking (EOT) were significantly and negatively correlated with recall accuracy for positive and negative words (*r*s range from −.270 to −.430). Correlations with neutral words were not significant and the factor DIF was not correlated with the immediate recall of any type of words. Importantly, correlations remained significant while controlling for current mood states (PANAS).

Study 2: Mixed lists. The median-spilt in the mixed lists condition created groups of 21 Low alexithymia (LA) scorers (TAS-20 total score ≤ 45; Mean TAS-20 = 39.95; SE = 0.79) and 23 High alexithymia (HA) scorers (TAS-20 total score > 45, Mean TAS-20 = 54.96; SE = 1.49). As in Majerus and D'argembeau (2011, Experiment 3), we first compared immediate recall performance for emotion-frequent (or Neutral rare) lists (i.e. two neutral words embedded within four negative or four positive) and emotion-rare lists (i.e. two negative or two positive words embedded within four neutral). We first ran a repeated-measures analysis of variance on the accuracy of immediate recall with the two-level factor of Type of lists (emotion-frequent lists vs. emotion-rare lists) as the within-subject variable, and alexithymia levels (Alexithymia level: Low vs. High) as a between-subject factor. As in Majerus and D'argembeau (2011, Experiment 3), we observed that emotion-rare lists ($M = 0.80$, $SE = 0.02$) containing a minority of emotion words were better recalled than emotion-frequent lists ($M = 0.79$, $SE = 0.02$), $F(1, 42) = 4.17$, $p < .02$, $\eta^2 = .09$. No effect of alexithymia group emerged in the mixed lists, $F(1, 42) < 1$, $p = .33$, $\eta^2 = .02$. Nor was there any interaction between alexithymia group and Type of list, $F(1, 42) < 1$, $p = .60$, $\eta^2 = .01$. Hence, because it was previously shown that this advantage for emotion-rare lists was due to the rare words embedded in frequent words, we ran a second ANOVA comparing recall performance of the two emotion words in the emotion-rare lists (embedded among four neutral words) to the two neutral words embedded in emotion-frequent lists (among four emotion-frequent words). So we ran a repeated measure analysis of variance on the accuracy of immediate recall with a 3 level between-subjects factor of Type of rare words (Rare Neutral vs. Rare Negative vs. Rare Positive) and alexithymia levels (Alexithymia level: Low vs. High) as a between-subject factor. We found, as in Majerus and D'argembeau (2011, Experiment 3), a highly significant effect of the Type of rare words, $F(2, 41) = 5.33$, $p < .01$, $\eta^2 = .21$, which supports the preferential attentional grabbing effect of emotion words. This effect showed that recall performance was worse for rare neutral words ($M = 0.79$, $SE = 0.02$) than for both rare positive words ($M = 0.82$, $SE = 0.02$) and rare negative words ($M = 0.82$, $SE = 0.02$), which did not differ from each other. However, as previously found, no effect of alexithymia group emerged in the mixed lists, $F(1, 42) < 1$, $p = .33$, $\eta^2 = .02$. Nor was there any interaction between alexithymia group and Type of list, $F(2, 41) < 1$, $p = .75$, $\eta^2 = .01$.

We also ran the same regression analyses in the mixed list condition as in the pure list condition. We first entered age and gender in a block of predictors. We included PA and NA in the regression model in a second block. Finally, the Alexithymia total score was introduced in a third block. We ran the regression on rare and frequent neutral and emotion words. The hierarchical multiple regressions revealed that none of the independent variables (predictors) contributed significantly to the regression for neutral and emotion words. All the *F*s were smaller than 1, n.s. and, regarding alexithymia, illustrated in Table 2 all the standardised βs were non-significant ($-0.101 < \beta s > -.051$, all $ps > .50$). Consistent with the lack of an alexithymia effect in the mixed list condition, illustrated in Table 3, no significant or even marginally significant correlations were observed in the mixed lists condition (all $p > .15$).

Discussion

In the present research, participants were involved in an short-term memory task in which they had to listen and recall lists of six words. In Study 1, the lists were composed of words belonging to the same valence (i.e. pure lists condition) and in Study 2 the lists were composed of neutral and emotional words (i.e. mixed lists condition).

The results of Study 1 first confirm that, in pure lists, emotion words, and more particularly positive ones, were better recalled than neutral words (Majerus & D'argembeau, 2011). For Majerus and D'argembeau (2011), in pure lists, the impact of emotional valence on STM performance was discussed as an effect of lexico-semantic long-term memory (LTM) organisation. In other words, when participants have to store and to immediately recall pure lists of words, the organisation of LTM determines STM effectiveness.

Importantly, as expected, we found the main effect of alexithymia which hampered recall performance in pure lists. This only partly confirmed our hypothesis since Alexithymia levels did not significantly interact with the type of words, but rather, there was a more general deficit for short-term recall of words in pure lists in HA. This reasonably suggests a more general deficit of LTM organisation and support in HA. Very few studies have found a general memory deficit in HA. To our knowledge, only one study has found a global deficit in long-term memory for neutral words in HA (Nielson & Meltzer, 2009). In that study, participants had to repeat aloud 30 neutral words and were instructed to intentionally remember the list. Following this encoding stage, they performed an immediate free recall task and a 24-h delayed memory test. Interestingly, the 30 HA participants recalled fewer neutral words than the 30 LA participants during the immediate free recall but no difference appeared 24-h later. The authors proposed that alexithymia might inhibit short-term, but not long-term retrieval (Nielson & Meltzer, 2009). Therefore, together with the present findings in the pure list condition, this suggests either poor encoding or an immediate retrieval deficit in HA.

This influence of HA memory accuracy for words was also confirmed by the hierarchical regressions and partial negative correlations. While the relationship between alexithymia and memory for neutral words was not significant, those involving positive and negative words reached significance. For Majerus and D'argembeau (2011), in pure lists, the STM advantage for emotion words is supposedly due to two main influences. First, emotional words form a specific semantic category that is richer compared to neutral words. Second, semantic representations for emotional words are more easily accessed than that of neutral words. Therefore, in HA, it seems that mental lexical representations are not organised in a similar manner as in LA, leading to (1) a global reduction of STM performance for words and (2) an unbalanced disadvantage for emotion words, particularly positive, words compared to neutral words. Different explanations may be suggested. First, the global deficit found in HA might relate to deficits in executive functions (See Vermeulen et al., 2018 for a review). As a matter of fact, alexithymia affects verbal fluency and impairs processing speed and abstraction (Vermeulen et al., 2018). Second, even if we need to be careful when drawing conclusions about neutral words because no interaction emerged from the analysis of variance, alexithymia seems to particularly influence memory for emotion words as observed in by the regression and correlational data. None of the regressions or correlations involving neutral words reached significance.

As already mentioned previously, regarding mental lexical representations, people scoring high on alexithymia might be unable to link their feelings with memories (Taylor et al., 1997). This proposal fits perfectly with Bucci's (1997) idea that high alexithymia scorers develops weak links between symbolic (e.g. words) and subsymbolic representations (e.g. somatic information) of their past affective experiences (see also Taylor & Bagby, 2004). Collectively, these later models as well as our findings are consistent with the recently proposed attention-appraisal model of alexithymia (Preece, Becerra, Allan, Robinson, & Dandy, 2017). In this emotion regulation model of alexithymia, Preece et al. (2017) suggest a four-stage Situation–Attention–Appraisal–Response valuation system, whereby a single stimulus, a more complex event, or even an emotional response is valuated (evaluated) regarding its personal significance. In this model, Preece et al. (2017) suggest that alexithymia can occur due to poorly organised or integrated emotion schemas, what they call ability deficit. However, for Preece et al. (2017) alexithymia may also represent an avoidant emotional regulation strategy. This avoidance deficit occurs at the emotional response stage of the valuation (of stimuli) system. Avoidance alexithymia can be observed when people avoid focusing their resources on the emotional response (attention stage of response valuation) or when people avoid integrating current input about a stimulation (appraisal stage) into their emotion schemas. In other words, ability deficits relate to the poorly integrated emotion schemas in high alexithymia scorers. This deficit mainly relates to DIF and DDF facets of alexithymia. With underdeveloped schemas, people are unable to process adequately the most important aspects of their emotional response but they can also barely differentiate or interpret the patterns of information about their emotional responses in order to create a specific evaluation (e.g. I feel sad) rather than a diffuse or general one (e.g. I am upset). Avoidance deficits are related to the emotion regulation strategy used in alexithymia. Avoidance deficit relates to avoidant emotion regulation strategy and relates to EOT in this model.

In the present study, ability deficits might be involved in the less accurate memory performances observed as alexithymia scores increase. Indeed, the poorly integrated emotion schemas in HA might have reduced the influence of the richness of emotion categories as suggested by Majerus and D'argembeau (2011). Majerus and D'argembeau (2011) suggest that emotion words are better memorised because emotion categories are richer than neutral ones. This explanation is coherent with the density hypothesis (Unkelbach, Fiedler, Bayer, Stegmüller, & Danner, 2008). The density hypothesis elucidates easier and faster processing of positive compared to negative information (Unkelbach et al., 2008). Concretely, they claim that there exists a greater similarity between different positive stimuli than between different negative stimuli. This greater similarity creates a greater density of positive information within a multidimensional space, like the circumplex model of affect (Russell, 1980). In this view, "joyful" and "lovely" are more similar than "sad" and "ugly," and accordingly, are jointly stored closer together. With underdeveloped schemas and their ability deficit, HA people are potentially less able to quickly access emotion categories and to differentiate the closely related items within these categories. This may explain why HA was more negatively associated with positive than negative words.

Interestingly, the factor DIF did not predict or correlate with memory for words. Only DDF for positive words and EOT for both positive and negative words negatively predicted memory performance. This result might be related to the different types of alexithymia the literature has identified. For instance, Ueno, Maeda, and Komaki (2014) found two different clusters of alexithymic profiles. The first one involves highly neurotic participants with high levels of DIF, and the second involves low openness and high levels of EOT. The fact that the present findings showed mainly a relation between EOT and memory for emotion words might relate to the proneness in high EOT participants to be less open to experience and to rather use suppression (or avoidance) as a regulation strategy (see Preece et al., 2017). Also, Preece et al. (2017) identified two sub-types of alexithymia depending on the processing stage that was involved. While DIF and DDF are mainly involved during the appraisal stage, EOT is mainly involved during the attention stage. As we used verbal material, the poorly differentiated schemas in high DDF participants may have hampered memory for emotion words. On the other hand, as high EOT suppress or avoid emotional material this could explain the negative relationship observed between memory for emotion words and EOT.

Conversely, in mixed lists, where emotional and neutral words are intermingled in the same sequence and in which there exists an emotional capture by negative and positive words, no effect of alexithymia was observed. This is in line with other research showing that relevant information might normally capture attentional resources and LTM memory of high alexithymia scorers (Meltzer & Nielson, 2010). However, it might be suggested that our results differ between groups due to the heterogeneity of the groups. Indeed, we did not control for general intelligence or education. However, we believe this is quite unlikely since all the participants were normal people, mostly undergraduate university students, who were randomly assigned to one of the two conditions. Moreover, age, gender and affect were controlled in the present studies.

To conclude, the present research is the first examining short-term memory performance for neutral and emotion words in alexithymia. We used two different validated experimental designs to investigate the impact of long-term memory organisation (pure lists,

Study 1) and attentional capture by emotion (mixed lists, Study 2). First, in the two studies, we replicated initial findings of an emotional advantage for emotion words, mainly positive ones, by Majerus and D'argembeau (2011). Second, we found that long-term memory organisation in HA affected short-term memory performance as shown by their global STM deficit in pure lists. To our knowledge, the present research is the first that shows evidence of impaired mental representation or organisation of neutral words in the STM of HA those. Future studies examining the semantic organisation of emotional and neutral material in an isolated fashion, as in pure lists, are very welcome.

Acknowledgements

The author wishes to thank Natalina Ventura for her idea and help in collecting the data andalso wishes to thank Giorgia Panayiotou and an anonymous reviewer for their helpful comments on a previous version of the manuscript.

Disclosure statement

No potential conflict of interest was reported by the author.

Data availability statement

The data that support the findings of this study are openly available in Zenodo at http://doi.org/10.5281/zenodo.1967085

Cite Data Set as: Nicolas Vermeulen (2019). Alexithymia disrupts verbal short-term memory [Data set]. Zenodo. http://doi.org/10.5281/zenodo.1967085

References

Bagby, R. M., Parker, J. D. A., & Taylor, G. J. (1994a). The twenty-item Toronto alexithymia scale—I. Item selection and cross-validation of the factor structure. *Journal of Psychosomatic Research*, *38*, 23–32.

Bagby, R. M., Taylor, G. J., & Parker, J. D. A. (1994b). The twenty-item Toronto alexithymia scale—II. Convergent, discriminant, and concurrent validity. *Journal of Psychosomatic Research*, *38*, 33–40.

Bayot, M., Pleyers, G., Kotsou, I., Lefèvre, N., Sauter, D. A., & Vermeulen, N. (2014). Joint effect of alexithymia and mood on the categorization of nonverbal emotional vocalizations. *Psychiatry Research*, *216*, 242–247.

Bucci, W. (1997). Symptoms and symbols: A multiple code theory of somatization. *Psychoanalytic Inquiry*, *17*(2), 151–172.

Cohen, J. (1988). *Statistical power analysis for the behavioral sciences* (2nd ed.). Hillsdale, NJ: Lawrence Earlbaum Associates.

Distefano, R. A., & Koven, N. S. (2012). Dysfunctional emotion processing may explain visual memory deficits in alexithymia. *Personality and Individual Differences*, *52*, 611–615.

Franz, M., Schaefer, R., Schneider, C., Sitte W., & Bachor, J. (2004). Visual event-related potentials in subjects with alexithymia: Modified processing of emotional aversive information? *American Journal of Psychiatry*, *161*, 728–735.

Gaudreau, P., Sanchez, X., & Blondin, J. P. (2006). Positive and negative affective states in a performance-related setting – Testing the factorial structure of the PANAS across two samples of French-Canadian participants. *European Journal of Psychological Assessment*, *22*, 240–249.

Loas, G., Parker, J. D. A., Otmani, O., Verrier, A., & Fremaux, D. (1997). Confirmatory factor analysis of the French translation of the 20-item Toronto Alexithymia Scale. *Perceptual and Motor Skills*, *85*, 1018–1018.

Majerus, S., & D'argembeau, A. (2011). Verbal short-term memory reflects the organization of long-term memory: Further evidence from short-term memory for emotional words. *Journal of Memory and Language*, *64*, 181–197.

Meltzer, M. A., & Nielson, K. A. (2010). Memory for emotionally provocative words in alexithymia: A role for stimulus relevance. *Consciousness and Cognition*, *19*, 1062–1068.

Meriau, K., Wartenburger, I., Kazzer, P., Prehn, K., Lammers, C.-H., van der Meer, E., … Heekeren, H. R. (2006). A neural network reflecting individual differences in cognitive processing of emotions during perceptual decision making. *Neuroimage*, *33*, 1016–1027.

Mueller, J., Alpers, G., & Reim, N. (2006). Dissociation of rated emotional valence and Stroop interference in observer-rated alexithymia. *Journal of Psychosomatic Research*, *61*, 261–269.

Nielson, K. A., & Meltzer, M. A. (2009). Modulation of long-term memory by arousal in alexithymia: The role of interpretation. *Consciousness and Cognition*, *18*(3), 786–793.

Preece, D., Becerra, R., Allan, A., Robinson, K., & Dandy, J. (2017). Establishing the theoretical components of alexithymia via factor analysis: Introduction and validation of the attention-appraisal model of alexithymia. *Personality and Individual Differences*, *119*, 341–352. doi:10.1016/j.paid.2017.08.003

Russell, J. A. (1980). A circumplex model of affect. *Journal of Personality and Social Psychology*, *39*, 1161–1178.

Swart, M., Kortekaas, R., & Aleman, A. (2009). Dealing with feelings: Characterization of trait alexithymia on emotion regulation strategies and cognitive-emotional processing. *Plos One*, *4*(6), e5751. doi: 10.1371/journal.pone.0005751.

Takahashi, J., Hirano, T., & Gyoba, J. (2015). Effects of facial expressions on visual short-term memory in relation to alexithymia traits. *Personality and Individual Differences*, *83*, 128–135.

Taylor, G. J., & Bagby, R. M. (2000). An overview of the alexithymia construct. In R. Bar-On & J. D. A. Parker (Eds.), *The handbook of emotional intelligence* (pp. 40–67). San Francisco, CA: Jossey-Bass.

Taylor, G. J., & Bagby, R. M. (2004). New is in alexithymia research. *Psychotherapy and Psychosomatics*, *73*, 68–77.

Taylor, G. J., Bagby, R. M., & Parker, J. D. A. (1997). *Disorders of affect regulation. Alexithymia in medical and psychiatric illness*. Cambridge: Cambridge University Press.

Ueno, M., Maeda, M., & Komaki, G. (2014). Different subgroups of high scorers on the TAS-20 based on the big five personality traits. *Personality and Individual Differences*, *68*, 71–76.

Unkelbach, C., Fiedler, K., Bayer, M., Stegmüller, M., & Danner, D. (2008). Why positive information is processed faster: The density hypothesis. *Journal of Personality and Social Psychology, 95*(1), 36–49. doi:10.1037/0022-3514.95.1.36

Vermeulen, N., Domachowska, I., & Nielson, K. A. (2018). Memory and executive functions in alexithymia. In O. Luminet, R. M. Bagby, & G. J. Taylor (Eds.), *Alexithymia: Advances in research, theory, and clinical practice* (pp. 78–89). Cambridge: Cambridge University Press.

Vermeulen, N., & Luminet, O. (2009). Alexithymia factors and memory performances for neutral and emotional words. *Personality and Individual Differences, 47*, 305–309.

Vermeulen, N., Luminet, O., & Corneille, O. (2006). Alexithymia and the automatic processing of affective information: Evidence from the affective priming paradigm. *Cognition & Emotion, 20*, 64–91.

Vermeulen, N., Luminet, O., De Sousa, M. C., Campanella, S. (2008). Categorical perception of anger is disrupted in alexithymia: Evidence from a visual ERP study. *Cognition & Emotion, 22*, 1052–1067.

Watson, D., Clark, L. A., & Tellegen, A. (1988). Development and validation of brief measures of positive and negative affect – The PANAS scales. *Journal of Personality and Social Psychology, 54*, 1063–1070.

Alexithymic traits predict the speed of classifying non-literal statements using nonverbal cues

Lorna S. Jakobson and Pauline M. Pearson

ABSTRACT

There is increasing interest in exploring the impact of alexithymia on interpersonal interactions. This study explored relationships between alexithymia and the complex mentalising skills needed to infer how a speaker intended a non-literal statement to be understood. A sample of university students ($N = 70$) viewed videotaped exchanges and attempted to classify remarks as literal, sarcastic, jocular, or white lies. Alexithymia was not associated with less consistent labelling of statement types. However, after accounting for variance due to verbal intelligence and sex, we found that those who reported more difficulties identifying their own feelings needed more time to distinguish between different statement types on the basis of the speaker's nonverbal cues. These findings highlight the value of examining response times, and of accounting for individual differences in specific alexithymic traits, when assessing social perception and cognition.

Alexithymia is a personality trait characterised by an externally focused, logical, thinking style; a limited ability to fantasise; and difficulties interpreting, describing, and regulating one's emotions (Nemiah, Freyberger, & Sifenos, 1976). Though opinions are mixed, some argue that individuals with alexithymia also have an impairment in theory of mind (ToM) – i.e. the ability to make inferences about other people's mental states (see Grynberg, Berthoz, & Bird, 2018). These impairments could impact socio-perceptual processes (e.g. decoding of nonverbal cues) and/or the cognitive operations (related to language and reasoning) that, according to the two-systems account of ToM (Apperly & Butterfill, 2009; Frith & Frith, 2008), underlie our ability to understand others' emotions (affective ToM) and engage in cognitive perspective taking (cognitive ToM).

Recent research suggests that individuals with alexithymia show atypical physiological responses to emotional body postures (Borhani, Borgomaneri, Làdavas, & Bertini, 2016). Alexithymia is also associated with impairments in the ability to detect, recognise, and label briefly-presented facial expressions (see Luminet & Zamariola, 2018), and to process prosodic cues and nonverbal vocalisations such as crying or laughter (see Welding & Samur, 2018). Difficulties experienced by those with alexithymia in processing these socio-perceptual cues have been linked to atypical activation of sensorimotor pathways (e.g. Ihme et al., 2014) and emotional embodiment (Scarpazza & di Pellegrino, 2018), which could interfere with the ability to simulate another's mental state (Ondobaka, Kilner, & Friston, 2017).

Despite this evidence that the socio-perceptual route to ToM may be compromised in those with alexithymia, studies utilising a range of behavioural measures of ToM skills have generally not supported a link. Thus, individuals with alexithymia have not been found to show impaired ability to attribute mental states to geometric shapes that move in particular ways, or to fictional characters (e.g. Milosavljevic et al., 2016). Of greater relevance to the current study is research investigating the complex perceptual and cognitive processes that underlie our ability to detect whether a speaker intends a statement to be taken literally. Several groups have argued that alexithymia does not disrupt this ability (Gramaglia et al., 2016) unless the statements in question can best be understood by making appropriate inferences about the speaker's affective state (Oakley, Brewer, Bird, & Catmur, 2016). However, it is important to note that this work has relied exclusively on accuracy measures. It may be that other variables, such as response time (RT), would be more sensitive to such problems. Indeed, Olkoniemi, Strömberg, and Kaakinen (2019) have recently reported that those scoring high (vs. low) in alexithymia are slower, but not less accurate, in categorising written sarcastic statements. This suggests that they find it difficult to identify local inconsistencies in the written message and resolve its intended meaning. It is not known whether they are also slower at processing spoken sarcasm, but here inconsistencies can occur not only between the words spoken, but also between verbal and nonverbal cues.

The current study

We studied individuals' ability to recognise when – and in what way – a speaker was being insincere. We began by acknowledging (a) that under normal circumstances, both cognitive and affective ToM skills support these abilities (e.g. Shamay-Tsoory & Aharon-Peretz, 2007); and (b) that the acquisition and deployment of these mentalising skills depends, in part, on an individual's ability to process and integrate a range of contextual, language-based, and nonverbal cues both quickly and accurately.

In completing our task, participants viewed videos depicting speakers making sincere or insincere statements and had to judge if each statement was meant to be taken literally, was said in jest or sarcastically, or was a white lie. In half of the videos, participants could support their inferences using a combination of nonverbal cues (from face, body, and voice) and verbal information regarding the speaker's true opinions (*context*), whereas in the remaining videos only nonverbal cues were available (*no context*). We expected that it would be harder, overall, for participants to distinguish between different statement types when they were forced to rely solely on transient nonverbal cues. In addition, however, we expected that those reporting stronger alexithymic traits would need more time to make their judgments, especially in the more difficult *no context* condition.

We used hierarchical regression to examine which characteristics predicted how quickly and accurately our participants could perform the task. We first assessed how well Verbal IQ and participant sex predicted task performance. The former variable was important as the task requires verbal processing; the latter variable was of interest as past research suggests that males and females differ in how they evaluate nonliteral statements (e.g. Rothermich & Pell, 2015). Next, we assessed whether adding measures of specific alexithymic traits *improved* prediction of accuracy and/or RTs. We focused here on the traits of externally oriented thinking (EOT), difficulty identifying feelings (DIF), and difficulty describing feelings (DDF). Demers and Koven (2015) note that there are large individual differences in how strongly these aspects of alexithymia are expressed. As DIF and DDF are strongly associated with emotional knowledge deficits (see Luminet & Zamariola, 2018), and higher DDF scores predict slower identification of some facial expressions (Ihme et al., 2014), we predicted that DIF and DDF would be better predictors of performance on our experimental task than EOT, after accounting for variance due to verbal IQ and participant sex.

Materials and methods

Participants

Participation was limited to individuals with Verbal IQs ≥ 80 to rule out the possibility that poor performance in some cases might reflect a general cognitive delay or difficulties in understanding task instructions. The final sample included 34 males ($M_{age} = 20.6$ years, $SD = 4.0$) and 36 females ($M_{age} = 20.5$ years, $SD = 5.3$) recruited from an introductory psychology course. All were native English speakers with no reported history of developmental or language-related deficits. All gave informed consent and were compensated by earning credit toward a course requirement.

Materials and procedure

General procedure

Participants completed select subtests of the Wechsler Abbreviated Scale of Intelligence, Second Edition (WASI-II; Wechsler, 2011), the experimental task, and the 20-item Toronto Alexithymia Scale (TAS-20). The University of Manitoba Psychology/Sociology Research Ethics Board approved the testing protocol, which was carried out in compliance with relevant guidelines and regulations.

Verbal IQ

Verbal IQ was estimated using the Verbal Composite score from the WASI-II. This composite is computed using the Vocabulary and Similarities subtests, which were administered and scored according to standard procedures. Verbal IQ was expressed as a standard score ($M = 100$, $SD = 15$), determined using published norms.

Toronto Alexithymia Scale (TAS-20)

The TAS-20 (Parker, Taylor, & Bagby, 2003) is a 20 item self-report measure with three subscales measuring DIF, DDF, and EOT. For each item, participants respond using a 5-point Likert scale ranging from *Strongly disagree* to *Strongly agree*. The TAS-20 is a valid and reliable measure of alexithymia (Parker et al., 2003).

Experimental task

The 40 experimental videos used in the experimental task comprise part of the RISC database (Rothermich & Pell, 2015). Each video depicted an interaction between two people: one (the *questioner*) poses a question, and the other (the *target*) answers. The interactions were relatively neutral in valence and low in intensity. The target's literal responses were phrased either positively (e.g. compliments) or negatively (e.g. criticisms). Non-literal statements included white lies and sarcastic responses meant to be interpreted either negatively (sarcasm) or in a positive light (jocular statements). (See Rothermich & Pell for sample scripts.) In half of the videos of each type the interaction was preceded by a short segment in which the target informs a third party of his/her true opinion on a particular topic before the questioner arrives. When watching these vignettes, participants can use this information to decide whether a non-literal interpretation of the target's response to the question is warranted. The other half of the vignettes do not include this verbal contextual information. Because the actual words used in the target responses on a given topic are closely matched across conditions, participants in the no context condition have to rely on nonverbal cues to make judgments.

The task was programmed in e-Prime. Stimuli were presented on a computer monitor, at a viewing distance of approximately 57 cm. The displays were 23 cm high but varied in width. In the original videos the questioner was sometimes off-screen. To standardise the displays, we cropped the videos in which s/he was present, to ensure that only the target was visible. Although this eliminated some proxemic cues, it also maximised the chance that participants would focus their attention on the target during the crucial exchange, as they might when engaged in a 1:1 conversation. Each video lasted approximately 20 seconds.

Participants viewed two practice videos, and then completed two counterbalanced blocks of 20 trials. Each block included four examples of each type of statement (i.e. literal positive, literal negative, jocular, sarcastic, and white lie) – two with and two without verbal context. After viewing each video, participants indicated (via key press) which of five labels most accurately described the type of statement the speaker had made, and RT was recorded. Trial order was pseudo-randomised to ensure that no more than two trials of the same type appeared consecutively. After the final trial, participants responded to the following open-ended question: *Which cues did the actors shown use to signal their intentions (i.e. vocal tone, facial expressions etc.)?*

Results

Verbal IQ and alexithymia measures

Verbal IQ scores had a mean of 101.5 (*SD* 8.7) and ranged from 84 to 123. Mean scores on the TAS-20 were as follows: $M_{\text{Total}} = 47.2$ (*SD* 10.2); $M_{\text{DDF}} = 13.2$ (*SD* 4.4); $M_{\text{DIF}} = 14.9$ (*SD* 5.0); and $M_{\text{EOT}} = 19.1$ (*SD* 4.9). Verbal IQ was negatively correlated with TAS-20 Total scores [$r(70) = -.29$, $p = .014$] and with EOT scores [$r(70) = -.28$, $p = .018$], with medium effect size.

Labelling statement type

Participants' responses to the open-ended question confirmed that they were sensitive to a range of nonverbal cues. Use of facial cues and eye behaviour was reported most frequently (43%), followed by use of vocal cues (e.g. changes in pitch, laughter; 39%), gestures and body movements (16%), and other/ambiguous cues (e.g. "overreactions"; 2%). These cues were not, however, always interpreted in the same way (see Table 1). Participants performed quite well when verbal context was available (see hits, along the diagonal in the upper matrix). Here, the most frequent error involved failing to detect the positive, humorous intent of jocular statements and labelling them as sarcastic. Accuracy was lower and mislabelling errors were more varied when participants had to rely solely on nonverbal cues to make their judgments (see lower matrix). Median RTs were also slower in the no context condition [$F(1,69) = 42.81$, p

Table 1. Percentage of time each label was applied to each type of statement.

			Statement type			
			Literal	Sarcastic	Jocular	White lie
Label applied	Context	Literal	93.4	0.4	4.6	7.9
		Sarcastic	1.6	91.1	20.7	1.8
		Jocular	0.4	3.2	70.7	0.7
		White lie	4.6	5.4	3.9	89.6
	No context	Literal	75.0	2.1	9.6	9.6
		Sarcastic	5.9	77.5	35.4	14.3
		Jocular	14.5	1.8	54.6	3.2
		White lie	4.6	18.6	0.4	72.9

Note: Responses to positive and negative literal items were pooled.

$<.001$, $\eta_p^2 = .383$; *Mdn* $RT_{context} = 2521$ ms, 95% CI [2273, 2768] vs. *Mdn* $RT_{no\ context} = 3388$ ms, 95% CI [2972, 3804]] suggesting that participants found statements made in this condition more difficult to interpret, as expected.

To account for both hits and labelling errors in subsequent analyses, we computed unbiased recognition (H_u) scores (after Wagner, 1993). These scores account for response bias and are insensitive to imbalances in the number of stimuli included in different classes. Scores can take values between 0 (indicating that a particular label was never applied) to +1 (indicating that a stimulus of a given type was always correctly labelled and that the category label was never misapplied). For each condition, we computed an overall H_u score and separate mean scores for the literal and non-literal items.

Relationships between alexithymia and the ability to identify statement type

We conducted separate hierarchical regressions predicting mean H_u scores and median RTs in each condition. We focused on performance with non-literal statements because (a) these were of greater theoretical interest; and (b) the mean H_u score for non-literal statements was almost perfectly correlated with the overall H_u score, in both conditions [$r(70) \geq .97$, large effect size]. In each analysis, verbal IQ and sex were entered at Step 1, and the three TAS-20 subscale scores at Step 2. Before proceeding we confirmed that variance inflation factor (VIF) scores were well below 10 (all ≤ 1.26, $M = 1.20$) and that tolerance levels were above .20 (all $\geq .79$), indicating that multicollinearity was not an issue (Field, 2013). The results appear in Table 2. We had a large enough sample to detect a medium effect ($f^2 = .17$) related to the addition of the TAS measures at Step 2 with power of .80.

Verbal IQ accounted for significant variance in H_u accuracy when verbal context was available [Model 1, $F(2,67) = 3.94$, $p = .024$. $f^2 = 0.17$]. This was also the case in the no context condition but adding DDF scores at Step 2 significantly improved prediction in this case [Model 2, $F(5,64) = 2.88$, $p = .021$, $f^2 = 0.22$]. Unexpectedly, participants who reported *more* difficulty describing their own feelings performed more accurately in this condition.

The main question addressed in the present report was whether alexithymic traits might influence how quickly participants could evaluate non-literal statements. When verbal context was available, median RTs were not predicted by any of the study variables. In the no context condition, however, median RTs were positively associated with DIF scores, after accounting for variance related to verbal IQ and sex [Model 2, $F(5,64) = 3.33$, $p = .010$, $f^2 = 0.26$]. This suggests that, although people exhibiting problems with emotional introspection may succeed (or even *excel*) at interpreting non-literal speech in some circumstances, they need additional time to decode the speaker's intention on the basis of nonverbal cues.

When TAS-20 Total scores were substituted for subscale scores in these regressions they accounted for unique variance in accuracy, but not RT (data not shown). This is important to note, as it suggests that the use of this composite measure may obscure important relationships between specific aspects of alexithymia and ToM.

Discussion

Consistent with earlier reports (e.g. Gramaglia et al., 2016), we found that alexithymia was not associated with *impaired* accuracy in discerning a speaker's intentions. Indeed, after accounting for variance due to Verbal IQ and sex, we found that higher DDF scores predicted greater accuracy in the no context

Table 2. Linear models of significant predictors of task performance for non-literal statements by condition.

Dependent variable	Condition			*b*	*SE B*	*β*	*p*
H_u accuracy	Context[a]	Step 1	(Constant)	0.05	0.25		0.854
			VIQ	**0.01**	**0.00**	**0.34**	**0.007**
			Sex	−0.02	0.04	−0.05	0.656
		Step 2	(Constant)	−0.17	0.31		0.578
			VIQ	**0.01**	**0.00**	**0.36**	**0.005**
			Sex	0.00	0.05	−0.01	0.929
			DIF	0.00	0.00	0.13	0.297
			DDF	0.00	0.01	0.12	0.366
			EOT	0.00	0.00	0.00	0.975
H_u accuracy	No context[b]	Step 1	(Constant)	0.04	0.26		0.877
			VIQ	0.01	0.00	0.24	0.062
			Sex	−0.06	0.05	−0.15	0.215
		Step 2	(Constant)	−0.37	0.32		0.247
			VIQ	**0.01**	**0.00**	**0.29**	**0.021**
			Sex	−0.03	0.05	−0.09	0.454
			DIF	0.00	0.00	0.08	0.509
			DDF	**0.01**	**0.01**	**0.32**	**0.014**
			EOT	0.00	0.00	0.02	0.863
Median RT	No context[c]	Step 1	(Constant)	4380.95	2676.21		0.106
			VIQ	−25.70	27.39	−0.12	0.351
			Sex	**1060.45**	**473.43**	**0.28**	**0.028**
		Step 2	(Constant)	2383.32	3171.88		0.455
			VIQ	−23.45	27.24	−0.11	0.393
			Sex	**1334.98**	**462.29**	**0.35**	**0.005**
			DIF	**151.96**	**47.50**	**0.39**	**0.002**
			DDF	−20.19	54.79	−0.05	0.714
			EOT	−33.26	47.59	−0.08	0.487

Note: VIQ = verbal IQ. Toronto Alexithymia Scale: Difficulty Identifying Feelings (DIF), Difficulty Describing Feelings (DFF) and Externally Orienting Thinking (EOT) subscales.
[a] $R^2 = .105$ for Step 1; $\Delta R^2 = .040$ for Step 2.
[b] $R^2 = .058$ for Step 1; $\Delta R^2 = .125$ for Step 2.
[c] $R^2 = .071$ for Step 1; $\Delta R^2 = .135$ for Step 2.

condition. One possible explanation for this result relates to the finding that, in non-clinical (student) samples, both DDF and DIF scores are positively related to two aspects of sensory processing sensitivity: ease of excitation and having lower sensory thresholds (Liss, Mailloux, & Erchull, 2008). Those who scored high on DDF may have found the complexity of dynamic displays engaging; if so, any extra effort they may have expended in processing them may have enhanced their performance. Of course, had more "emotionally charged" interactions been shown, these individuals might have been more easily overwhelmed by them than their peers, resulting in less accurate task performance.

Importantly, we found that individuals scoring high on the DIF scale needed *more time* to make judgments in the no context condition. It will be important to try to replicate this effect in future research, and determine the cause(s) of this sluggish responding. We suspect that it relates to difficulties with processing of nonverbal cues, although problems integrating inferences arising from socio-perceptual processing with those arising from cognitive operations related to language and reasoning may also have played a role. Pexman (2008) argues that this type of integration is essential for understanding sarcasm. Clearly, not being able to perform these processes rapidly could negatively impact on the success of everyday social interactions.

Overall, our findings emphasise the importance of examining the relationship between task performance and specific aspects of alexithymia, reflected in subscale scores. It may be that one's particular "alexithymia profile" plays a key role in determining the extent to which one experiences difficulties on a given task (e.g. Goerlich-Dobre, Votinov, Habel, Pripfl, & Lamm, 2015). Subtyping research has been hampered by the fact that several popular alexithymia assessment instruments do not adequately sample deficits in emotional reactivity and fantasising. Assessing difficulties in these areas may allow one to account for variance in mentalising abilities, above and beyond that attributed to difficulties in identifying feelings. In short, focusing on specific dimensions or subtypes of alexithymia is likely to advance our understanding of how it relates to ToM, and to social functioning more generally. This basic research may have important clinical implications, given the high prevalence of alexithymia in a variety of clinical conditions (Taylor, Bagby, & Parker, 1997).

Despite its strengths, the present study had some limitations. First, alexithymia was measured through self-report, but pragmatic language skill was evaluated through a performance-based measure. This might have weakened observed relationships. Future work might incorporate an observation scale and/or objective, performance-based measures to assess alexithymic traits. Second, although our displays had good ecological validity, their complexity made it impossible to determine how accurately specific cues were processed. Finally, because our focus was on on-line processing, we did not explore how alexithymia might impact the extent to which social inferences are modulated by past experience. Investigating both bottom-up and top-down processes should be an important objective of future research, in addition to determining how expressive (rather than receptive) nonverbal skills may contribute to the interpersonal difficulties that reportedly affect those with alexithymia.

As a final note, it is important to highlight the fact that although Verbal IQ was negatively correlated with alexithymia (see also Grynberg et al. 2012), it also accounted for unique variance in how accurately non-literal statements were categorised. Indeed, Verbal IQ was the only significant predictor of accuracy in the context condition. Here, information about the target's true opinion can be processed before the target's response is even uttered, assuming one has good language comprehension skills. As comprehension of neutral words appears to be preserved in alexithymia (see Welding & Samur, 2018), they may have relied on verbal reasoning to detect the mismatch with what was said later. Participant sex also accounted for unique variance in how quickly judgments were made in the no context condition. Given these results, we urge researchers interested in exploring relationships between alexithymia and pragmatic language skills to consider the impact of verbal ability and sex in their studies.

Conclusions

Making inferences about a speaker's intentions is complex and requires both affective and cognitive ToM. We have shown that individuals who report difficulties identifying their own feelings need more time to make these judgments. These findings add to the literature demonstrating the importance of accounting for natural variation in specific alexithymic traits when conducting research exploring social perception and cognition. The results highlight the importance of employing tasks that are adequately challenging and cannot be solved using verbal reasoning alone, examining relationships between performance and specific dimensions or subtypes of alexithymia, accounting for variance related to verbal ability and sex, and incorporating RT measures in studies of this kind.

Acknowledgements

The research was supported by the Natural Sciences and Engineering Research Council of Canada under grant 138829–13 (to LSJ). We would like to thank Dr. Marc Pell (Neuropragmatics and Emotion Lab, McGill University) for providing the stimuli for the experimental task used in this study, and acknowledge the contributions of Zofia Kozub, Colleen Hare, and Sarah Rigby.

Disclosure statement

No potential conflict of interest was reported by the authors.

Funding

The research was supported by the Natural Sciences and Engineering Research Council of Canada under grant 138829-13 (to LSJ).

Data availability statement

Data associated with this paper are available at https://doi.org/10.5203/FK2/1CE8UZ.

ORCID

Lorna S. Jakobson http://orcid.org/0000-0002-0849-5090
Pauline M. Pearson http://orcid.org/0000-0002-9491-8976

References

Apperly, I. A., & Butterfill, S. A. (2009). Do humans have two systems to track beliefs and belief-like states? *Psychological Review, 116*, 953–970. doi:10.1037/a0016923

Borhani, K., Borgomaneri, S., Làdavas, E., & Bertini, C. (2016). The effect of alexithymia on early visual processing of emotional body postures. *Biological Psychology, 115*, 1–8.

Demers, L. A., & Koven, N. S. (2015). The relation of alexithymic traits to affective theory of mind. *The American Journal of Psychology, 128*, 31–42.

Field, A. (2013). *Discovering statistics using IBM SPSS Statistics* (4th ed.). Los Angeles: Sage.

Frith, C. D., & Frith, U. (2008). Implicit and explicit processes in social cognition. *Neuron, 60*, 503–510. doi:10.1016/j.neuron.2008.10.032

Goerlich-Dobre, K. S., Votinov, M., Habel, U., Pripfl, J., & Lamm, C. (2015). Neuroanatomical profiles of alexithymia dimensions and subtypes. *Human Brain Mapping, 36*, 3805–3818.

Gramaglia, C., Ressico, F., Gambaro, E., Palazzolo, A., Mazzarino, M., Bert, F., … Zeppegno, P. (2016). Alexithymia, empathy, emotion identification and social inference in anorexia nervosa: A case-control study. *Eating Behaviors, 22*, 46–50.

Grynberg, D., Berthoz, S., & Bird, G. (2018). Social and interpersonal implications of alexithymia. In O. Luminet, R. M. Bagby, & G. J. Taylor (Eds.), *Alexithymia: Advances in research, theory, and clinical practice* (pp. 174–189). New York, NY: Cambridge University Press.

Grynberg, D., Chang, B., Corneille, O., Maurage, P., Vermeulen, N., Berthoz, S., & Luminet, O. (2012). Alexithymia and the processing of emotional facial expressions (EFEs): Systematic review, unanswered questions and further perspectives. *PLoS One, 7* (8), e42429.

Ihme, K., Sacher, J., Lichev, V., Rosenberg, N., Kugel, H., Rufer, M., … Suslow, T. (2014). Alexithymia and the labeling of facial emotions: Response slowing and increased motor and somatosensory processing. *BMC Neuroscience, 15*, 40.

Liss, M., Mailloux, J., & Erchull, M. J. (2008). The relationships between sensory processing sensitivity, alexithymia, autism, depression, and anxiety. *Personality and Individual Differences, 45*, 255–259.

Luminet, O., & Zamariola, G. (2018). Emotion knowledge and emotion regulation in alexithymia. In O. Luminet, R. M. Bagby, & G. J. Taylor (Eds.), *Alexithymia: Advances in research, theory, and clinical practice* (pp. 49–77). New York, NY: Cambridge University Press.

Milosavljevic, B., Carter Leno, V., Simonoff, E., Baird, G., Pickles, A., Jones, C. R., … Happé, F. (2016). Alexithymia in adolescents with autism spectrum disorder: Its relationship to internalising difficulties, sensory modulation and social cognition. *Journal of Autism and Developmental Disorders, 46*(4), 1354–1367.

Nemiah, J. C., Freyberger, H., & Sifenos, P. E. (1976). Alexithymia: A view of the psychosomatic process. In O. W. Hill (Ed.), *Modern trends in psychosomatic medicine, Vol. 3* (pp. 430–439). London: Butterworths.

Oakley, B. F., Brewer, R., Bird, G., & Catmur, C. (2016). Theory of mind is not theory of emotion: A cautionary note on the reading the mind in the eyes test. *Journal of Abnormal Psychology, 125*(6), 818–823.

Olkoniemi, H., Strömberg, V., & Kaakinen, J. K. (2019). The ability to recognise emotions predicts the time-course of sarcasm processing: Evidence from eye movements. *Quarterly Journal of Experimental Psychology, 72*(5), 1212–1223.

Ondobaka, S., Kilner, J., & Friston, K. (2017). The role of interoceptive inference in theory of mind. *Brain and Cognition, 112*, 64–68.

Parker, J. D. A., Taylor, G. J., & Bagby, R. M. (2003). The 20-item Toronto Alexithymia Scale–III: Reliability and factorial validity in a community population. *Journal of Psychosomatic Research, 55*, 269–275.

Pexman, P. M. (2008). It's fascinating research: The cognition of verbal irony. *Current Directions in Psychological Science, 17*, 286–290.

Rothermich, K., & Pell, M. D. (2015). Introducing RISC: A new video inventory for testing social perception. *PLoS ONE, 10* (7), 1–24.

Scarpazza, C., & di Pellegrino, G. (2018). Alexithymia, embodiment of emotions and interoceptive abilities. In R. J. Teixeira, B. Bermond, & P. P. Moormann (Eds.), *Current developments in alexithymia – A cognitive and affective deficit* (pp. 35–51). Hauppauge, NY: Nova Science Publishers.

Shamay-Tsoory, S. G., & Aharon-Peretz, J. (2007). Dissociable prefrontal networks for cognitive and affective theory of mind: A lesion study. *Neuropsychologia, 45*, 3054–3067. doi:10.1016/j.neuropsychologia.2007.05.021

Taylor, G. J., Bagby, R. M., & Parker, J. D. A. (1997). *Disorders of affect regulation: Alexithymia in medical and psychiatric illness*. Cambridge: Cambridge University Press.

Wagner, H. L. (1993). On measuring performance in category judgment studies of nonverbal behavior. *Journal of Nonverbal Behavior, 17*(1), 3–28.

Wechsler, D. (2011). *Wechsler abbreviated scale of intelligence* (2nd ed.). San Antonio, TX: Psychological Corporation.

Welding, C., & Samur, D. (2018). Language processing in alexithymia. In O. Luminet, R. M. Bagby, & G. J. Taylor (Eds.), *Alexithymia: Advances in research, theory, and clinical practice* (pp. 90–103). New York, NY: Cambridge University Press.

OPEN ACCESS

Getting lost in a story: how narrative engagement emerges from narrative perspective and individual differences in alexithymia

Dalya Samur, Mattie Tops, Ringailė Slapšinskaitė and Sander L. Koole

ABSTRACT
The present research examines how narrative engagement, or the extent to which people immerse themselves into the world of a story, varies as a function of narrative perspective and individual differences in alexithymia. The authors hypothesised that narrative engagement would be higher when people assume a first-person (rather than third-person) perspective and for people lower (rather than higher) on alexithymia. In an online study ($N = 541$) and a lab study ($N = 55$), participants with varying levels of alexithymia read first- and/or third-person narrated texts and then rated their narrative engagement. As expected, first-person stories evoked more narrative engagement than third-person stories, and global alexithymia was negatively correlated with narrative engagement. Narrative perspective did not interact with cognitive facets of alexithymia (i.e. difficulties identifying, verbalising, and understanding feelings). However, narrative perspective did interact with affective facets of alexithymia (i.e. emotionalising and fantasising): First-person (rather than third-person) stories elicited more narrative engagement at lower levels of affective alexithymia, but not at higher levels of affective alexithymia. The interaction effect was significant in Study 1; the interaction was significant in Study 2 after controlling for trait absorption. Together, these findings suggest that alexithymia is linked to difficulties in mentally simulating narrative worlds.

When people are reading a story, they vary in the degree to which they become mentally engrossed by the world that is described in the narrative. Such differences in narrative engagement relate to people's unique ability to transcend the here and now and project themselves into distant times and places (Macrae, Christian, & Miles, 2014). By leading people to construct mental models of a fictional social world, narrative engagement contributes to the development of social-emotional skills, such as empathy and social inference (Mar & Oatley, 2008), which are vital in social life. Furthermore, narrative engagement increases reading enjoyment (Busselle & Bilandzic, 2009), thereby contributing to the development of literacy skills and their associated cognitive competencies (Mol & Bus, 2011). It is therefore important to learn more about the psychological processes that underlie narrative engagement.

In the present article, we examine how narrative engagement emerges from the interplay between the linguistic properties of a narrative and individual dispositions of the person who is processing the narrative. Narratives display varying linguistic properties, and some of these properties are likely to evoke more engagement than others. One important linguistic property is whether a story is told from a first-person or a third-person perspective (Borghi, Glenberg, & Kaschak, 2004). In addition, some people may be more prone to get mentally immersed into narratives than others. Here, we address the potential role of individual differences in alexithymia, which relate to difficulties in social-emotional processing (Grynberg et al., 2012). In the following paragraphs, we begin by discussing how narrative perspective may influence narrative engagement. Next, we turn to alexithymia, and consider whether and how it may shape narrative engagement along with narrative perspective. Finally, we present two studies that were designed to test our theoretical analysis.

Narrative engagement and perspective taking

Narrative engagement may be defined as a phenomenon in which readers are mentally simulating the world of a story and become psychologically absorbed in that world (Green & Brock, 2000). The theoretical notion of engagement into a narrative was originally conceived by Gerrig (1993) to understand how people are psychologically impacted by stories (Green & Brock, 2002; van Laer, De Ruyter, Visconti, & Wetzels, 2014). Using travel as a metaphor for reading, Gerrig conceptualised narrative transportation as a state of detachment from the world of origin that the reader (symbolically, the "traveller") experiences by being carried away by the story. Other researchers have further developed this theory and extended it to other contexts, for instance, to understand how people may become persuaded by a story (Green & Brock, 2002), why children become interested in reading outside of school (Jensen, Bernat, Wilson, & Goonewardene, 2011), and how reading fiction may evoke empathy (Bal & Veltkamp, 2013).

To achieve a state of narrative engagement, the reader has to become mentally attuned to the intentions and subjective experiences of the narrator and/or character (Busselle & Bilandzic, 2009). This attunement is likely to be facilitated when the narrative takes the viewpoint of the main character in the narrative. One important linguistic tool for such character and narrator conflation is using the pronoun "I" for the spectator in a first-person perspective, rather than using the pronouns "he or she" as in a third-person perspective. First-person stories symbolically put the reader in the narrators' shoes, which increases the likelihood that readers become psychologically invested in the story (Oatley, 1999; Stanzel, 1984). Hence, adopting a first-person perspective can be expected to generally evoke more narrative engagement than adopting a third-person perspective.

Consistent with the aforementioned notion, research has shown that leading people to take a first-person (rather than third-person) perspective enhances cognitive and emotional identification with narrative events (Gerrig, 1993; Green & Brock, 2000; Macrae et al., 2014). For example, Papeo and colleagues (2011) measured their participants' brain activation in motor areas, while they were reading action verbs and non-action verbs in first-person and third-person perspectives. The results showed that reading action verbs in a first-person perspective, rather than a third-person perspective, led to increased activation in motor areas of the brain. Another study examined the effects of narrative perspective in an emotionally relevant context (Christian, Parkinson, Macrae, Miles, & Wheatley, 2015). Specifically, participants read painful scenarios that were written in either a first-person or third-person perspective. Scenarios in the first-person perspective, compared to scenarios in the third-person perspective, elicited greater activity in the brain areas related to emotional awareness, visual imagery, and body ownership.

The aforementioned studies suggest that a first-person perspective, at least on an implicit level, leads readers to engage in more mental simulation of a story than a third-person narrative perspective. Given that narrative engagement is presumably based on such mental simulations, it follows that readers may experience higher levels of engagement for stories that are told from a first-person perspective rather than a third-person perspective. As far as we know, this notion has been empirically tested in only one study to date. In this study, participants were asked to read literary stories that were written from either a first or a third person perspective (Hartung, Burke, Hagoort, & Willems, 2016). The findings showed that participants reported higher narrative engagement during stories that were written in a first-person perspective than for stories written in a third-person perspective. Thus, there are both theoretical and empirical reasons to believe that first-person stories evoke more narrative engagement than third-person stories.

Alexithymia and narrative processing

Besides the linguistic properties of a narrative, narrative engagement may also be influenced by individual differences in narrative processing. One relevant individual difference here is alexithymia. Alexithymia, literally "no words for feelings", is a personality dimension that was introduced by Sifneos (1973) to characterise a sub-group of psychiatric patients who displayed marked difficulties in expressing their feelings, a formal manner of speaking, and restricted imagination. People vary in their levels of alexithymia, and these variations can be assessed with well-validated self-report questionnaires such as the Toronto Alexithymia Scale (Bagby, Taylor, & Parker, 1994) and the Bermond-Vorst Alexithymia Questionnaire (Vorst & Bermond, 2001). The latter scale distinguishes between cognitive and affective facets of alexithymia. The cognitive facet of alexithymia relates to difficulties in identifying, analysing, and verbalising of emotions. The affective facet of alexithymia relates to differences in emotional arousability ("emotionalising"), and differences in imagination ("fantasising"). The combined scores on the cognitive and affective scales index a person's overall level of alexithymia.

The relation between alexithymia and language processing has been understudied (Hobson, Brewer, Catmur, & Bird, 2019; Welding & Samur, 2018), which seems surprising given that linguistic difficulties belong to the core of the alexithymia construct. Nevertheless, empirical studies have shown that people with higher (rather than lower) levels of alexithymia use fewer and less complex emotion language (Roedema & Simons, 1999; Wotschack & Klann-Delius, 2013) and that the former people display reduced sensitivity to the emotional qualities of speech at a neurophysiological level (Goerlich et al., 2012). Moreover, people with higher (rather than lower) levels of alexithymia have difficulties with more complex forms of linguistic processes (Welding & Samur, 2018).

Additional research has linked alexithymia to difficulties in narrative processing. One consistent finding in the literature is that people with higher (rather than lower) levels of alexithymia display poorer empathic abilities (Grynberg, Luminet, Corneille, Grèzes, & Berthoz, 2010) and reduced perspective-taking ability (Moriguchi et al., 2007). Based on these and related findings Samur, Luminet, and Koole (2017) hypothesised that people with higher (rather than lower) levels of alexithymia are likely to find it harder to process narratives. Consistent with this, Samur et al. observed in three independent samples (combined $N = 1{,}283$) that alexithymia is associated with lower reading frequency. Reduced reading frequency among people with higher levels of alexithymia was partly mediated by mentalising skills, that is, understanding what is on other people's minds (2017). Another study found that alexithymia is negatively associated with reading comprehension, even after controlling for demographic variables and conceptually related personality traits like trait absorption and openness to experience (Samur & Koole, 2020). These two paths, namely mentalising and reading comprehension, have been examined separately so far, which makes it difficult to conclude on the underlying mechanisms.

In view of the aforementioned considerations, it seems likely that people with higher (rather than lower) alexithymia will be less prone to narrative transportation. Thus, the effects of alexithymia are the theoretical opposite of the effects of adopting a first-person (rather than third-person) perspective. To our knowledge, no studies to date have examined whether alexithymia might interact with narrative perspective in shaping narrative processing.

The present research and hypotheses

In the present research, we conducted two studies to investigate how narrative engagement emerges from narrative perspective and individual differences in alexithymia. In Study 1, we examined a large online sample of American participants ($N = 541$) from varying age groups and social backgrounds (Samur, Tops, & Koole, 2018). In Study 2, we investigated a smaller group of Dutch university students ($N = 55$) in a behavioural laboratory, an environment that enabled more control over participants' reading experience.

In both studies, participants rated their levels of narrative engagement during texts using a validated scale (Green & Brock, 2000; Kuijpers, Hakemulder, Tan, & Doicaru, 2014). Moreover, participants rated the Bermond-Vorst Alexithymia Questionnaire (BVAQ; Vorst & Bermond, 2001). We chose the BVAQ because, unlike the more widely used Toronto Alexithymia Scale, it covers both cognitive and affective facets of alexithymia. The affective facet of alexithymia (i.e. the emotionalising and fantasising scales) is conceptually more closely related to narrative transportation than the cognitive facet of alexithymia. Consequently, we expected stronger effects for the affective facet than for the cognitive facet of alexithymia. In both studies, we further statistically controlled for a trait absorption, to ensure that our observed effects were specific to alexithymia, and not a general deficiency in absorption skills.

In line with the previous literature (Hartung et al., 2016), we predicted that participants would display more narrative engagement for stories that were written in a first-person perspective than for stories that were written in a third-person perspective. Furthermore, we predicted that participants with higher levels of alexithymia would display less narrative engagement than participants with lower levels of alexithymia. Finally, we explored the interplay between narrative perspective taking and alexithymia on narrative engagement. In this regard, we had three competing predictions. First, according to the *independence hypothesis*, narrative perspective and alexithymia would have independent effects on narrative engagement. Second, alexithymia and narrative perspective may interact in a non-linear manner. Such a nonlinear interaction may take one of two forms. First, people with higher levels of alexithymia may be insufficiently motivated to engage themselves with a narrative. If this is correct, a first-person (rather than a third-person) story may be especially helpful for people with higher levels of alexithymia, given that a first-person perspective increases engagement with the text. We refer to this as the *motivational support hypothesis*. Alternatively, however, it is possible that people with higher (rather than lower) levels of alexithymia are deficient in the required skills to increase their narrative identification. This would mean that people with higher levels of alexithymia may be unable to increase their narrative engagement, and hence will be less sensitive to variations in narrative perspective. We refer to the latter as the *functional impairment hypothesis*.

Study 1

Study 1 examined a large online sample of American participants ($N = 541$) of varying levels of alexithymia (Samur et al., 2018). Some of the participants ($N = 215$) read a fictional story that was written from a first-person perspective, whereas other participants ($N = 326$) read a fictional story that was written from a third-person perspective. We predicted that stories written from a first-person perspective would evoke more narrative engagement than stories written from a third-person perspective. In addition, we predicted that participants that have higher levels of alexithymia would experience less narrative engagement than participants low in alexithymia. Finally, we explored whether (and, if so, how) narrative perspective and alexithymia might interact in predicting narrative engagement.

Method

Participants and design

In Study 1, we drew from a previously published online study (Samur et al., 2018). Participants were recruited using Amazon's Mechanical Turk service, which is a widely used internet platform among social scientists for online data collection (Paolacci, Chandler, & Ipeirotis, 2010). The data acquired via this service has been shown to be equally valid and reliable as those obtained using traditional methods (Buhrmester, Kwang, & Gosling, 2011; Hauser & Schwarz, 2016). In this service, researchers can determine which level of prior performance approval of participants is sufficient to qualify for participating in the study. High approval rate of a participant tends to produce better quality data. Therefore, we followed the common protocol to include participants with more than 95% approval rate (Peer, Vosgerau, & Acquisti, 2014).

The complete dataset from the online study by Samur et al. (2018) included 1,087 participants. From this dataset, only the conditions where participants read a fiction story were selected ($N = 558$). Of the latter group, only the participants who completed a narrative engagement scale were included in the final sample of the present study ($N = 541$; 296 Females; $M_{age} = 36.21$, $SD_{age} = 11.83$). There were fourteen stories in total with a mixture of either first-person or third-person perspective. Participants were grouped into one of the conditions according to the perspective of the story that they have read: first-person story ($N = 215$) or third-person story ($N = 326$).

Procedure and materials

After providing informed consent, participants read one fictional story that was drawn from the set of 14 stories. Next, participants completed the scales to assess alexithymia, transportation, and trait absorption, which were embedded among other questionnaires. A full report of the studies can be found in Samur et al. (2018).

The fictional narratives were drawn from short stories and excerpts from novels that were used in previous research (Kidd & Castano, 2013; Samur et al., 2018). The first author (DS) recoded these fourteen texts into two groups based on their narrative perspective: First-person and third-person stories. Narrative perspective was decided by examining the use of pronouns by the narrator: using the pronoun "I" for first-person perspective and the pronouns "he or she" for third-person perspective. In all the texts, the pronoun used by the narrator has remained same from the beginning until the end of the story. In the final set, there were six texts that were written in a first-person perspective, and eight texts that were in a third-person perspective. The mean of included texts was 3,310 words. All texts in each group were checked by the author to ensure that there were no clear differences between two groups in terms of theme and valence. The full list including the title and author information of all texts can be found in the Supplementary Materials S1.

To measure narrative engagement, we asked participants to complete the Transportation Scale (Green & Brock, 2000), which measures narrative engagement as a construct of imagery, emotion and attention. The scale included 11 text-invariant items that we used following previous research (Jensen et al., 2011; Murphy, Frank, Chatterjee, & Baezconde-Garbanati, 2013). In this scale, participants rated their reading experience (e.g. "I could picture myself in the scene of the events described in the narrative") using a 7-point Likert scale, ranging from "strongly disagree" to "strongly agree". After recoding the reversed items, we averaged all responses. This scale had satisfactory reliability ($\alpha = .79$).

We used the Bermond – Vorst Alexithymia Questionnaire (BVAQ) to measure individual differences in alexithymia (Vorst & Bermond, 2001). The BVAQ consists of 40 items that are divided into five subscales: emotionalising (8 items) (e.g. "When something unexpected happens, I remain calm and unmoved."), fantasising (8 items) (e.g. "I have few daydreams and fantasies."), identifying (8 items) (e.g. "When I am tense, it remains unclear from which of my feelings this comes."), analysing (8 items) (e.g. "I hardly ever consider my feelings.") and verbalising (8 items) (e.g. "I find it difficult to express my feelings."). Participants responded to the statements with a 5-point Likert scale, ranging from "this in no way applies" to "this definitely applies". We reported our results on total BVAQ scores, which had satisfactory reliability ($\alpha = .89$), as well as in two facets: affective alexithymia ($\alpha = .84$) and cognitive alexithymia ($\alpha = .88$).

We included the Fantasy subscale from Interpersonal Reactivity Index (Davis, 1980), as a well-validated measure of trait absorption (Davis, Luce, & Kraus, 1994). This scale was used since it relates to individual differences in absorption into the feelings and actions of characters in fictional context. Participants responded to the statements with a 5-point Likert scale, ranging from "strongly disagree" to "strongly agree". The scale has 7 items (e.g. *I really get involved with the feelings of the characters in a novel)* and showed satisfactory reliability in Study 1 ($\alpha = .85$).

Results and discussion

The means and standard deviations of all measures are displayed in Table 1. The correlations between measures are displayed in Table 2. We performed our analyses using global alexithymia scores, as well as the separate scores of the affective and cognitive facets of alexithymia and their respective subscales. Affective and cognitive facets of alexithymia were moderately positively correlated, $r = .37$, $p < .001$. Thus, the affective and cognitive facets of alexithymia had some overlap, but not so much to be redundant with another. Notably, the cognitive facet of alexithymia has three subscales and the affective facet has two subscales. Analysis at the subscale level yielded a similar pattern as the analysis at the facet level. These correlations can be found in Table 3.

We found no significant relation between reading time and alexithymia scores, $r = -.10$, $p = .48$. Further descriptive results of the alexithymia subscales and

Table 1. Means and standard deviations of measures in Studies 1 and 2.

	Mean	Standard deviation
Experiment 1		
Alexithymia Total Score	99.74	21.02
Alexithymia Affective facet	40.47	10.65
Alexithymia Cognitive facet	59.27	14.66
IRI Fantasy	3.58	.86
Transportation	4.36	.91
Experiment 2		
Alexithymia Total Score	100.24	18.82
Alexithymia Affective facet	40.47	9.51
Alexithymia Cognitive facet	59.76	15.62
IRI Fantasy	3.49	.78
SWAS Attention	3.82	1.11
SWAS Transportation	3.23	1.14
SWAS Emotional Engagement	3.68	1.10
SWAS Mental Imagery	4.62	1.04

Note: SWAS: Story World Absorption Scale.

Table 2. Correlations between alexithymia, absorption, and transportation in Studies 1 and 2.

	Study 1	Study 2			
	Transportation Scale	SWAS Mental Imagery	SWAS Emotional Engagement	SWAS Attention	SWAS Transportation
Alexithymia Total Score	−.37**	−.27*	−.19	−.14	−.05
Alexithymia Affective facet	−.32**	−.36**	−.16	−.11	−.15
Alexithymia Cognitive facet	−.30**	−.10	−.13	−.10	.03
IRI Fantasy	.40**	.45**	.51**	.44**	.38**

Note: SWAS: Story World Absorption Scale.

Table 3. Correlations between BVAQ facets, and narrative engagement.

	Study 1	Study 2			
	Transportation Scale	SWAS Mental Imagery	SWAS Emotional Engagement	SWAS Attention	SWAS Transportation
Fantasising	−.29**	−.21	−.15	−.20	−.29*
Emotionalising	−.23**	−.36**	−.10	.03	.05
Verbalising	−.21**	−.13	−.22	−.18	−.04
Identifying	−.19**	−.09	.01	−.08	.00
Analysing	−.31**	−.02	−.07	.03	.12

Note: SWAS: Story World Absorption Scale.

IRI fantasy scale can be found in Supplementary Materials S2.

After examining the correlations between variables, we conducted an Analysis of Variance (ANOVA) to examine the effects of narrative perspective and alexithymia on narrative engagement. In line with our predictions, participants who had read a first-person story (M = 4.50, SD = .87) reported more narrative engagement than participants who had read a third-person story (M = 4.26, SD = .92), $F(1, 538) = 10.11$, $p = .002$, $\eta^2 = .02$. The latter effect is graphically displayed in Figure 1. The engagement levels for each story can be found in the Supplementary Materials S1. Also as predicted, the alexithymia total scores were negatively correlated with narrative engagement, $F(1, 538) = 84.73$, $p < .001$, $\eta^2 = .14$. The latter effect is graphically displayed in Figure 2.

There was no interaction effect between global alexithymia scores and narrative perspective on engagement levels, $F(2, 537) = 1.12$, $p = .29$. However, follow-up analyses yielded different results for the cognitive and affective facets of alexithymia. First,

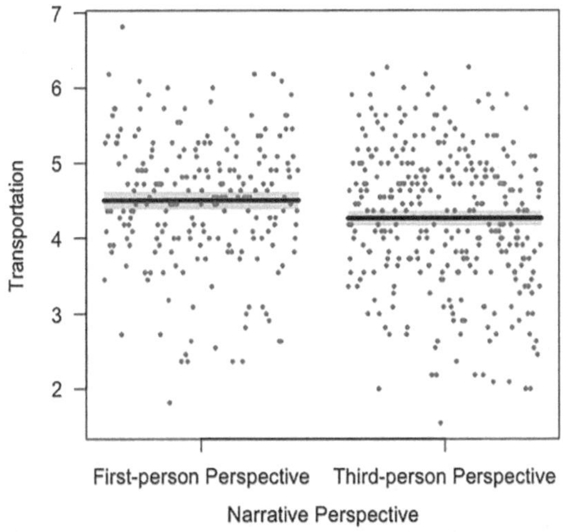

Figure 1. Transportation Scale, the measure of narrative engagement, as a function of narrative perspective.

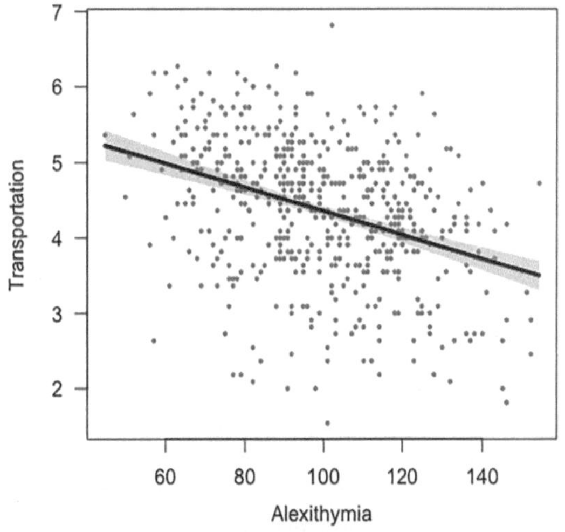

Figure 2. Transportation, the measure of narrative engagement, as a function of total Alexithymia scores.

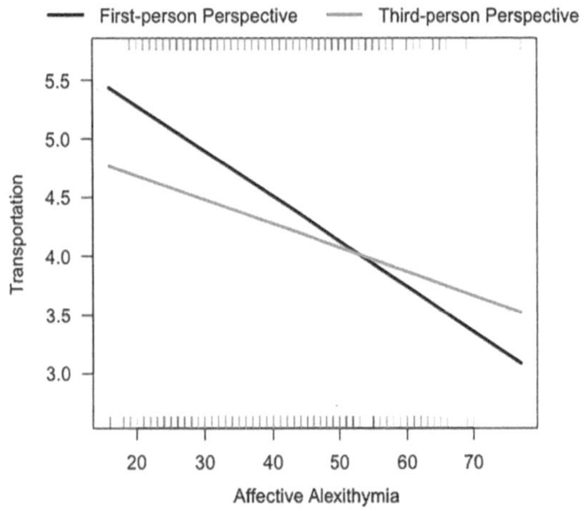

Figure 3. Transportation, the measure of narrative engagement, as a function of narrative perspective and affective Alexithymia.

we examined the effect of the cognitive facet of alexithymia. There were significant main effects of cognitive alexithymia, $F(1, 538) = 52.69$, $p < .001$, $\eta^2 = .09$, and narrative perspective, $F(1, 538) = 10.07$, $p = .002$, $\eta^2 = .02$, but there was no interaction effect ($F(1, 537) = .53$, $p = .47$). When we included absorption as a covariate, the interaction effect remained non-significant, $F < 1$, $p > .05$.

Next, we turned to the affective facet of alexithymia. The main effect of affective alexithymia, $F(1, 538) = 60.11$, $p < .001$, $\eta^2 = .10$, and the main effect of narrative perspective, $F(1, 538) = 9.15$, $p = .003$, $\eta^2 = .02$, were significant. Moreover, the interaction between affective alexithymia and perspective was also significant ($F(1, 537) = 6.30$, $p = .01$, $\eta^2 = .01$). The latter effect is visually displayed in Figure 3. Participants with low alexithymia reported more narrative engagement when they had read a first-person story than when they had read a third-person story. By contrast, participants with low alexithymia were unaffected by narrative perspective. The interaction effect held even after we statistically controlled for IRI fantasy, $F(1, 536) = 6.25$, $p = .01$, $\eta^2 = .01$.

Study 2

The results of Study 1 confirmed our predicted main effects of narrative perspective and alexithymia on narrative engagement and provided initial exploratory evidence for an interaction between narrative perspective and the affective facet of alexithymia. However, the data for Study 1 were originally collected for a different purpose (Samur et al., 2018), which meant that participants were not randomly assigned to different narrative perspectives. It therefore remained important to conduct a study that was explicitly a priori designed to examine the effects of narrative perspective and alexithymia on narrative engagement. We designed Study 2 to this end. In Study 2, we took additional steps to improve our methodology.

First, Study 2 used a new set of four pre-tested fiction stories, two that were written in a first-person perspective and two that were written in a third-person perspective. Second, Study 2 used a within-subjects design, which increases statistical power and thus the sensitivity of our experiment. The latter was useful because we were not able to run as many participants for Study 2 as we did for Study 1. Third, we conducted Study 2 in a lab environment, which reduced the influence of potentially interfering influences (e.g. interruptions, noise) and afforded more control over participants' reading experience.

Fourth, we used a more versatile engagement scale in Study 2. This scale was specifically built to measure the deictic shift from real world to the narrative world using four distinct facets: Mental imagery, emotional engagement, transportation and attention. Notably, the engagement scale from Study 1 included items corresponding predominantly on mental imagery and mix of items from attention and emotional engagement subscales of the engagement measure from Study 2.

Method

Participants and design

Fifty-five participants (30 Females; $M_{age} = 21.85$, $SD_{age} = 7.38$) were recruited from the Vrije Universiteit Amsterdam, who were rewarded with either study credits or money for their voluntary participation. Since the design has been changed in multiple ways, the sample size for Study 2 is calculated for a medium effect size on the basis of within-group comparison.

Procedure and materials

Upon arrival in the laboratory, participants were greeted by a female experimenter, who led them to individual cubicles and seated participants behind a desk-top computer. The remainder of the experiment was computer-administered. First, participants filled out the BVAQ. Next, participants were introduced to the reading assignments (four in total). Every participant read two stories that were written in a first-person perspective and two stories that were written in a third-person perspective. The order of the stories was randomised. For each text, participants filled out the Story World Absorption Scale (Kuijpers et al., 2014). After the reading assignments, participants filled out the IRI fantasy scale, and Toronto Alexithymia Scale in a randomised order. Finally, participants provided their demographic data, and were debriefed, thanked and rewarded for their participation.

Eight stories were selected for a pilot study (N = 20) according to their length and perspective of narrative. In the pilot, participants were asked to evaluate complexity, and emotional arousal of each story. Based on the pilot study, we chose four stories, two written in a first-person perspective and two written in a third-person perspective. The two categories were matched for word count, complexity, and emotional arousal levels. The mean of included texts was 1,101 words. In the present study, every participant read four stories that were written in either a first-person or a third-person perspective.

To measure their narrative transportation, participants filled out the Story World Absorption Scale (SWAS; Kuijpers et al., 2014). It combines four subscales: attention (e.g. "The story gripped me in such a way that I could close myself off for things that were happening around me"), transportation (e.g. "When I was finished with reading the story it felt like I had taken a trip to the world of the story"), emotional engagement (e.g. "I felt how the main character was feeling"), mental imagery (e.g. "When I was reading the story I could see the situations happening in the story being played out before my eyes"). The SWAS items had satisfactory reliability for each story (Story 1, $\alpha = .96$; Story 2, $\alpha = .94$; Story 3, $\alpha = .96$; Story 4, $\alpha = .95$).

For the measure of alexithymia and trait absorption, we used the same scales as in Study 1, namely, the BVAQ and IRI fantasy. Both scales had satisfactory reliability (respectively, $\alpha = .88$ and $\alpha = .83$).

We also used Toronto Alexithymia Scale with 20 items (Kooiman, Spinhoven, & Trijsburg, 2002) to make a comparison with the other alexithymia scale results, namely BVAQ. The latter has three subscales: difficulty identifying feelings (e.g. "I am often confused about what emotion I am feeling."), difficulty describing feelings (e.g. "It is difficult for me to find the right words for my feelings."), and externally oriented thinking (e.g. "I prefer to analyze problems rather than just describe them."). Participants responded using 5-point Likert scales, ranging from "strongly disagree" to "strongly agree". It had satisfactory reliability ($\alpha = .83$).

Results and discussion

The means and standard deviations of all measures are displayed in Table 1. The correlations between measures are displayed in Table 2. As in Study 1, we performed all analyses using global alexithymia scores, as well as cognitive and affective facets of alexithymia. The correlations between alexithymia subscales, as measured by BVAQ, and narrative engagement, including all SWAS subscales can be found in Table 3. Consistent with Study 1, only fantasising subscale is significantly correlated with SWAS Transportation and emotionalising subscale with SWAS Mental Imagery. We found no significant relation between reading time and alexithymia scores, $r = .02$, $p = .54$. Further descriptive results of IRI fantasy scale can be found in Supplementary Materials S2.

The correlation between the cognitive and affective facets of alexithymia was directionally positive but non-significant, $r = .07$, $p > .05$. The previous literature indicates that the correlation between the cognitive and affective facets of alexithymia tends to be small (Bermond et al., 2007) or non-existent (Bermond, Oosterveld, & Vorst, 2015). The cognitive facet of the BVAQ was strongly correlated with the Toronto Alexithymia Scale, $r = .88$, $p < .001$. By contrast, the affective facet of the BVAQ was uncorrelated with the Toronto Alexithymia Scale, $r = .07$, $p > .05$. This pattern of correlations between the BVAQ facets and the Toronto Alexithymia Scale is consistent with previous findings in the literature (Vorst & Bermond, 2001). The complete correlations table for the subscales of BVAQ and Toronto Alexithymia Scale can be found in Supplementary Materials S3. The correlations between Toronto Alexithymia Scale, and SWAS subscales can be found in Supplementary Materials S3.

Next, we conducted a series of ANOVAs to examine the effects of narrative perspective and alexithymia, as measured by BVAQ, on narrative engagement. Consistent with Study 1, participants who had read first-person stories (M = 4.18, SD = 1.12) reported more narrative engagement, as indicated by a higher SWAS total score, than participants who had read third-person stories (M = 3.33, SD = 1.07), $F(1, 54) = 47.95$, $p < .001$, $\eta^2 = .47$. The effect of narrative perspective was significant for all four subscales of the SWAS, *Fs* > 19, *ps* < .001.

Global alexithymia scores, as measured by BVAQ, were unrelated to the SWAS overall scores, $F(1, 53) = 1.76$, $p = .19$. However, separate analyses for the SWAS subscales revealed that, global alexithymia scores were correlated with the mental imagery subscale of the SWAS (see Table 2). Next, we checked whether the effects of total alexithymia scores on mental imagery interacted with narrative perspective. In the latter analysis, the main effect of narrative perspective fell to non-significance, $F(1, 53) = 1.48$, $p = .23$, $\eta^2 = .02$ and the main effect of alexithymia remained significant, $F(1, 53) = 4.02$, $p = .05$, $\eta^2 = .07$. Importantly, as in Study 1, total alexithymia scores did not show an interaction effect with narrative perspective on mental imagery, $F(1, 53) = .18$, $p = .68$ (Figures 4 and 5).

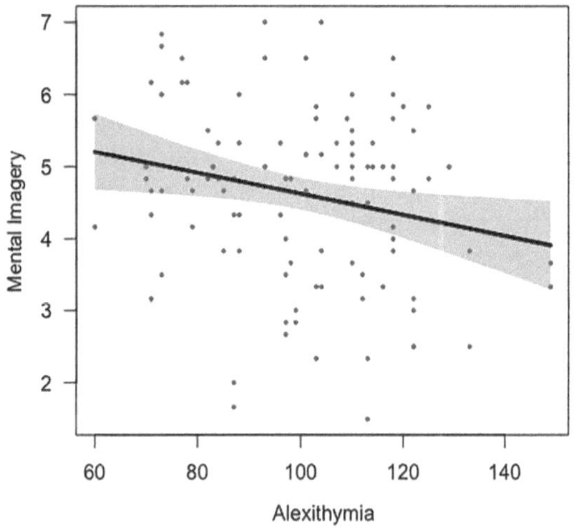

Figure 5. Mental imagery scores of the SWAS as a function of Alexithymia.

Next, as in Study 1, we also conducted separate analyses for the affective and cognitive facets of alexithymia. First, we examined whether the effect of the cognitive facet of alexithymia on mental imagery depends on the narrative perspective. The main effect of cognitive alexithymia was not significant, $F(1, 53) = .55$, $p = .46$, while the main effect of perspective was significant, $F(1, 53) = 6.96$, $p = .01$, $\eta^2 = .12$. There was also no significant interaction between cognitive alexithymia and narrative perspective, ($F(1, 53) = 2.45$, $p = .12$, $\eta^2 = .04$). The latter result remained non-significant after we controlled for IRI fantasy ($F(1, 52) = 2.31$, $p = .14$, $\eta^2 = .04$).

Finally, we examined whether affective alexithymia interacted with narrative perspective in predicting narrative transportation. While the main effect of affective alexithymia was significant ($F(1, 53) = 7.84$, $p = .007$, $\eta^2 = .12$), the main effect of narrative perspective fell to non-significance, $F(1, 53) = .43$, $p = .51$. The affective alexithymia facet had a marginal interaction with narrative perspective in the expected direction ($F(1, 53) = 2.98$, $p = .09$) (see Figure 4). The latter effect became statistically significant after we

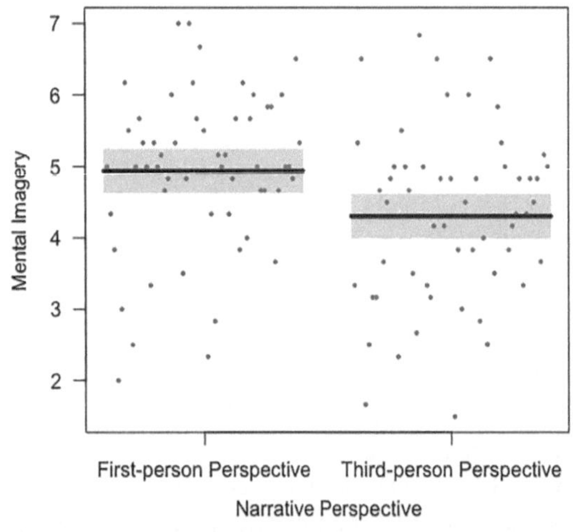

Figure 4. Mental imagery scores of the SWAS as a function of narrative perspective.

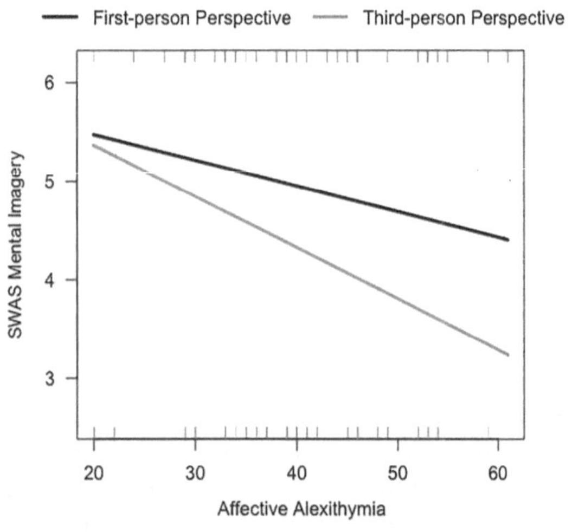

Figure 6. SWAS mental imagery as a function of narrative perspective and affective Alexithymia.

controlled for IRI Fantasy scale as a covariate, $F(1, 52) = 7.42$, $p = .009$, $\eta^2 = .12$. To make sure these findings were not due to inflation of regression parameters, which is also referred to as collinearity (Dormann et al., 2013), we performed additional checks by calculating variance inflation factor (VIF) for regression models including affective alexithymia, IRI fantasy and mental imagery scores. All trials yielded VIF factors less than 2, which is below the accepted threshold (< 10) (Figure 6).

General discussion

In the present article, we examined how narrative engagement emerges from narrative perspective and individual differences in alexithymia. In Study 1, which used a large online sample (N = 541) with a between-subjects design, and Study 2, which was a small-scale experimental study (N = 55) with a within-subjects design, we found strongly converging findings that were largely consistent with our theoretical predictions. First, as expected, first-person stories evoked more engagement than third-person stories. Second, alexithymia was negatively associated with the extent to which participants were mentally immersed into a story. Third, narrative perspective interacted with the affective subscales, but not the cognitive subscales of alexithymia. The latter effect signified that first-person stories evoked more engagement than third-person narratives among participants with lower levels of affective alexithymia, whereas narrative perspective had no effect among participants with higher levels of affective alexithymia.

The present studies are among the first to provide direct evidence for a link between alexithymia and narrative engagement, where people with higher (rather than lower) levels of alexithymia are less likely to become mentally immersed into a narrative world. The lower levels of mental engagement in alexithymia cast new theoretical light on recent findings that people with higher (rather than lower) alexithymia are prone to read less in their daily lives (Samur et al., 2017; Samur & Koole, 2020). Moreover, the fantasising subscale of alexithymia is found to be consistently associated with narrative transportation in both studies. Narrative transportation is a process that increases readers' engagement with a narrative (Gerrig, 1993; Green & Brock, 2002; van Laer et al., 2014). Hence, the limited propensity in imaginative ability is likely to make reading less rewarding (Busselle & Bilandzic, 2009). The present findings thereby help to explain why people with higher (rather than lower) alexithymia are likely to read less in everyday life.

By studying the effects of alexithymia alongside the effects of narrative perspective, the present studies further illuminate one of the potential mechanisms whereby alexithymia may influence narrative engagement. In Study 1, we found that the cognitive facet of alexithymia and narrative perspective had a main effect on narrative engagement. The main effect of cognitive alexithymia was non-significant in Study 2, but this was likely because of the small sample size of that study. The implication seems to be that cognitive alexithymia and narrative perspective influence narrative engagement through independent mechanisms. The prior literature has consistently linked cognitive alexithymia to deficits in mentalising skills (Grynberg et al., 2012; Moriguchi et al., 2006). We therefore tentatively suggest that mentalising deficits in cognitive alexithymia may lower narrative engagement irrespective of whether people adopt a first-person or a third-person perspective. However, measuring mental attunement using different methodologies, such as open-ended questions on character's inner world, may reveal the link between cognitive alexithymia and narrative engagement further.

Unlike cognitive alexithymia, affective alexithymia did interact with narrative perspective. Specifically, both studies showed that first-person stories elicited more narrative engagement than third-person stories among people low in alexithymia, but this effect was absent among people with higher levels of alexithymia. This interaction suggests that affective alexithymia is specifically linked to functional impairments in mentally simulating someone else's perspective. These findings are in line with previous evidence that affective alexithymia is predictive of lower activations at the neural substrates of mental imagery (van der Velde et al., 2013). Given that the findings in Study 2 showed that the interaction was most pronounced for the facets of narrative engagement that are involved with mental imagery, the inability to generate mental imagery lies at the heart of the reading problems of people with higher (rather than lower) levels of affective alexithymia. Therefore, future research should focus on the story content, such as the level of abstractness or the amount of emotional dynamics of the characters, that may explain these differences. More concrete stories can perhaps lead to higher levels of narrative engagement among people with higher levels of alexithymia.

The dissociable effects of the affective and cognitive facets of alexithymia on narrative engagement are of interest for the broader alexithymia literature. Notably, there is an ongoing debate surrounding the definition of the alexithymia construct and the comprising facets (Watters, Taylor, Quilty, & Bagby, 2016). While some scholars find affective dimension of alexithymia problematic at a conceptual level, others would argue that fantasising and emotionalising concepts are part of the original construct (Bermond et al., 2007; Vorst & Bermond, 2001). According to the latter, whereas the cognitive facets seem to be linked with brain areas related to automatic emotion processing, including perception and recognition of emotion, the affective facets of alexithymia are associated with areas guiding conscious experience of emotion and emotion control (Goerlich-Dobre, Votinov, Habel, Pripfl, & Lamm, 2015). The present findings suggest that the differences between the affective and cognitive facets of alexithymia may have a particular significance for mental simulation processes in reading. Cognitive facets of alexithymia might be related to mental simulations on implicit levels which, for example, are activated when one is watching someone performing an action (Grèzes, Frith, & Passingham, 2004). By contrast, the affective facets of alexithymia may be associated with more explicit forms of mental simulation which, for example, become activated when one deliberately imagines another person's emotions (Ruby & Decety, 2004).

The present research inevitably has limitations. First, the present set of two studies were heterogeneous in terms of their design, sample size, and study environment. Although the findings of the present studies converged in their most important respects, it remains desirable to conduct more better controlled replications of the present work including exhaustive checks on story content (e.g. theme, valence), the linguistics checks, such as the consistency of the use of first- or third-person perspective pronouns, and reading comprehension. Second, the present studies assessed narrative engagement using self-report measures that were administered after the reading experience. To control for possible memory distortions, it would be important to measure engagement while people are reading. Although self-report measures tend to disrupt reading flow when administered during reading, recent work indicates that it is possible to derive an index of narrative engagement from the activation of visual imagery areas of the brain (Christian et al., 2015). The latter methodology would provide an important complement to the present research. Third, the present studies were limited to a single session of reading, and thus remain silent about any effects lasting after reading. For example, the effect of persuasive messages after an immersive reading (Green & Brock, 2002) might be less on people with higher (rather than lower) levels of alexithymia. There is also some suggestive evidence that repeatedly experiencing narrative engagement may lead to enhancements of social-cognitive processing (Bal & Veltkamp, 2013). It thus would be of interest to extend the present studies to include longitudinal designs in future work.

Despite these caveats, the findings that links alexithymia to perspective-taking and mental imagery from the present research provide arguably the most direct evidence to date that links alexithymia to deficiencies in mental simulation. This link is highly theoretically meaningful in view of modern theories of embodied cognition (Barsalou, 2008) and embodied emotion (Niedenthal, 2007), which accord a central role to mental simulation (Barsalou, Santos, Simmons, & Wilson, 2008; Niedenthal, 2007). Embodiment theories have already been successfully applied to understand the language comprehension and the acquisition of reading skills (Glenberg, Witt, & Metcalfe, 2013). From this perspective, inability to generate mental simulations may be a common factor that explains the problems of people with higher (rather than lower) levels of alexithymia in dealing with their emotions, in relating with other people, and with narrative processing. Although much more work remains to be done, the present research suggests that further studying embodied mental simulations may provide important answers to the myriad problems that are connected with alexithymia.

Disclosure statement

No potential conflict of interest was reported by the author(s).

Funding

The authors gratefully acknowledge the support of a Consolidator Grant from the European Research Council (ERC-2011-StG_20101124) to Sander L. Koole and a Research Talent Grant from the Netherlands Organization for Scientific Research (NWO-406-14-097) to Dalya Samur and Sander L. Koole.

References

Bagby, R. M., Taylor, G. J., & Parker, J. D. (1994). The twenty-item Toronto Alexithymia Scale—II. Convergent, discriminant, and concurrent validity. *Journal of Psychosomatic Research, 38*(1), 33–40.

Bal, P. M., & Veltkamp, M. (2013). How does fiction reading influence empathy? An experimental investigation on the role of emotional transportation. *PloS One, 8*(1), 1–12.

Barsalou, L. W. (2008). Grounded cognition. *Annual Review of Psychology, 59*, 617–645.

Barsalou, L. W., Santos, A., Simmons, W. K., & Wilson, C. (2008). Language and simulation in conceptual processing. In M. De Vega, A. M. Glenberg, & A. C. Graesser (Eds.), *Symbols, embodiment, and meaning* (pp. 245–283). Oxford: Oxford University Press.

Bermond, B., Clayton, K., Liberova, A., Luminet, O., Maruszewski, T., Ricci Bitti, P. E., ... Wicherts, J. (2007). A cognitive and an affective dimension of alexithymia in six languages and seven populations. *Cognition & Emotion, 21*(5), 1125–1136. doi:10.1080/02699930601056989

Bermond, B., Oosterveld, P., & Vorst, H. C. (2015). Measures of alexithymia. In G. J. Boyle, D. H. Saklofske, & G. Matthews (Eds.), *Measures of personality and social psychological constructs* (pp. 227–256). London: Academic Press.

Borghi, A. M., Glenberg, A. M., & Kaschak, M. P. (2004). Putting words in perspective. *Memory & Cognition, 32*(6), 863–873.

Buhrmester, M., Kwang, T., & Gosling, S. D. (2011). Amazon's mechanical Turk. *Perspectives on Psychological Science, 6*(1), 3–5. doi:10.1177/ 1745691610393980

Busselle, R., & Bilandzic, H. (2009). Measuring narrative engagement. *Media Psychology, 12*(4), 321–347. doi:10.1080/15213260903287259

Christian, B. M., Parkinson, C., Macrae, C. N., Miles, L. K., & Wheatley, T. (2015). When imagining yourself in pain, visual perspective matters: The neural and behavioral correlates of simulated sensory experiences. *Journal of Cognitive Neuroscience, 27*(5), 866–875.

Davis, M. H. (1980). *Interpersonal Reactivity Index*. New York: Edwin Mellen Press.

Davis, M. H., Luce, C., & Kraus, S. J. (1994). The heritability of characteristics associated with dispositional empathy. *Journal of Personality, 62*(3), 369–391.

Dormann, C. F., Elith, J., Bacher, S., Buchmann, C., Carl, G., Carré, G., García Marquéz, J. R., et al. (2013). Collinearity: A review of methods to deal with it and a simulation study evaluating their performance. *Ecography, 36*(1), 27–46.

Gerrig, R. (1993). *Experiencing narrative worlds: On the psychological Activities of reading*. New Haven, CT: Yale UP.

Glenberg, A. M., Witt, J. K., & Metcalfe, J. (2013). From the revolution to embodiment. *Perspectives on Psychological Science, 8* (5), 573–585.

Goerlich-Dobre, K. S., Votinov, M., Habel, U., Pripfl, J., & Lamm, C. (2015). Neuroanatomical profiles of alexithymia dimensions and subtypes. *Human Brain Mapping, 36*(10), 3805–3818.

Goerlich, K. S., Aleman, A., & Martens, S. (2012). The sound of feelings: Electrophysiological responses to emotional speech in alexithymia. *PLoS ONE, 7*(5), e36951. doi:10.1371/journal.pone.0036951

Green, M. C., & Brock, T. C. (2000). The role of transportation in the persuasiveness of public narratives. *Journal of Personality and Social Psychology, 79*(5), 701–721. doi:10.1037/0022-3514.79.5.701

Green, M. C., & Brock, T. C. (2002). In the mind's eye: Transportation-imagery model of narrative persuasion. In T. C. B. M. C. Green & J. J. Strange (Eds.), *Narrative impact: Social and cognitive foundations* (pp. 315–341). Mahwah, NJ: Lawrence Erlbaum Associates.

Grèzes, J., Frith, C., & Passingham, R. E. (2004). Brain mechanisms for inferring deceit in the actions of others. *Journal of Neuroscience, 24*(24), 5500–5505.

Grynberg, D., Chang, B., Corneille, O., Maurage, P., Vermeulen, N., Berthoz, S., & Luminet, O. (2012). Alexithymia and the processing of emotional facial expressions (EFEs): systematic review, unanswered questions and further perspectives. *PloS One, 7* (8), e42429.

Grynberg, D., Luminet, O., Corneille, O., Grèzes, J., & Berthoz, S. (2010). Alexithymia in the interpersonal domain: A general deficit of empathy? *Personality and Individual Differences, 49* (8), 845–850.

Hartung, F., Burke, M., Hagoort, P., & Willems, R. M. (2016). Taking perspective: Personal pronouns affect experiential aspects of literary reading. *PLOS ONE, 11*(5), e0154732. doi:10.1371/journal.pone.0154732

Hauser, D. J., & Schwarz, N. (2016). Attentive Turkers: MTurk participants perform better on online attention checks than do subject pool participants. *Behavior Research Methods, 48*(1), 400–407. doi:10.3758/s13428-015-0578-z

Hobson, H., Brewer, R., Catmur, C., & Bird, G. (2019). The role of language in Alexithymia: Moving towards a multiroute model of Alexithymia. *Emotion Review, 11*(3), 247–261.

Jensen, J. D., Bernat, J. K., Wilson, K. M., & Goonewardene, J. (2011). The delay hypothesis: The manifestation of media effects over time. *Human Communication Research, 37*(4), 509–528. doi:10.1111/j.1468-2958.2011.01415.x

Kidd, D. C., & Castano, E. (2013). Reading literary fiction improves theory of mind. *Science, 342*(6156), 377–380. doi:10.1126/science.1239918

Kooiman, C. G., Spinhoven, P., & Trijsburg, R. W. (2002). The assessment of Alexithymia. *Journal of Psychosomatic Research, 53*(6), 1083–1090.

Kuijpers, M. M., Hakemulder, F., Tan, E., & Doicaru, M. (2014). Exploring absorbing reading experiences: Developing and validating a self-report world absorption. *Scientific Study of Literature, 4*(1), 89–122.

Macrae, C. N., Christian, B. M., & Miles, L. K. (2014). Imagination and behavioral control. In J. P. Forges & E. Harmon-Jones (Eds.), *Motivation and Its Regulation* (pp. 97–112). New York: Psychology Press.

Mar, R. A., & Oatley, K. (2008). The function of fiction is the abstraction and simulation of social experience. *Perspectives on Psychological Science, 3*(3), 173–192.

Mol, S. E., & Bus, A. G. (2011). To read or not to read: A meta-analysis of print exposure from infancy to early adulthood. *Psychological Bulletin, 137*(2), 267–296.

Moriguchi, Y., Decety, J., Ohnishi, T., Maeda, M., Mori, T., Nemoto, K., ... Komaki, G. (2007). Empathy and Judging other's pain: An fMRI study of Alexithymia. *Cerebral Cortex, 17*(9), 2223–2234. doi:10.1093/cercor/bhl130

Moriguchi, Y., Ohnishi, T., Lane, R. D., Maeda, M., Mori, T., Nemoto, K., … Komaki, G. (2006). Impaired self-awareness and theory of mind: An fMRI study of mentalizing in alexithymia. *Neuroimage, 32*(3), 1472–1482.

Murphy, S. T., Frank, L. B., Chatterjee, J. S., & Baezconde-Garbanati, L. (2013). Narrative versus Nonnarrative: The role of identification, transportation, and emotion in reducing health disparities. *Journal of Communication, 63*(1), 116–137. doi:10.1111/jcom.12007

Niedenthal, P. M. (2007). Embodying emotion. *Science, 316*(5827), 1002–1005.

Oatley, K. (1999). Meetings of minds: Dialogue, sympathy, and identification, in reading fiction. *Poetics, 26*(5-6), 439–454. doi:10.1016/S0304-422X(99)00011-X

Paolacci, G., Chandler, J., & Ipeirotis, P. (2010). Running Experiments on Amazon Mechanical Turk. *Judgment and Decision Making, 5*(5), 411–419.

Papeo, L., Corradi-Dell'Acqua, C., & Rumiati, R. I. (2011). "She" is not like "I": The tie between language and action is in our imagination. *Journal of Cognitive Neuroscience, 23*(12), 3939–3948.

Peer, E., Vosgerau, J., & Acquisti, A. (2014). Reputation as a sufficient condition for data quality on Amazon Mechanical Turk. *Behavior Research Methods, 46*(4), 1023–1031. doi:10.3758/s13428-013-0434-y

Roedema, T. M., & Simons, R. F. (1999). Emotion-processing deficit in alexithymia. *Psychophysiology, 36*, 379–387.

Ruby, P., & Decety, J. (2004). How would you feel versus how do you think she would feel? A neuroimaging study of perspective-taking with social emotions. *Journal of Cognitive Neuroscience, 16*(6), 988–999.

Samur, D., & Koole, S. L. (2020). Profiling booklovers: Personality correlates of reading motivation, reading comprehension, and reading frequency. Manuscript in preparation.

Samur, D., Luminet, O., & Koole, S. L. (2017). Alexithymia predicts lower reading frequency: The mediating roles of mentalizing ability and reading attitude. *Poetics*, doi:10.1016/j.poetic.2017.09.002

Samur, D., Tops, M., & Koole, S. L. (2018). Does a single session of reading literary fiction prime enhanced mentalizing performance? Four replication experiments of Kidd and Castano (2013). *Cognition and Emotion*, 1–15. doi:10.1080/02699931.2017.1279591

Sifneos, P. E. (1973). The Prevalence of 'Alexithymic' Characteristics in Psychosomatic patients. *Psychotherapy and Psychosomatics, 22*, 255–262.

Stanzel, F. K. (1984). *A theory of narrative*. Cambridge: Cambridge University Press.

van der Velde, J., Servaas, M. N., Goerlich, K. S., Bruggeman, R., Horton, P., Costafreda, S. G., & Aleman, A. (2013). Neural correlates of alexithymia: A meta-analysis of emotion processing studies. *Neuroscience & Biobehavioral Reviews, 37*(8), 1774–1785. doi:10.1016/J.NEUBIOREV.2013.07.008

van Laer, T., De Ruyter, K., Visconti, L. M., & Wetzels, M. (2014). The extended transportation-imagery model: A meta-analysis of the antecedents and consequences of consumers' narrative transportation. *Journal of Consumer Research, 40*(5), 797–817.

Vorst, H. C. M., & Bermond, B. (2001). Validity and reliability of the Bermond–Vorst Alexithymia Questionnaire. *Personality and Individual Differences, 30*(3), 413–434. doi:10.1016/S0191-8869(00)00033-7

Watters, C. A., Taylor, G. J., Quilty, L. C., & Bagby, R. M. (2016). An examination of the topology and measurement of the alexithymia construct using network analysis. *Journal of Personality Assessment, 98*(6), 649–659.

Welding, C., & Samur, D. (2018). Language processing in alexithymia. In O. Luminet, R. M. Bagby, & G. Taylor (Eds.), *Alexithymia: Advances in research, theory, and clinical practice* (pp. 90–103). Cambridge: Cambridge University Press.

Wotschack, C., & Klann-Delius, G. (2013). Alexithymia and the conceptualization of emotions: A study of language use and semantic knowledge. *Journal of Research in Personality, 47*(5), 514–523. doi:10.1016/J.JRP.2013.01.011

Index

Page numbers in **bold** refer to tables and those in *italic* refer to figures.